The Neuropsychology of Epilepsy

CRITICAL ISSUES IN NEUROPSYCHOLOGY

Series Editors

Antonio E. Puente
University of North Carolina, Wilmington

Cecil R. Reynolds
Texas A & M University

Current Volumes in this Series

A Continuation Order Plan is available for the series. A continuation order will bring delivery of each new volume immediately upon publication. Volumes are billed only upon actual shipment. For further information, please contact the publisher.

The Neuropsychology of Epilepsy

Edited by

Thomas L. Bennett

Colorado State University
Fort Collins, Colorado

Plenum Press • New York and London

Library of Congress Cataloging-in-Publication Data

The Neuropsychology of epilepsy / edited by Thomas L. Bennett.
      p.   cm. -- (Critical issues in neuropsychology)
    Includes bibliographical references and index.
    ISBN 0-306-43948-4
    1. Epilepsy. 2. Clinical neuropsychology.   I. Series.
    [DNLM: 1. Epilepsy--psychology. 2. Epilepsy--therapy.
  3. Neuropsychology.   WL 385 N4934]
  RC372.N42 1992
  616.8'53--dc20
  DNLC/DLC
  for Library of Congress   91-45703
                                                           CIP

ISBN 0-306-43948-4

© 1992 Plenum Press, New York
A Division of Plenum Publishing Corporation
233 Spring Street, New York, N.Y. 10013

Printed in the United States of America

For Becky, Nancy, and my other patients,
who have taught me so much about life with epilepsy
and
For Jackie, Dean, Shannon, Brian, and Laurie,
who have always supported me in all my endeavors

Contributors

Michael Anton • Epi-Care Center, Baptist Memorial Hospital, and Semmes-Murphey Clinic, Departments of Neurosurgery and Psychiatry, University of Tennessee-Memphis, Memphis, Tennessee

Thomas L. Bennett • Department of Psychology, Colorado State University, Fort Collins, Colorado

Howard W. Blume • Department of Surgery, Beth Israel Hospital, Boston, Massachusetts

Bryan E. Connell • Carolinas Epilepsy Center, Carolinas Medical Center, Charlotte, North Carolina

Ruben C. Gur • Brain Behavior Laboratory, Department of Psychiatry, University of Pennsylvania School of Medicine, Philadelphia, Pennsylvania

Sandra D. Haynes • Department of Psychology, Colorado State University, Fort Collins, Colorado

Bruce P. Hermann • Epi-Care Center, Baptist Memorial Hospital, and Semmes-Murphey Clinic, Departments of Neurosurgery and Psychiatry, University of Tennessee-Memphis, Memphis, Tennessee

Gail S. Hochanadel • Department of Neurology, Lahey Clinic Medical Center, Burlington, Massachusetts

D. Brian Kester • Brain Behavior Laboratory, Department of Psychiatry, University of Pennsylvania School of Medicine, Philadelphia, Pennsylvania

DeLee Lantz • Departments of Anatomy and Psychiatry, U.C.L.A. School of Medicine, Los Angeles, California, and Neuropsychology Research, Veterans Administration Medical Center, Sepulveda, California

Gregory P. Lee • Department of Psychiatry, and Section of Neurosurgery, Department of Surgery, Medical College of Georgia, Augusta, Georgia

David W. Loring • Section of Behavioral Neurology, Department of Neurology, Medical College of Georgia, Augusta, Georgia

Gerald C. McIntosh • Rehabilitation Department and Life Skills Rehabilitation Center, Poudre Valley Hospital, Fort Collins, Colorado

Kimford J. Meador • Section of Behavioral Neurology, Department of Neurology, Medical College of Georgia, Augusta, Georgia

Dan M. Mungas • Alzheimer's Disease Diagnostic and Treatment Center, University of California, Davis Medical Center, Sacramento, California

Michael J. O'Connor • Division of Neurosurgery, University of Pennsylvania School of Medicine, Philadelphia, Pennsylvania

Lindsey J. Robinson • Brain Behavior Laboratory, Department of Psychiatry, University of Pennsylvania School of Medicine, Philadelphia, Pennsylvania

Kimberlee J. Sass • Section of Neurological Surgery, Department of Surgery, Yale University School of Medicine, New Haven, Connecticut

Andrew J. Saykin • Brain Behavior Laboratory, Department of Psychiatry, University of Pennsylvania School of Medicine, Philadelphia, Pennsylvania

Donald L. Schomer • Department of Neurology, Beth Israel Hospital, Boston, Massachusetts

Dennis D. Spencer • Section of Neurological Surgery, Department of Surgery, Yale University School of Medicine, New Haven, Connecticut

Susan S. Spencer • Department of Neurology, Yale University School of Medicine, New Haven, Connecticut

Michael R. Sperling • Department of Neurology, University of Pennsylvania School of Medicine, Philadelphia, Pennsylvania

Paul A. Spiers • Clinical Research Center, Massachusetts Institute of Technology, Cambridge, Massachusetts

Paul Stafiniak • Brain Behavior Laboratory, Department of Psychiatry, University of Pennsylvania School of Medicine, Philadelphia, Pennsylvania

M. B. Sterman • Departments of Anatomy and Psychiatry, U.C.L.A. School of Medicine, Los Angeles, California, and Neuropsychology Research, Veterans Administration Medical Center, Sepulveda, California

Michael Westerveld • Section of Neurological Surgery, Department of Surgery, Yale University School of Medicine, New Haven, Connecticut

Steve Whitman • Center for Urban Affairs and Policy Research, Northwestern University, Evanston, Illinois

Preface

This was an exciting project to work on, and I attempted to obtain a broad sampling of current research on the neuropsychology of epilepsy. Because the emphasis of the book takes a neuropsychological perspective on epilepsy, the coverage is not redundant with previous texts on this topic. The book is organized around three themes, although individual chapters certainly often extend beyond the part in which they are located. The three major topics are the nature of epilepsy, cognitive and emotional consequences of epilepsy, and treatment approaches to epilepsy and outcome.

In Part I, following a historical overview of epilepsy in Chapter 1 by Sandra D. Haynes and me, Gerald C. McIntosh presents a conceptualization of the epilepsies from a neurologist's perspective. The characteristics of seizure types are discussed, and the etiology of secondary epilepsies is described. Epileptic syndromes are considered. McIntosh outlines clinical seizure patterns associated with seizures originating from different cortical regions.

Bruce P. Hermann and colleagues continue the section on the nature of epilepsy by considering the multiplicity of forces that infringe on people with epilepsy, and they consider epilepsy from a psychosocial perspective. They describe major categories of risk factors for psychological and social problems for persons with epilepsy and then describe two empirical studies, one with adults and one with children, that investigate the influence of these factors on psychosocial adjustment. In Chapter 4, the final chapter in Part I, Hermann and Connell continue the discussion on the nature of epilepsy by discussing nonepileptic or "pseudo-" seizures. They emphasize the fact that the diagnosis of nonepileptic seizures (NES) versus epileptic seizures (ES) can be a very difficult venture. Epilepsy can be manifested by unusual and even bizarre attacks, and patients with epilepsy may show normal interictal and even ictal scalp recordings.

The cognitive and emotional consequences of epilepsy are described in Part II of the book. This section begins with Chapter 5, in which I discuss the cognitive effects of epilepsy and anticonvulsant medications. Two themes emerge in this chapter. First, epilepsy can itself produce cognitive deficits. However, the nature and extent of the deficits depend on seizure type and frequency, age at onset and duration of the disorder, and etiology of the seizure disorder. Second, anticonvulsant medications can themselves produce cognitive deficits, and this makes the process of determining the effects of epilepsy, *per se*, on cognitive processes even more difficult.

In the next chapter, Paul A. Spiers and his colleagues provide a neuroanatomical model, supported by fascinating case histories, to account for their view that temporolimbic epilepsy can yield behavioral alterations. Ictal and interictal manifestations of temporolimbic epilepsy are described, and it is argued that certain predictable long-term changes in behavior may occur as a result of a seizure focus in this region of the brain. Dan M. Mungas further addresses this issue next in the book in his comprehensive report of research that used cluster analysis to determine if there are subgroups of patients with epilepsy who are homogeneous according to specific patterns of behavior. In contrast to Spiers and his colleagues, Mungas concludes that there does not appear to be a specific syndrome of behavior that can be identified in temporolimbic epilepsy. Needless to say, this issue remains far from settled.

In the final chapter of Part II, Lindsey J. Robinson and Andrew J. Saykin discuss the psychological and psychosocial outcome of anterior temporal lobectomy. Robinson and Saykin point out that past inquiries have suffered from a number of methodological flaws including subject selection, methods of measuring outcome, consideration of potential mediating variables, and use of appropriate control groups. Indeed, when appropriate control subjects were used in their own research, both nonoperated and operated subjects showed reductions in psychopathology at the second testing, even though the control subjects continued to experience frequent seizures.

The focus of Part III is on treatment approaches to epilepsy and outcome results. This section begins with a chapter by Gerald C. McIntosh that describes medical treatment of the epilepsies. In that chapter he describes the use of phenytoin, phenobarbital, primidone, valproic acid, ethosuximide, and carbamazepine in seizure control. Supplemental use of benzodiazepine-type anticonvulsants is discussed as well. The mechanisms and actions of these drugs and efficacy by seizure type are also considered, as are guidelines for initiation and cessation of anticonvulsant drug therapy.

M. B. Sterman was the first to suggest that EEG biofeedback might reduce the incidence of seizures in people with poorly controlled epilepsy, and over the years, he has made important contributions to this topic, from both an application and a theoretical standpoint. In his chapter with DeLee Lantz, he reports a secondary benefit of seizure reduction following EEG biofeedback training: Patients whose seizures were reduced in frequency demonstrated an improvement in cognitive processes as indexed by their neuropsychological test scores.

Wada testing, the administration of sodium amobarbital via the left or right carotid to produce temporary unilateral hemispheric dysfunction, is an indispensable part of the preoperative evaluation of patients who are candidates for epilepsy surgery. During the temporary inactivation of the hemisphere, the effects of the proposed surgery on language and memory processes can be assessed. In Chapter 11, Loring, Meador, and Lee discuss criteria and validity issues related to this procedure.

As described in Chapter 12, David W. Loring and his colleagues have made a major contribution to the presurgical evaluation of potential lobectomy patients with epilepsy through their development of depth electrode assessment procedures in the hippocampus. Patients are unilaterally stimulated through these electrodes. The stimulation temporarily disrupts mesial temporal lobe functioning, and learning ability is evaluated during this reversible lesion. As a result, the capacity of the hippocampus contralateral to the proposed surgery to support new learning can be assessed.

In Chapter 13, Saykin and his colleagues present a selective review of neuropsychological changes after anterior temporal lobectomy. The chapter concludes with the presentation of data from a series of recent studies conducted in their center examining changes in memory, language, and musical processing following this surgical intervention. In the final chapter of this book, Sass and colleagues discuss the neuropsychology of corpus callosotomy for epilepsy. Most patients tolerate the procedure well, but mild declines in isolated areas of cognitive function are common, and severe declines can occur. The authors review the factors that can alter neuropsychological function following corpus callosotomy.

Throughout the book, the authors communicate their excitement about research on the neuropsychology of epilepsy. Directions for future research are proposed. Their findings strengthen the long-held view that the experimental study of people with epilepsy is one of our best ways to understand the mechanisms by which the brain regulates human behavior.

This book began at the suggestion of Cecil R. Reynolds, one of the editors of this series. I had written a chapter about epilepsy for the 1989 *Handbook of Clinical Child Neuropsychology* (Plenum) and he suggested this work as a follow-up. I appreciate Cecil's encouragement to undertake this project. I am also very appreciative of the contributing authors, and others who were not directly connected to the book, for their support, encouragement, and many suggestions.

The influence of John M. Rhodes has always been felt in my research and textbook writing in the fields of physiological psychology and clinical neuropsychology. Jack was trained as a clinical psychologist at the University of Southern California before going to France to learn neuropsychology from the great European epileptologists about 30 years ago. I had the good fortune to be Jack's student in the mid- to late-1960s at the University of New Mexico, where he introduced me to neuropsychology and the EEG analysis of behavior. His influence imprinted the view on me that psychology will never understand behavior unless it understands how the human brain regulates behavior. He also passed on to me a message that Henri Gastaut had impressed on him during his studies in France: "If you want to understand the human brain, you must understand the human epileptic." This book helps to underscore Gastaut's belief.

Thomas L. Bennett

Fort Collins, Colorado

Contents

**Part II.   COGNITIVE AND EMOTIONAL CONSEQUENCES OF
             EPILEPSY**

Chapter 13
NEUROPSYCHOLOGICAL CHANGES AFTER ANTERIOR TEMPORAL
   LOBECTOMY: ACUTE EFFECTS ON MEMORY, LANGUAGE,
   AND MUSIC 263

Andrew J. Saykin, Lindsey J. Robinson, Paul Stafiniak, D. Brian Kester,
Ruben C. Gur, Michael J. O'Connor, and Michael R. Sperling

Chapter 14
THE NEUROPSYCHOLOGY OF CORPUS CALLOSOTOMY FOR
   EPILEPSY 291

Kimberlee J. Sass, Susan S. Spencer, Michael Westerveld,
and Dennis D. Spencer

I

The Nature of Epilepsy

Historical Perspective and Overview

SANDRA D. HAYNES and THOMAS L. BENNETT

The history of epilepsy is both fascinating and complex. Progress over the millennia in discovering the nature and manifestations of epilepsy, however, has been slow. What follows is a brief overview of the history of epilepsy. The material contained in this summary is based on the works of several authors who have produced scholarly works on the history of epilepsy, and much of the material is based on the work of Oswei Temkin (1971). His book, *The Falling Sickness*, remains the most detailed and scholarly work on the history of epilepsy to date.

Throughout history, human beings have attributed disease to naturalistic causes, to mystical causes, or to some combination of these two etiologies. The dominant view at any given time appears to depend on the zeitgeist of the time, on previously established facts concerning disease in general or the specific disease in question, and on the superficial manifestations of the disease. Epilepsy is an extreme exemplar of this phenomenon. Persons afflicted with epilepsy commonly manifest both physical and psychological symptoms, easily allowing for either physiological or mystical explanations of cause. This has contributed to our incomplete understanding of epilepsy.

Because of the varied, frightening, and awesome manner in which this disorder manifests, the etiology of epilepsy has often been seen as mystical. Indeed, superstitious belief has at times stifled the search for the cause and treatment of epilepsy. On the other hand, highly accurate naturalistic descriptions of this disorder can be found dating as far back as 400 B.C., when Hippocrates argued that the bizarre sensations, emotions, and behaviors associated with epilepsy were actually the symptoms of a brain disorder. Unfortunately, the early insight of the Hippocratic

SANDRA D. HAYNES and THOMAS L. BENNETT • Department of Psychology, Colorado State University, Fort Collins, Colorado 80523.

The Neuropsychology of Epilepsy, edited by Thomas L. Bennett. Plenum Press, New York, 1992.

authors has been continually discounted and clouded by superstitious beliefs. Thus, throughout human history, the true nature of epilepsy has been shrouded in ignorance. Even today, with great advances in our understanding of epilepsy, many persons maintain mystical origins for epilepsy. Ignorance surrounding epilepsy, however, extends beyond those believing in mystical etiologies. Persons with epilepsy often face discrimination from employers and insurance companies and are refused driving privileges, entrance into military service, and, in some states, marriage licenses (Blumer & Benson, 1982).

It is not surprising that as the accepted etiology of epilepsy vacillated between naturalistic and spiritual causes, the treatment of persons with epilepsy has also vacillated between naturalistic healers (e.g., neurologists and psychiatrists) and spiritual healers (e.g., magicians and religious healers). Recently, neuropsychologists have begun to contribute to the treatment of epilepsy. Because of the neurological problems, psychosocial difficulties, and personality changes that often accompany this disorder, neuropsychologists are in a unique position to treat these symptoms while simultaneously providing the patient with an integrated treatment program designed to accommodate individual circumstances.

ANCIENT MEDICINE

Possession by an evil spirit or demon and being cursed by a god were the most common etiologies attributed to epilepsy. A description of an attack closely resembling an epileptic seizure appears in an Akkadian text of 2000 B.C. An exorcist was employed to avert this seizure. The seizure was apparently attributed to the god Sin (Fulton, 1959; Temkin, 1971). This suggests that satanic possession is one of the oldest alleged causes of epilepsy (Taylor, 1958). Likewise, the Homeric Greeks believed that the Olympian or celestial gods inflicted or averted diseases at will. Thus, their medicine was based on mysticism and superstition, with disease being something to be feared (McHenry, 1969). Additionally, scanty evidence prior to the time of Hippocrates reveals that prehistoric man treated epilepsy by trephining, presumably to release evil spirits.

HIPPOCRATES, GALEN, AND ANTIQUITY

The first definitive works on diseases can be found in the Hippocratic writings (460–370 B.C.). The first writing about epilepsy is found in these works, in a chapter entitled "On the Sacred Disease" (Temkin, 1971; McHenry, 1969; O'Leary & Goldring, 1976). This chapter is often considered one of the best written chapters in all of the Hippocratic works, and some authors believe that it contains a more accurate description of epilepsy than any other medical writings until the 17th century (Levine, 1971). Penfield (1958), who devoted much of his life to the study of the pathology and treatment of epilepsy (Clarke & Dewhurst, 1972), goes so far as to assert that "On the Sacred Disease" contained the most accurate description of the brain until the writings of John Hughlings Jackson in the 19th century. He observed that the quality of this writing demonstrates that it could have been done only by a person who carefully studied epilepsy and the disorder's associated seizures.

Magical beliefs surrounding disease were popular in ancient Greece, and many of these were detailed in the Hippocratic text. Discounting such beliefs, the author argued that gods were not responsible for afflicting diseases, including epilepsy. In fact, the author of "On the Sacred Disease" contended that holy and pure gods were not capable of doing evil things to people's bodies. Instead, Hippocrates stated that epilepsy is a natural disease with causes like other natural diseases. Hippocrates believed that epilepsy is a heritable disease and that seizures originated in the brain (Levine, 1971; McHenry, 1969). The author asserted that the brain was responsible for both normal and abnormal psychological functions. Thus, the symptoms of epilepsy could be accounted for as a function (or dysfunction) of brain activity. Hippocrates recognized that seizures may result in death, especially in younger children, that children can outgrow the disease, that the disorder can worsen over time, and that epilepsy can manifest in animals as well as man. The aura preceding a seizure is also alluded to.

The primary seizures described in this work were generalized, convulsive seizures, but unilateral seizures were also described (Levine, 1971; McHenry, 1969; Temkin, 1971). The name "great disease" was used in this writing, a term later translated in French as "*grand mal*" (Masland, 1974; Temkin, 1971). Obviously, these observations demonstrate a great understanding of epilepsy.

In accordance with the medical views of 400 B.C., however, the author of "On the Sacred Disease" attributed seizures to an excess of phlegm that rushed into the blood vessels of the brain, filled the ventricles, and created a buildup of pressure, which was released via a seizure. Epilepsy, then, was believed to afflict those individuals who were naturally "phlegmatic" rather those who were naturally "choleric." A sudden rush of phlegm, as all movements of other humors believed to cause disease, could be set off by cold, sun, and winds, all things considered "divine" (McHenry, 1969). Thus, despite great insight, this Hippocratic treatise was still partially a product of its time, as it maintained that epilepsy, like other diseases, had a mystical and a natural quality (Temkin, 1971).

Nonetheless, Hippocrates argued that epilepsy is not primarily the product of supernatural power, and, therefore, there was no need to treat the disease with magic. Indeed, Hippocrates reasoned that holding onto misconceptions about epilepsy prevented rational treatment of the disorder. Thus, the treatment for epilepsy that he advocated was the use of personal care and ancient pharmaceutical therapies. Treatment included strict diet, exercise, good amounts of sleep, sexual abstinence, change of scenery, and avoidance of anger. The chance of recovery was believed to increase if one could find meaningful work. Such remedies were similar to those used by physicians for many diseases during antiquity. In addition to these general treatments, specific treatments were directed at the locus of the aura. Pharmacological treatments were based on reason if not on accurate information. The quality of the disease had to be uncovered and then treated with a herbal remedy of opposite qualities. Since epilepsy was cold and moist because of its "phlegmatic" quality, treatment of this disorder required hot and dry substances. By employing these remedies, Hippocrates believed that epilepsy could be cured like all natural diseases (Levine, 1971; Temkin, 1971).

In another Hippocratic work entitled "Epidemics," specific neurological signs or symptoms associated with epilepsy were outlined, including suffocation, tongue biting, and incontinence. The epileptic cry resulting from expulsion of air against a partially closed larynx was also mentioned. It was reiterated that epilepsy occurred most frequently in early life, was a heritable disease, could be precipitated by a variety of causes, and that isolated seizures could occur without repetition (O'Leary & Goldring, 1976).

Public opinion of the time did not match the Hippocratic view. Rather than attributing epilepsy to natural causes, the popular belief was that epilepsy was caused by mystical powers. Specifically, it was believed that a supernatural force attacked the person's mind or senses, presumably because the epileptic seizure resembled the sudden overtaking of the body by a god. Thus, the Greek-rooted word *epilepsy*, meaning to seizure or attack, was used to describe this disorder (Siegel, 1968).

The title of the Hippocratic work, "On the Sacred Disease," reflected the popular conviction of mystical involvement. It is assumed that the word "sacred" was used for epilepsy because it implies possession by a god or demon. The first association of epilepsy with the moon began in antiquity, as some believed that seizures were brought on by disobedience to Selene, the goddess of the moon (Courville, 1951; Temkin, 1971). Additionally, the word "sacred" is akin to "taboo," echoing the belief that a person afflicted with epilepsy was to be avoided (Levine, 1971). A seizure was considered a bad omen, and the god or demon causing the seizure was to be feared and avoided. If one kept away from the person with epilepsy, it was believed, the demon could not enter one's own body. Avoidance of the individual with epilepsy was especially important when he or she was experiencing a seizure. The person with epilepsy was considered unclean and was not to be touched. No one would eat with this person, and often the afflicted was banned from her or his own home (Temkin, 1971).

Despite the recommendations set forth by Hippocrates, treatment of epilepsy was often left to magic or supernatural means. Treatments were many and varied, ranging from herbal remedies, especially mistletoe and peony, to the more magical treatments associated with the wearing of amulets and the drinking of human blood, to cauterization of the head in several places. Even Greek physicians, who tended to reject demonic etiologies, believed in the effectiveness of amulets and religious healings, and in the influence of the cycles of the moon increasing the likelihood of seizures (Temkin, 1971).

Galen, a scholar of the Hippocratic writings, provided descriptions of the symptoms associated with epilepsy that were extremely accurate. However, like Hippocrates he held the erroneous belief that the cause of epilepsy was humoral distribution. He held fast to the beliefs that epilepsy was caused by too much phlegm in the brain and that, the third and fourth ventricles were the sites for this buildup, which eventually led to blockage. Galen, like Hippocrates, never attempted to demonstrate such blockage (Siegel, 1968). Therefore, since neither of these authors presented anatomic support for this belief (largely because of the reluctance of the Greeks to perform human dissections and, thus, autopsies), the attribution of epilepsy to phlegm appears to be arbitrary (Siegel, 1968; McHenry, 1969). Also in line with Hippocrates, Galen believed that epilepsy could be cured (Temkin, 1971).

In his writings, Galen commented extensively on the Hippocratic works, including "On the Sacred Disease." At times, Galen's commentaries have been criticized as verbose, speculative, and of little practical value (McHenry, 1969). Nonetheless, Galen accurately claimed that seizures resulted from hyperirritability of the brain, especially in those areas that control voluntary movement. He believed that overstimulation of "all of the nerves" caused convulsions of the entire body and that overstimulation of just "one nerve" controlling a single limb caused convulsions of only part of the body. In this way, Galen accounted for epilepsies characterized by generalized versus partial seizures. Galen argued that epilepsy did not always involve convulsions. These other types of attacks, which we today call "absence seizures," were called "little epilepsy." He believed that if epilepsy did not affect consciousness, the focus was in the "cervical spine" (Siegel, 1968). Because of the symptom of aura, Galen believed that epilepsy could originate in organs other than the brain. Irritation could begin in a peripheral organ such as the stomach and move to the brain, causing a convulsion (McHenry, 1969; Siegel, 1968).

On the basis of his observations, Galen identified three types of epilepsy; those originating in the brain (similar to grand mal seizures), those originating from the periphery (akin to Jacksonian seizures), and those originating from the internal organs ("epilepsy by sympathy"). Thus, he initiated the first classification system for epilepsy (Masland, 1974; Siegel, 1968). He coined the term *aura*, meaning breeze, to describe the subjective event felt by the person with epilepsy prior to a seizure. He did so after hearing a patient describe this episode as a cool breeze running through his body. He also noted that people who experience repeated seizures seem to show permanent personality changes (Temkin, 1971).

MAGICIANS AND PHYSICIANS OF THE MIDDLE AGES

Medieval times were a stagnant period for medical inquiry. Few advances were made in medicine, largely because of a reversion to attributing disease etiology to possession by gods (McHenry, 1969).

During the Middle Ages epilepsy became known as the "falling sickness" or "falling evil," terms used for all diseases in which the patient suddenly fell. The person with epilepsy was called "demoniacus" or "lunaticus" depending on attribution of cause, demonic possession or cycles of the moon.

Intrusive demonic possession became the prominent theory of cause for epilepsy among physicians and lay people alike. Unlike antiquity, when possession was never considered intrusive, the practice of exorcism became a popular treatment. Belief in intrusive demonic possession was spread by biblical report of the healing of a person stricken with an epileptic seizure by Jesus Christ (Mark 14:29; Matthew 14:20; Luke 37:43). This supported the position that the etiology of epilepsy was demonic possession, and, consequently, most medical opinions proposed during antiquity were shunned (Temkin, 1971). Thus, the mistaken beliefs first expressed and then renounced by the Greeks were being reintroduced and propagated under the influence of the Christian church (Courville, 1951).

During the Middle Ages, epilepsy became more closely associated with the cycles of the moon, along with other disorders considered "lunacies"; thus epilepsy was equated with mental illness. Like other diseases with periodic disturbances, epilepsy was believed to be caused by the goddess of the moon and was sometimes called the disease of the moon. It was believed that epilepsy could be caught by standing in the light of a full moon and that seizures were more prevalent during the full moon (Courville, 1951; Temkin, 1971).

As the accepted etiology of epilepsy became more magical, treatment became more magical or religious. Many saints and sages were credited with having the ability to counteract the effects of epilepsy. Three of the most prominent were Gaspar, Melchior, and Balthazar, the wise men said to have visited Jesus (Murphy, 1959). It was believed that by whispering these men's names, epilepsy could be cured (Lennox, 1939).

In the Middle Ages, epilepsy was still regarded as contagious, and the stricken individual was often placed in isolation (McHenry, 1969). Persons with epilepsy were banished from their homes and were spat upon in the streets. This practice was believed to prevent infection by a demon. Hence, the Romans popularly called epilepsy "the disease that is spit upon," and this action further promoted the myth of possession. The Roman view of disease as retribution by a god made ill persons, including those with epilepsy, responsible for their illness. Epilepsy was especially shameful and repulsive because it was believed that the individual was actually possessed by a demon (Temkin, 1971).

Many physicians in post-Hippocratic years left written descriptions of epilepsy, although few physicians of medieval times stand out as rational. Nonetheless, some advances in our understanding of epilepsy were made during this period, and many authors worked to assure that previous work would be preserved.

One of the most accurate descriptions of epilepsy by modern standards was left by Aretaeus of Cappadocia in the second or third century A.D. He differentiated between nervous and mental disorders, assigning epilepsy to the former category. He described various forms of the aura before the seizure, noting that it could take one of several forms including fetid odors, luminous circles of diverse color, noises in the ear, tremors, and sensations in the hands and feet (Temkin, 1971).

Lennox (1939, 1940, 1941) acknowledged three physicians of the Middle Ages for their work on epilepsy: John of Gaddesden, Antonius Guainerius, and Bernard of Gordon. John of Gaddesden (approximately 1280–1361) gave one of the most thorough accounts of epilepsy as well as other diseases in his book, *Rosa Medicinae*. In this work, John of Gaddesden elaborated on Galen's seizure classification system. He claimed that there were different types of epilepsy. He saw epilepsy as beginning through a "secret cause" in the head. In contrast to epilepsy, catalepsy began in an extremity, either hand or foot, or other organ of the body except the stomach. Analepsy began in the stomach and moved to the head (Lennox, 1939). Antonius Guainerius were born close to the turn of the 15th century. Lennox (1940) commended Antonius Guainerius for his clarity in setting forth the knowledge of the time on epilepsy in writing.

Bernard of Gordon, who lived at nearly the same time as Antonius Guainerius, also studied epilepsy. He was the first to distinguish apoplexy from epilepsy. His distinction was that the paroxysm of epilepsy was short-lived, whereas the paroxysm of apoplexy was long-lived and could progress to death. In this, Bernard of Gordon may have confused apolexy with status epilepticus. Further, he maintained that epilepsy was caused by an occlusion of a "nonprincipal" ventricle, whereas apoplexy was caused by an occlusion of a "principal" ventricle. He also suggested that the moon, sun, and winds, corrupted semen or menstrual blood, loud noises and bright lights, worms, and other strange events could produce epileptic seizures. He advocated the use of "Hail Marys" and spitting as preventive measures. However, he shunned the use of amulets for treating epilepsy, a common treatment for the disorder at that time (Lennox, 1941).

THE RENAISSANCE

During the Renaissance new facts about anatomy were being discovered and applied to diseases, including epilepsy. Old systems of medicine were being questioned and abandoned (McHenry, 1969). Physicians and priests began debating the belief in demonic possession as an etiology for epilepsy. Often the notion of possession creating epilepsy was rejected. The most common stance, however, was that epilepsy characterized by generalized seizures was of natural causes, whereas epilepsy characterized by absence attacks or partial seizures was caused by demonic possession or hysteria (Temkin, 1971).

By approximately 1600, the concept of symptomatic epilepsy was formed, showing that epilepsy could be triggered by head injury and that seizures could occur as the result of diseases such as syphilis. This formulation helped to demonstrate that epilepsy was not caused by demonic possession and aided in determining differential diagnosis between epilepsy and hysteria (Temkin, 1971).

Nevertheless, the belief in demonic possession was slow to fade among both lay people and physicians alike. Epilepsy continued to be looked on as a difficult disease to treat. The person afflicted was to be pitied (Temkin, 1971).

FRANÇOIS LE BOE, THOMAS WILLIS,
THE IATROCHEMISTS, THE IATROPHYSICISTS, AND
THE SEVENTEENTH AND EIGHTEENTH CENTURIES

The reported exorcism performed by Jesus Christ on a boy with epilepsy insured that most physicians throughout the 17th century would support the notion that epilepsy was caused by demonic possession. Changes in the conception of epilepsy and therapeutic treatment did occur, however, especially in the realm of the iatrochemists and iatrophysicists.

François le Boe, better known as Sylvius (1614–1672), was a major proponent of iatrochemistry. He espoused the theory that "acid vapors" caused epilepsy by irritating the animal spirits contained in the spinal cord, thereby causing convulsions, and in the brain, thereby causing psychiatric symptoms. Sylvius recommended treating epilepsy with basic salts to counteract the acid vapors. Sylvius' theory, however, lacked a sound foundation in physiology or pathology (O'Leary & Goldring, 1976; Temkin, 1971).

The noted physician and lecturer Thomas Willis (1621–1672) also espoused a chemical theory of epilepsy. According to Willis, muscular movement was caused by the mixing of two vitriolic chemical particles in the muscle tissue. When these substances traveling in the blood accumulated in the cerebral cortex, they spilled over into the meninges and moved progressively throughout the brain and spinal cord. This action irritated the nerves and caused the vitriol chemicals in the muscles to "explode." Both the psychological and physical symptoms of epilepsy were explained in this way. Willis also believed that such spirits could attack specific nerves, causing convulsions in different parts of the body. He believed that seizures could be triggered by anger, passion, terror, joy, drunkenness, exercise, changes in the season, and other things that may cause agitation in humans. He supported the idea that epilepsy was heritable, but only in some cases. He described incontinence as releasing of the sphincters as a result of interference with the control centers in the brain. Perhaps his most important contributions to the understanding of epilepsy, however, were in two areas. First, he recognized that the aura associated with a seizure did not begin in the peripheral organ of the sensation but rather in the brain. He also described the loss of memory and intellectual capabilities in persons with epilepsy, although he attributes such loss to accumulation of vitriol matter in the cerebral cortex between seizures (Dewhurst, 1980; Streeter, 1922; Temkin, 1971).

Unlike the iatrochemists, the iatrophysicists were reluctant to give chemical forces full credit for causing epilepsy. According to the iatrophysicists, all actions were purposeful and controlled by a living soul that ruled the body. Irritation of nerves could cause seizures, but only after an idea or emotion produced the irritation. Iatrophysicists justified this stance by noting the number of persons manifesting psychological disturbances who also suffered from epilepsy (O'Leary & Goldring, 1976; Temkin, 1971).

Seventeenth century treatment of epilepsy remained much the same as it had been since medieval times. Myths and ancient remedies regarding epilepsy and its treatment emigrated with the Pilgrims, to colonial America, where they were met with a similar set of beliefs held by the American Indians (Blanton, 1931; Vogel, 1970).

One of the major advances of the 18th century, however, was the beginning of the use of crude chemical preparations to treat epilepsy, even though many of them were not based on sound physiological or chemical footing. It was also in this century that Tissot first described petit mal seizures, although he initiated a new myth—that masturbation was a primary cause of epilepsy (O'Leary & Goldring, 1976).

ADVANCES IN PSYCHIATRY AND NEUROLOGY DURING THE NINETEENTH CENTURY AND THE CONTRIBUTIONS OF JOHN HUGHLINGS JACKSON

With the prison reforms of the 19th century, persons with epilepsy were moved from prisons to asylums with the insane. In time, separate wards were established for persons with epilepsy in the asylums. Gradually, under the initial recommendation of Etienne Dominique Esquirol (1722–1840), they were moved to separate institutions designed for the care and study of persons with epilepsy. One of the most famous of these wards restricted to women was run by Jean Martin Charcot. Charcot developed a classification system that attempted to differentiate hysteria from epilepsy. He believed that there was an anatomic substrate for both epilepsy and hysteria, but he asserted that these were independent disorders (McHenry, 1969).

The placement of persons with epilepsy in special wards and hospitals bolstered epilepsy as a valid topic of research in the medical community. By the late 1800s, journals such as *Brain* had printed hundreds of articles on the topic of epilepsy. Research was aided by the advances made in the study of neurology over the previous centuries (Haymaker & Schiller, 1970; McHenry, 1969). Later in the 18th century it was realized that institutionalized persons usually presented with far worse symptoms than those not requiring hospitalization. For a true picture of epilepsy, therefore, research had to extend beyond the hospitalized (Temkin, 1971).

Epilepsy became viewed as a naturalistic disease, and the idea of demonic possession began to fade. Epilepsy was divided into two major categories according to seizure type—grand mal for full-blown convulsive seizures and petit mal for all other forms of seizures. A French physician, Louis Florentine Calmeil (1798–1895), coined the term "absence" to distinguish between brief mental confusions and epileptic seizures. Calmeil introduced the term status epilepticus to describe an uncontrollable series of seizures that often resulted in death (O'Leary & Goldring, 1976). Epileptic vertigo became the term used to describe mental changes caused by epilepsy. Partial seizures were being described by the psychiatrists Morel and Falret (Haymaker & Schiller, 1970; McHenry, 1969). Yet in 1861, J. Russell Reynolds tried to restrict the use of the word epilepsy to idiopathic epilepsy, creating the use of the word epileptiform to describe symptomatic epilepsy. Auras were being divided into the categories of sensory, psychic, and motor.

The significance of auras was further clarified by William Gowers in his 1881 classic, *Epilepsy and Other Chronic Convulsive Diseases*. In this book, he outlined the vast knowledge gained on etiology, pathology, diagnosis, prognosis, and treatment of epilepsy to date. Statistics were employed in Gowers's book and in other arenas in the study of epilepsy to determine the influence of heredity, age of onset, and etiology (Gowers, 1881/1963). Autopsies were being performed on the brains of persons with epilepsy, often yielding confusing results, as there did not appear to be a single major site for abnormalities in such persons. Bromide of potassium was introduced by Sir Charles Locock in 1857 as the first anticonvulsant drug. It was touted as the cure for epilepsy and obviously failed. Thus, in the 1800s epilepsy came to be viewed more scientifically than ever before (Temkin, 1971).

Intellectual deterioration and deficits in memory and attention in persons with epilepsy were noted by Gowers (1881/1963). Personality changes associated with epilepsy were also being noted; among these were hyposexuality, mania, and bouts of rage. With knowledge of interictal personality changes in persons with epilepsy came the potential for abuse. Furor epilepticus became a major concern, with many believing that the person with epilepsy was capable of hideous acts during such angry fits. Criminals now found it profitable to pose as sufferers of epilepsy (Temkin, 1971).

Edouard Brown-Sequard spent much of his later life searching for the cause and proper treatment of epilepsy. It was one of his students, John Hughlings Jackson (1835–1911), however, who became famous for his work on epilepsy. Jackson, a prominent neurologist, were also interested in psychology and philosophy. He is often referred to as the "father of English neurology." Early in his career, Jackson began writing about epilepsy. Jackson accurately described epilepsy as an abnormal local discharge of the nerve tissue (Haymaker & Schiller, 1970).

Rather than focus on the study of generalized seizures as his predecessors had done, Jackson began his study of epilepsy by investigating the simplest form of epilepsy, unilateral seizures. Jackson demonstrated that symptoms of seizures could start in the periphery and march up a limb and that unilateral seizures could generalize. These seizures became popularly known as "Jacksonian seizures." Jackson called these seizures "uncinate seizures" or "middle-level fits" because they originated in the motor regions or middle level of the cerebral system (Haymaker & Schiller, 1970; Taylor, 1958).

Jackson described such seizures as attacks that usually commenced locally in the face, hand, or foot but did not always remain local. Seizures could affect only one side of the body or the entire body. When the seizure spread, consciousness was lost. If the seizure did not spread, consciousness was not necessarily lost but was merely limited or altered. Jackson believed that a seizure could be aborted by pulling or pressing on the part of the body where the convulsion began. He believed that focal convulsions were caused by a discharging lesion originating from damaged nerve cells, especially in the corpus striatum (McHenry, 1969). Jackson differentiated these sensory auras from the psychic auras his patients called intellectual auras or dreamy stages by asserting that these different seizure types arose from different systems within the brain (Taylor, 1958).

Jackson raised the idea that any disorder of the brain that gave rise to seizures could be considered genuine epilepsy. He asserted that epilepsy is not a single disorder but could take different forms. Jackson argued that local convulsions are true convulsions. This idea was not well received in many medical circles. Many neurologists, supporting Reynolds' system of calling only idiopathic epilepsy true epilepsy, rejected Jacksonian seizures as true epilepsy because of the repeated confirmation of damage to the temporal lobes at autopsy in persons suffering from this type of disorder. Thus, Jackson was one of the first to identify physical loci of epileptic seizure focus and to describe accurately the spread of seizure activity from an abnormal discharge of specific cells. He was able to use this conceptual model to explain why seizures varied in severity.

Jackson also used clinical observation in his research, and he noted common personality changes in persons with epilepsy and advocated an entirely new way to view epilepsy. He believed that researchers should study the nature of the convulsion, the march of the convulsion, and the postictal condition of the person. By so doing, one could obtain information about the region of seizure focus, the nature of the disturbance, and the pathological cause. Jackson also did much to disprove phrenology in his study of epilepsy (Taylor, 1958).

EMIL KRAEPELIN, HENRI GASTAUT, THE RISE OF NEUROPSYCHOLOGY, AND THE TWENTIETH CENTURY

Early in the 20th century, treatment of epilepsy came more under the realm of neurologists than psychiatrists. Far less faith was placed in mystical and religious healers. More anticonvulsants came into use, and today there are approximately 15 prescribed separately or in various combinations (Rodin, 1984). Seizure classification systems became more and more refined as a greater number of seizure types were recognized and more knowledge about the neuropathology of epilepsy was accumulated (Masland, 1974).

Because of the emphasis on the neurological aspects of epilepsy, many of the behavioral and emotional aspects of the disease were being ignored. In Europe during the first part of the 20th century, however, Emil Kraepelin listed epilepsy as one of the three major categories of insanity (Blumer, 1984). He recognized the two different types of epilepsy acknowledged at the time, grand mal and petit mal, and that these types had different behavioral and emotional manifestations. Among these were hallucinations, grandiose delusions, religiosity, rapid, often dramatic mood changes, memory lapses, anxiety, violence, and delirious states prior to seizures or as a result of a seizure, which could last hours to days. Although Kraepelin wrongly classified epilepsy as insanity, he advocated the need for psychiatric attention for people with epilepsy.

In 1937, Gibbs, Gibbs, and Lennox reinitiated the study of Jacksonian seizures, renaming them psychomotor seizures. In a series of studies from 1951 to 1953, Henri Gastaut had collected evidence using the EEG to link the origin of such seizures to the temporolimbic or rhinencephalic region. He also listed personality changes common to patients with this seizure type and their anatomic basis. He found that these personality changes were almost directly opposite to those seen in temporal lobe ablation studies (Kluver–Bucy syndrome). Such changes included diminished activity, hyposexuality, and hyposocial behavior with intermittent periods of irritability that may culminate in angry outbursts. This offered strong anatomic evidence for the epileptic personality reported by others (Blumer, 1984).

With increased understanding of the origin and neuropathology of epilepsy, much research since the mid 1950s has refocused on the cognitive, personality, and psychosocial consequences of epilepsy. As a result, psychologists, and neuropsychologists in particular, have played an increasingly important role in the study, assessment, and treatment of epilepsy. Using sensitive neuropsychological tests, neuropsychologists have identified specific interictal cognitive impairments in attention, memory, language, reasoning ability, and psychomotor ability in persons with epilepsy (Dodrill, 1978). Such techniques have helped in the understanding of the progression of neuropathology of epilepsy. Retraining programs and the teaching of compensatory measures specific to an individual's level of functioning have been found to aid in minimizing the effects of such impairments (Bennett & Krein, 1989). Trimble and Thompson (1986) advocate the use of neuropsychological assessment of cognitive function prior to and after medication changes to minimize detrimental effects of the medication on cognition. Specific personality changes associated with epilepsy have been suggested as well (e.g., Blumer & Benson, 1982). Techniques utilized in the neuropsychological practice such as psychotherapy, biofeedback, and education can be valuable tools in helping the person with epilepsy cope with the personality changes, stresses, and psychosocial problems that accompany epilepsy.

REFERENCES

Bennett, T. L., & Krein, L. K. (1988). The neuropsychology of epilepsy: Psychological and social impact. In C. R. Reynolds & E. Fletcher-Janzen (Eds.), *Handbook of clinical child neuropsychology* (pp. 419–441). New York: Plenum Press.

Blanton, W. B. (1931). *Medicine in Virginia in the eighteenth century*. Richmond, VA: Garrett & Massie.

Blumer, D. (1984). The psychiatric dimension of epilepsy: Historical perspective and current significance. In D. Blumer (Ed.), *Psychiatric aspects of epilepsy* (pp. 1–65). Washington, D.C.: American Psychiatric Press.

Blumer, D., & Benson, D. F. (1982). Psychiatric manifestations of epilepsy. In D. F. Benson & D. Blumer (Eds.), *Psychiatric aspects of neurologic disease, Volume 2* (pp. 25–48). New York: Grune & Stratton.

Clarke, E., & Dewhurst, K. (1972). *An illustrated history of brain function*. Berkeley, CA: University of California Press.

Courville, C. B. (1951). Epilepsy in mythology, legend, and folktale. *Bulletin of the Los Angeles Neurological Society, 16*, 213–224.

Dewhurst, K. W. (1980). *Thomas Willis Oxford Lectures*. Oxford: Sandford Publications.

Dodrill, C. B. (1978). A neuropsychological battery for epilepsy. *Epilepsia, 19*, 611–623.

Fulton, J. F. (1959). History of focal epilepsy. *International Journal of Neurology, 1*, 21–33.

Gibbs, F. A., Gibbs, E. L., & Lennox, W. G. (1937). Epilepsy: A paroxysmal cerebral dysrhythmia. *Brain, 60*, 377–388.

Gowers, W. R. (1963). *Epilepsy and other chronic convulsive diseases: Their causes, symptoms, and treatment*. London: Churchill. Original work published 1881.

Haymaker, W., & Schiller, F. (1970). *The founders of neurology*. Springfield, IL: Charles C. Thomas.

Lennox, W. G. (1939). John of Gaddesden on epilepsy. *Annals of Medical History*, *1*, 283–307.

Lennox, W. G. (1940). Antonius Guainerius on epilepsy. *Annals of Medical History*, *2*, 482–499.

Lennox, W. G. (1941). Bernard of Gordon on epilepsy. *Annals of Medical History*, *3*, 372–383.

Levine, E. B. (1971). *Hippocrates*. New York: Twayne.

Masland, R. L. (1974). The classification of the epilepsies: A historical review. In O. Magnus & A. M. Lorentz De Haas (Eds.), *Handbook of clinical neurology, Volume 15, The epilepsies* (pp. 1–29). New York: American Elsevier.

McHenry, L. C. (1969). *Garrison's history of neurology* Springfield, IL: Charles C. Thomas.

Murphy, E. L. (1959). The saints of epilepsy. *Wellcome Institute for the History of Medicine*, *3*, 303–311.

O'Leary, J. L., & Goldring, S. (1976). *Science and epilepsy: Neuroscience gains in epilepsy research*. New York: Raven Press.

Penfield, W. G. (1958). Hippocratic preamble: The brain and intelligence. In F. N. L. Poynter (Ed.), *The history and philosophy of knowledge of the brain and its functions* (pp. 1–4). Oxford: Blackwell.

Reynolds, J. R. (1861). *Epilepsy: Its symptoms, treatment, and relation to other chronic convulsive diseases*. London: Churchill.

Rodin, E. A. (1984). Epileptic and pseudoepileptic seizures: Differential diagnoses considerations. In D. Blumer (Ed.), *Psychiatric aspects of epilepsy* (pp. 179–195). Washington, DC: American Psychiatric Press.

Siegel, R. E. (1968). *Galen's system of physiology and medicine*. Basel: S. Karger.

Streeter, E. C. (1922). A note on the history of convulsive state prior to Boerhaave. *Association for Research in Nervous and Mental Disorders*, *7*, 5–29.

Taylor, J. (1958). *Selected writings of John Hughlings Jackson, Volume 1, On epilepsy and epileptiform convulsions*. New York: Basic Books.

Temkin, O. (1971). *The falling sickness*. Baltimore: Johns Hopkins University Press.

Trimble, M. R., & Thompson, P. J. (1986). Neuropsychological aspects of epilepsy. In I. Grant & K. M. Adams (Eds.), *Neuropsychological assessment of neuropsychological disorders* (pp. 321–346). New York: Oxford University Press.

Vogel, V. J. (1970). *American Indian Medicine*. Norman, OK: University of Oklahoma Press.

2

Neurological Conceptualizations of Epilepsy

GERALD C. McINTOSH

Epilepsy is a common neurological disorder, currently affecting over two million people in the United States. The generally accepted prevalence rate is five per 1000 when chronic epileptic disorders are considered. Approximately 2.2% of the population will have a single seizure some time in their lives (Epilepsy Foundation of America, 1975). The neurophysiological mechanisms active in epileptogenesis involve changes in membrane conductances and neurotransmitter function (Delgado-Escueta, Ward, Woodburg, & Porter, 1986a), and experimental models have been developed to correlate microstructural alterations with physiological and chemical observations.

Epilepsy may be studied by seizure type or by causation. Classification systems have been developed from both viewpoints. Associated symptom complexes have brought terminology depicting characteristic epileptic syndromes into general usage as well. Typical seizure patterns can be associated with specific cerebral localizations and with mechanisms of seizure induction. The clinical, electrocerebral, and imaging aspects in epileptic disorders and the differential diagnosis of epilepsy are other fields of ongoing study.

Epilepsy has been described in literature and known to mankind since antiquity. The Greeks were the first to use the word epilepsy to describe the circumstance in which someone was "seized by forces from without." The earliest text about epilepsy, written approximately 400 B.C. by Hippocrates, was entitled *On the Sacred Disease* (Sands, 1982). Society at that time often treated epileptics as individuals of special religious or social significance or often as victims of demonic possession (Schmidt & Wilder, 1968). As might be expected, typical generalized motor seizures

GERALD C. McINTOSH • Rehabilitation Department and Life Skills Rehabilitation Center, Poudre Valley Hospital, Fort Collins, Colorado 80524.

The Neuropsychology of Epilepsy, edited by Thomas L. Bennett. Plenum Press, New York, 1992.

were easier for a primitive culture lacking any scientific base to define in societal terms than partial or partial complex seizures accompanied by mannerisms rather than convulsive motor activity. Very little is seen in classical literature or premodern medicine on the topic of partial or partial complex seizures.

Clarity regarding the etiology and treatment of epilepsy lagged behind early advances in other areas of medicine. It was not until the end of the 19th century, with the writings of John Hughlings Jackson (Taylor, 1958), that the concept of a discharging epileptigenic focus was developed. Later, Gowers (1885/1964) organized the first classification of epilepsy into two major groupings, one with structural brain disease and the other with a generalized brain dysfunction leading to epilepsy. Behavioral aspects of seizures were difficult to interpret because motor abnormalities, as the observable alterations in consciousness, were necessary to make a clinical diagnosis. When a clinician could see only behavioral changes and mannerisms, a diagnosis of seizures was based on speculation (Goetz, 1987). Berger's (1929) initial description of electroencephalography (EEG) and developments that followed and continued in EEG correlation with epileptic disorders by Gibbs (Gibbs, Davis, & Lennox, 1936) and others allowed for the development of a more accurate understanding of the full scope of epilepsy and its effects on the human condition. Still, the unexpected intrusion of altered consciousness or specific neurological dysfunctions, even with the improved understanding of etiology and the developments in therapy that have occurred over the past 10 years, remains a devasting force in the lives of afflicted individuals.

BASIC MECHANISMS IN EPILEPTOGENESIS

This discussion of the neurophysiological mechanisms in epilepsy is limited to a concise review of currently accepted concepts. We refer the reader to a recent volume entirely dedicated to a review of these concepts should further detail seem necessary (Delgado-Escueta et al., 1986a). The basic scientific study of epilepsy addresses the cellular changes in membrane conductances and neurotransmitter alterations as they affect neuronal interaction in epileptogenesis. Experimental models for investigation of neurophysiological phenomena and the study of therapeutic mechanisms have also been developed and have become more sophisticated in recent years (Delgado-Escueta, Ferrendelli, & Prince, 1984). It seems that in the process of epileptogenesis either some neurons are discharging too easily because of alterations in membrane conductances or there is a failure of inhibitory neurotransmission. These distinctions in neurophysiological mechanism separate the focal and secondary generalized seizure mechanism from that of the primary generalized seizure.

The observable scalp electrode EEG finding that is considered to be a marker for epileptogenesis is the interictal spike. The actual discharge has been recognized to result from a neuronal "depolarization shift" with electrical synchrony in local cell populations (Goldensohn & Purpura, 1963) related in part to changes in membrane conductances. The ionic basis and biochemical substrate of this activation have been areas of considerable study but still leave many questions unanswered. Studies of the phenomena behind the interictal spike are aimed at better understanding of focal epileptogeneis. Scientific study of the effects of neurotransmitter (especially inhibitory neurotransmitter) function or dysfunction on primary generalized epileptogenesis has more recently been an area of considerable interest (Delgado-Escueta, Ward, Woodbury, & Porter, 1986b; Roberts, 1984). Still, the basic mechanisms of epileptogenesis in humans, although well understood in many specifics, have not yet been fully elucidated (Prince & Conners, 1986).

Methods of study in epileptogenesis have been directed at developing useful experimental models in order to compare microstructural changes with electrophysiological and biochemical observations (Delgado-Escueta et al., 1986b). These experimental models have been used in conjunction with the study of pharmacological and biochemical effects of anticonvulsants, bringing about effective gains in the understanding of epilepsy therapeutics (Macdonald & McLean, 1986). The electrophysiological models of epilepsy include kindling (McNamara, 1984), which refers to a phenomenon whereby repeated administration of an initially subconvulsive electrical stimulus results in a progressive intensification of seizure activity and focal irritative or electrical stimulation (Delgado-Escueto et al., 1986a). Animals with congenital photic or audiogenic convulsive responses serve as models for the primary generalized epilepsies (Delgado-Escueta et al., 1986b). In vitro models using brain-slice and cell-culture techniques mainly to study excitability of nerve cells have also been used extensively in efforts to bring about improved understanding of differences in membrane conductance between normal physiological states and epileptogenesis (Prince & Conners, 1984).

Anticonvulsant drugs are typically studied for their effectiveness in reducing repetitive firing, enhancing γ-aminobutyric acid (Roberts, 1984) (GABA, a major inhibitory neurotransmitter) responses, blocking maximal electrical seizures (MES), blocking pentylenotetrazole (PTZ, an epileptogenic chemical promoting disinhibition) seizures, and in clinical effectiveness (Macdonald & McLean, 1986).

Neurons can be stimulated to discharge repetitively in in vitro experimental situations. Most anticonvulsant drugs will make this phenomenon more difficult to induce. Reduction in repetitive neuronal firing serves as a quantitative measure of anticonvulsant effect (Delgado-Escueta et al., 1986a). Because GABA has been shown to be an inhibitory neurotransmitter, increases in GABA levels or availability imply potential suppression of epileptogenesis (Roberts, 1984). By using electrical shocks in experimental animals, a researcher can usually induce generalized seizures. This type of experimentally induced seizure is termed a maximal electrical seizure (MES). Blocking of this type of seizure is a general measure of anticonvulsant effectiveness (Macdonald & McLean, 1986). Pentylenotetrazole is a chemical that reduces normal electrocerebral inhibition. The exact mechanism of PTZ's disinhibition is not completely understood, but it probably works through a neurotransmittor mechanism. Blocking of PTZ seizures correlates with suppression of primary generalized seizures (Macdonald & McLean, 1986). In Chapter 9 the mechanism of action of specific anticonvulsants and each drug's effects as seen by these methods of study are further elaborated.

CLASSIFICATION OF SEIZURES

Gowers (1885/1964) was the first to develop a classification system for epilepsy. He not only conceived of two major groups of epileptics, those with structural brain disease and those with a more diffuse tendency toward seizures, but he also subdivided epilepsy by clinical seizure manifestation. Seizure classification did not progress much beyond the point of individual clinicians each introducing new and separate systems until the Commission on Classification and Terminology of the International League against Epilepsy (Dreifuss, Bancaud, Henriksen, Rubio-Donnadieu, Seino, & Penry, 1981) introduced a classification system for seizure type that is the major one currently in use. This system was recently revised (Dreifuss, Martinez-Lage, Roger, Seino-Wolf, & Dam, 1985) to include seizure syndromes, some of which are reviewed later in this chapter. The basis of this classification of seizure types is whether the seizures are localized (partial) in their origin or primarily generalized. Variations on this classification system, one of which is presented in Table 2.1, use a generally accepted organization pattern such that discharges of localized origin versus generalized discharges are the central factors involved in distinguishing seizure types in most classification systems (Rodin, 1987).

Partial and Partial Complex Seizures

Partial seizures usually consist of some specific motor, sensory, or psychic alterations (Penfield & Kristiansen, 1951). Often the psychic alteration, hence the frequently used term "psychomotor," is associated with automatisms consisting of stereotyped movements such as chewing, blinking, or lip smacking. The emotional content of the seizure-related psychic experience can be quite variable from individual to individual but tends to remain stereotyped for the particular epileptic person. The most common emotion is fear, but pleasure, sadness, and vague familiarity are also frequently reported. Sensory hallucinations or misperceptions may also be associated with epileptic ictal phenomena. These sensations may range throughout the spectrum of visual, gustatory, olfactory, auditory, or somatic perceptions. Motor phenomena that are either simple or complex may also be manifestations of these focal discharges. The specific neurological alterations correspond to the cerebral localization of the ictal discharge, and the progression of the symptoms indicates the spread of the abnormal electrocerebral activity. Should the activity become widespread enough, it will be associated with accompanying alterations in consciousness or frank secondary convulsive generalization. The subtypes alluded to above are included in the classifications of the system in Table 2.1. Later in this chapter we further review more specific seizure-associated neurological symptoms and their probable corresponding cerebral localizations.

A recent study on the distribution of seizure types done by epidemiologic survey of over 1200 epileptics over 15 years of age showed 56% to have parietal seizures, half of which showed secondary generalization, and 26.5% to have primary generalized

TABLE 2.1. Classification of Seizures and Syndromes:
The International Classification of Epileptic Seizures

I. Partial seizures
   A. Simple partial seizures
      1. With motor symptoms
      2. With somatosensory or special sensory symptoms
      3. With autonomic symptoms
      4. With psychic symptoms
   B. Complex partial seizures
      1. Beginning as simple partial seizures and progressing to impairment of consciousness
         a. With no other features
         b. With features as in I.A.1–4
         c. With automatisms
      2. With impairment of consciousness at onset
         a. With no other features
         b. With features as in I.A.1–4
         c. With automatisms
   C. Partial seizure evolving to secondarily generalized seizures
      1. Simple partial seizures evolving into generalized seizures
      2. Complex partial seizures evolving into generalized seizures
      3. Simple partial seizures evolving to complex partial seizures to generalized seizures
II. Generalized seizures
   A. Absence seizures
      1. Absence seizures
      2. Atypical absence seizures
   B. Myoclonic seizures
   C. Clonic seizures
   D. Tonic seizures
   E. Tonic–clonic seizures
   F. Atonic seizures
III. Unclassified epileptic seizures

seizures, 88% of those with generalized motor seizures (Keranen, Sillapaa, & Riekkinen, 1988).

Absence Seizures

The most common type of absence seizure is the so-called *petit mal*, which is associated clinically with a brief (5 to 30-sec) staring spell and a quite typical 3–3.5/sec spike–wave pattern on EEG. Absence seizures of this type occur in childhood, between the ages of 4 and 12, and seldom persist into adulthood (Niedermeyer, 1972). Rarer types of absence seizures include those seen typically in late adolescence and those seen in association with myoclonic jerking (Schmidt & Wilder, 1968).

Myoclonic Seizures

The primary myoclonic epilepsies are confined to infancy, with the exception of a rare benign juvenile form, and may be benign and self-limited or associated with mental retardation. Myoclonus may also be seen in toxic and metabolic states, most typically after anoxic cerebral insult (Lance & Adams, 1963) or in uremia (Zuckerman & Glaser, 1972), and in degenerative central nervous system diseases involving neuronal elements (Berkovic, Andermann, Carpenter, & Wolfe, 1986).

Generalized Motor Seizures

Generalized motor seizures, described as tonic, tonic–clonic, clonic, clonic–tonic–clonic, and atonic depending on the motor sequence observed with the seizure, are the most common of the primary generalized epilepsies (Niedermeyer, 1972). Some of the subtypes within this group may be familial and have been targets of genetic studies (Delgado-Escueta *et al.*, 1986b). The electroencephalographic abnormalities associated with specific epileptic syndromes have been the subject of major treatment in the literature of epilepsy and cannot be dealt with in any detail here. Suffice it to say that quite frequently a correlation of specific seizure type with specific EEG change can be made with some of the primary generalized epilepsies, whereas in the partial epilepsies, the interictal spike is the common EEG recorded event corresponding to the disorder.

ETIOLOGY OF SECONDARY EPILEPSIES

Causation in the secondary epilepsies can be divided into two general categories. First, there may be a structural brain disorder that initiates a seizure focus and hence partial seizures or partial seizures with secondary generalization. Alternatively, a metabolic or toxic disorder may reduce the threshold for depolarization, whereupon generalized convulsions may occur. Of course, an etiologic factor that lowers seizure threshold could initiate a discharge from an established epileptic focus as well.

Traumatic Cerebral Injury

Structural brain problems inducing epilepsy may be caused by a direct trauma from a head injury. There are more than one million persons in the United States each year who have had injuries associated with a loss of consciousness (Caveness, 1977), and approximately 10% of these individuals subsequently developed epilepsy (Caveness, 1976). Head injury is perhaps the most common single cause of focal epilepsy of known causation. There is an increased risk of developing seizures for up to 15 years after penetrating head injury, based on a follow-up study with Vietnam veterans (Weiss, Salazar, Vance, Grafman, & Jabbari, 1986). Another common cause of focal epilepsies that is also, in essence, traumatic is birth-related brain injury, usually from direct trauma at delivery or perinatal hypoxia. This type of epilepsy is frequently associated with motor dysfunction, that is, cerebral palsy (Perlstein & Gibbs, 1949). Direct causation with a discrete seizure focus is often speculative in these cases, although focal, possibly epileptogenic, lesions, frequently of temporal lobe localization, have been recognized in pathological studies of the brains of individuals with longstanding partial seizures where the etiology is suspected birth-related injury.

Brain Tumors

Brain tumors of all types may induce a seizure focus. Meningiomas, which are tumors of the connective tissue covering of the brain, are especially noted to be associated with seizures, whereas deeper tumors that do not involve the cortex are less likely to be associated with seizures. Partial, partial complex, and secondary generalized seizures are the common seizure types. The incidence of neoplasms in an epileptic population is variable, and rates depend on patient age and tumor classification (Epilepsy Foundation of American, 1975). More specific description of the association of cerebral neoplasms with epilepsy is beyond the scope of this discussion. Neurocutaneous disorders, such as neurofibromotosis and tuberous sclerosis, are typically associated with tumors and seizures. Tumor-related seizures are less common in infancy and childhood and more common in adults. The incidence of tumors in adult-onset epilepsy has been reported to be up to 15%, but no good surveys are available since computerized tomography (CT) and, more recently, magnetic resonance imaging (MRI) came into widespread use. Certainly, the incidence of neoplasms in persons with seizures of either adult or childhood onset is high enough to warrant studies in all patients presenting with new-onset partial, partial complex, or secondary generalized epilepsy.

Vascular Disorders

Structural lesions of vascular origin such as vascular malformations, hemorrhages, aneurysms, venous sinus thrombosis, and areas of ischemic infarction are associated with seizures with considerable frequency. These types of lesions can frequently be recognized with CT and MRI. In general, vascular disorders causing displacement of normal brain and those that are especially irritative to the cerebral cortex are likely to be epileptogenic. This is exemplified by the relatively high incidence of seizures with intracerebral hemorrhage and venous sinus thrombosis compared to the much lower incidence in ischemic cerebral infarction.

Infections

Infections in the central nervous system or cerebral spinal fluid may also be associated with partial and generalized seizures. The specific etiology in these cases may be related to a mix of structural and metabolic problems. Brain infection such as viral encephalitis, especially herpes simplex encephalitis, is associated with seizure activity. Infections with organisms other than viruses invading the brain parenchyma also cause focal electrocerebral discharges and hence seizures. Localized infections such as abscesses in subdural, epidural, and intraparenchymal locations are frequently recognized in association with seizures. Nonlocalized meningeal infections are uncommonly associated with seizures.

Toxic and Metabolic Disorders

Genetically derived metabolic disorders affecting neurons may cause primary generalized seizures but are quite rare disorders themselves. Acute metabolic abnormalities, especially those related to glucose, calcium, magnesium, and oxygen metabolism, are associated with seizure induction. Hypoglycemia has quite pronounced epileptogenic effects, as do hypocalcemia and hypoxia. Seizures may occur as toxic effects of heavy metals, in particular lead and magnesium. Certain medications, such as phenothiazines, antidepressants, central nervous system stimulants, narcotic analgesics, and bronchodilators, may induce seizures. Some so-called recreational drugs, especially amphetamines and cocaine, are known to cause seizures. Sedative–hypnotic and ethanol withdrawal will lower the seizure threshold and presents a setting typical for seizures of the primary generalized type. The exact mechanism whereby this occurs remains to be fully elucidated.

Table 2.2 provides a more inclusive list of potential etiologies for seizures.

TABLE 2.2.   Etiology of Seizures

I.	Congenital malformations present a birth
II.	Trauma
	A. Birth trauma—immediate and latent
	B. Head trauma in children and adults
III.	Neoplasm
	A. Associated with neurocutaneous syndromes
	B. Primary brain tumors
	C. Secondary brain tumors
IV.	Vascular
	A. Anoxic ischemic neonatal injury
	B. Arteriovenous malformation
	C. Vasculitis
	D. Ischemic cerebral infarction
	E. Intracerebral hemorrhage
	F. Subarachnoid hemorrhage
	G. Venous sinus thrombosis
V.	Infection
	A. Meningitis
	B. Brain abscess
	C. Subdural empyema
	D. Viral infections
	E. Fungal infections
	F. Parasitic infections
	G. Allergic reactions to infections or immunizations

EPILEPTIC SYNDROMES

Efforts to organize epilepsy into a useful system of epileptic syndromes have recently been realized (Dreifuss et al., 1985). The terminology developed with this proposal, which attempts to take into account characteristic clusters of symptoms associated with epilepsy, has not come easily into general usage (Rodin, 1987). We discuss several of these epileptic syndromes more specifically below. Characteristic epileptic syndromes promote more effective therapy through better anticonvulsant selection, but preoccupation with classification by epileptic syndrome will lead one to overlook the unifying thread of the common principles of epileptogenesis.

Certain epileptic conditions are relatively characteristic of specific age groups and are therefore worthy of discussion in that context. Age-determined epilepsies are typically characterized by specific seizure types, which can be correlated with particular EEG patterns and an anticipated prognosis. Unfortunately, attempts to generally characterize these disorders have failed, and we are left with a relatively large number of subtypes that are each seen infrequently in clinical settings. Perhaps at least some of these syndromes exist in a continuum rather than stereotyped specificity.

Neonatal Seizures and Infantile Spasms

Neonatal seizures may be benign and self-limited or at times severe when seen in association with major cerebral dysfunctions. Causation in the severe type is usually related to asphyxia at birth, congenital malformations, or massive infection. After the neonatal period, the majority with the severe form will develop typical infantile spasms first described by West (1841). The EEG in this disorder shows prominent disorganization called hypsarrhythmia and reflects severe diffuse electrocerebral and often accompanying structural impairment. In general, the prognosis and treatment perspective in infantile spasms remain poor (Lombroso, 1983). A benign form of infantile spasms not associated with typical EEG changes and brain abnormalities has also been recognized (Riikonen, 1983).

Lennox–Gastaut Syndrome

Lennox–Gastaut syndrome consists of the presence of slow (1–2.5/sec) spike-wave complexes on EEG in association with a mixed seizure picture and mental retardation or childhood dementia (Gastaut, Roger, Saulayrol, Tassinari, Regis & Dravet, 1966). The seizure type most typical of this syndrome is the akinetic drop attack, but a mixed variety of seizures is the usual case. Over half of the reported cases of Lennox–Gastaut syndrome are associated with a recognizable major brain disorder such as cerebral palsy, cerebral malformation, or progressively degenerative brain disease. In most of these cases the EEG has undergone a transition from a hypsarrhythmia pattern to a slow spike–wave pattern. The remainder of the cases have no evidence of underlying brain disease but a similar association of seizures, EEG changes, and disorders of cognition. The severity of cognitive impairment is associated with the presence of major brain disorder and the early onset of mixed seizures. When seizures begin after age of 10, even with the typical EEG changes, severe cognitive impairment is not usually present.

Generalized Epilepsies

The primary generalized epilepsies consist of a variety of generalized motor and generalized absence seizure types (Niedemeyer, 1972). Generalized synchronous paroxysmal EEG abnormalities are seen in association with generalized motor seizures with onset in late childhood and persistence into adult life. Drowsiness-induced seizures and seizures on awakening are typical. Photoconvulsive EEG changes are frequently recognized in this syndrome. A genetic predisposition appears to be present, but an inheritance pattern has not been further elucidated. Petit mal absence in association with 3/sec spike–wave discharges on EEG, usually without automatisms, is a well-recognized entity. Generalized motor seizures occur in association with typical absence seizures in 30–50% of these cases. Both seizures and 3/sec spike–wave discharges can be quite typically induced by hyperventilation. Petit mal does not usually persist into adult life and is not associated with cognitive dysfunction.

Primary generalized seizures with mixed generalized paroxysmal EEG changes do continue into adult life and are frequently associated with cognitive or personality disorders (Neidermeyer, 1972). This syndrome may represent a continuum with the idiopathic type of Lennox–Gastaut syndrome. Whether or not some of the specific epilepsy syndromes discussed above, as well as some not discussed, exist as distinct entities is a subject of continued debate by epileptologists. Although groupings of similar clinical patterns are at times helpful for purposes of therapy or establishing prognosis, the common principles of epileptogenesis are frequently more useful in a clinical and therapeutic consideration.

Febrile Convulsions

Febrile convulsions may well be the most common type of seizure, occurring in 3–4% of all healthy children between the ages of 6 months and 2 years (Neidermeyer, 1972). Brief generalized motor seizures occurring in neurologically normal children in association with a sudden rapid rise in body temperature are representative of this disorder. The EEG is normal with febrile convulsions. If the clinical or EEG picture differs from the presentation described above, then an underlying epileptic disorder may exist. Most would agree that in instances where epilepsy developed later in life, either there was a new secondary etiology or the abnormalities were overlooked when the febrile convulsions occurred.

CLINICAL SEIZURE PATTERNS ASSOCIATED WITH SPECIFIC CEREBRAL LOCALIZATIONS

Galen (130–200 A.D.) is said to have overheard an epileptic boy describe the sensation he felt just prior to an attack as a cool breeze, hence, "aura" in Latin. The word has stuck with us, although we now understand that these sensations are actually the clinical accompaniment of the initial seizure manifestations and not a "warning" as was taught previously.

Partial epilepsies are associated with typical seizure patterns depending on the localization of the initiating depolarization (Delgado-Escueta *et al.*, 1986b). An area of interest in the study of epilepsy has been observed clinical seizure patterns and their reflection of functional cortical anatomy. Clinical seizure manifestations are determined to a major extent by the site of the epileptogenic focus, and typical patterns tend to be seen with specific localizations. The most complete collection of this work is the anatomic studies of Penfield and Kristiansen (1951) and Penfield and Jasper (1954), but reports of similar associations still periodically appear in epilepsy literature. Future clinical correlation of seizure patterns using magnetic resonance imaging and positron emission tomography should complement these earlier anatomic studies.

Temporal Lobe Localization

Regional localization in temporal lobe epilepsy has been worked out in more detail than other partial epilepsies, perhaps because of the prominent frequency of temporal lobe seizures (Currie, Heathfield, Henson, & Scott, 1971). Auditory sensations precede other symptoms of seizure content in seizures originating from the superior temporal gyrus. The more posterior the localization is in the superior temporal gyrus, the more likely there will be accompanying vestibular symptoms such as dizziness or vertigo. Hippocampal discharge is associated with strange, often indescribable feelings and perceptional illusions. Amygdalar epilepsy may have a broad-range combination of symptoms including epigastric discomfort and nausea, facial pallor or flushing, pupillary dilation, fear, panic, and olfactory or gustatory hallucinations. Isolated olfactory sensations are reported in association with lesions of the uncus, but olfactory content as it often accompanies complex seizures has little value in localization beyond the general suggestion of a temporal lobe focus. Pure taste sensation is very rare as an initial seizure phenomenon but is said to suggest a perisylvian localization in the temporal lobe when seen in association with other complex sensations. Lateral and posterior temporal discharges produce auditory and visual hallucinations. Isolated fear as an initial seizure symptom seems to have no localizing value outside of suggesting the temporal lobe in general.

Insular seizures begin with vestibular hallucinations followed by autonomic symptoms or gastrointestinal symptoms. Palpitations are associated with perisylvian localization, both inferior frontal and temporal lobe. Piloerection with minimal gastric sensations was recently reported in association with mesial temporal lobe localization (Brogna, Lee, & Dreifuss, 1986).

Secondary generalization is said to be common in hippocampal seizures (more than 60%), less so with amygdalar seizures and insular seizures (less than 30%), and uncommon with lateral and posterior temporal seizures. However, with lateral and posterior temporal lobe localization, automatisms and amnesia are frequently seen as secondary phenomena rather than generalized motor seizures. Amygdalar and insular seizures are frequently associated with gradual loss of consciousness in association with oral automatisms, staring, and confusion prior to any generalized motor seizure activity.

Frontal Lobe Localization

Frontal lobe localization can also be associated with specific seizure phenomena frequently of focal motor character. The classic focal motor march or so-called Jacksonian seizure is usually localized to the precentral gyrus. Prefrontal motor areas are associated with postural changes, speech arrest, or vocalization and frequent urinary incontinence. Initial vocalization is localized to midfrontal regions adjacent to Broca's area. Discharges from Broca's area usually produce silence. Cingular gyrus seizures produce automatisms with sexual features and urinary incontinence. Forced thinking is another characteristic frontal lobe symptom, as is forced yawning at seizure onset. Orbital frontal seizures produce olfactory hallucinations often associated with automatisms. Frontal lobe discharges with dorsal–lateral localizations are frequently adversive, with forced but sometimes conscious tonic head turning away from the site of the lesion as a prominent initial feature, followed by partial motor or partial complex seizure activity. Inital unconscious adversive head movement with secondary generalization is also frequently encountered with lateral frontal localizations. Postictal motor paralysis is associated with frontal lobe seizures, especially of dorsal and lateral localizations.

Occipital and Parietal Lobe Localization

Occipital and parietal lobe epilepsies are seen much less frequently than either temporal or frontal lobe epilepsies. Occipital seizures are reported to be visual or partial complex with visual content (Ludwig & Ajmone-Marsan, 1975). Seizures from the occipital polar region tend to produce a pure color, light, or darkness prior to any secondary generalization. Parietal seizures are frequently somatosensory or visual with relatively frequent secondary generalization. Somatic sensations of various descriptions are associated with postcentral gyrus localization in a vast majority of cases (Ajmone-Marsan & Goldhammer, 1973). It is interesting that "pain" is said by Penfield and Jasper (1954) to have localization in the precentral gyrus in two cases where the seizure symptoms were reproduced by electrical stimulation. They speculated that the pain reported is associated with muscle contraction and therefore actually secondary to motor phenomenon.

In order to have an accurate and clinically useful understanding of the association of seizure phenomena and cerebral localization, it is essential to understand that the progression of symptoms in an epileptic seizure pattern may only give clinical information in reference to seizure spread, not necessarily initial localization, as the cerebral area of initial depolarization may yield few symptoms. For this reason, a wide variety of findings may be reported by an epileptic as a complex seizure evolves although the area of seizure initiation may be relatively silent.

REFLEX EPILEPSIES

Various modes of externally applied stimulation have been known to induce electrocerebral discharges, including primary generalized, focal, and focal with secondary generalization. Perhaps the most common are the visually induced seizures and convulsive EEG responses seen with photic stimulation of various types (Newmark & Penry, 1979). Cerebral hypocarbia has been known to generally induce seizure activity, and this can be easily achieved through hyperventilation. Specific reflex epilepsies imply induction of epileptogenesis by activation of cerebral localizations with specific activities.

Photic Stimulation and Hyperventilation

The most common type of reflex epilepsy is the visually induced seizure of the classic photoconvulsive type. However, photic responses on an EEG are not necessarily associated with visually induced seizures (Newmark & Penry, 1979). The mechanism involved in the photoconvulsive response has been studied extensively but is incompletely understood (Green, 1969). Most typically, photoconvulsive seizures are of the primary generalized type. Focal discharges, on the other hand, have been reported with eye opening (Iwato, Itoh, Mikami, & Arnano, 1980), with eye blinking (Rafal, Laxer, & Janowsky, 1986), and simple eye closure (DeMarco & Miottello, 1981). Children and rarely adults have been reported to induce photosensitive seizures purposefully, supposedly for the pleasurable sensations associated with the seizures (Faught, Falgout, Nidiffer, & Dreifuss, 1986). Individuals with self-induced seizures often have subnormal intelligence (Anderman, Berman, Cooke, Dickson, Gastaut, Kennedy, Margerison, Pond, Tizard, & Walsh, 1962). Seizure activity induced by television is another type of visually propagated epilepsy that has interestingly seemed to decline with improvements in television technology. Pattern-sensitive epilepsy suggests the correlation between paroxysmal EEG discharges and the relative numbers of synchronized cells firing with visual stimulus (Wilkins, Darby, & Binnie, 1979).

Hyperventilation with associated cerebral hypocarbia is another general epileptogenic induction mechanism. Hyperventilation is known to induce both 3/sec spike–wave petit mal and focal epileptogenic discharges (Servitz, Kristof, & Stejokova, 1981). Photic stimulation and hyperventilation are part of accepted clinical EEG protocol used to demonstrate epileptogenesis.

Specific Reflex Epilepsies

Seizure induction has also been reported with reading (Stevens, 1957; Mesri & Pagano, 1987), writing (Cirignotta, Zucconi, Mondini, & Lugaresi, 1986), language function (talking) (Devi & Iyer, 1985), mathematical calculations (Ingvar & Nyman, 1962), music (Berman, 1981), eating (Devi & Iyer, 1985), tooth brushing (Holmes, Blair, Eisenburg, Scheibaum, Margraf, & Zimmerman, 1982), tapping (Calderon-

Gonzalez, Hopkins, & McLean, 1966), voluntary movements (Lishman, Symonds, Whitly, & Willison, 1962), noise (Devi & Iyer, 1985), hot water immersion (Stensman & Ursing, 1971; Satishchandra, Shivaramakrishana, Kaliaperumal, & Schoenberg, 1988), startle (Devi & Iyer, 1985), and various sensory stimuli (Daube, 1966; Bencze, Troupin, & Prockop, 1988), presenting an interesting spectrum that is beyond the scope of our limited discussion. The possibility that complex mental stimuli may induce seizures is also an accepted concept but one that is difficult to bring to direct observation (Bencze *et al.*, 1988). Reenactment of the triggering situation may be helpful for diagnosis in confusing clinical situations (Fariello, Booker, Chun, & Orrison, 1983). The supposition is that activity in certain cerebral localizations in susceptible individuals will lead to a depolarization shift followed by spread of the electrocerebral discharge. The implications here for seizure control are obvious, but since these phenomena are so rarely observed, the therapeutic concept can only be infrequently applied (Vieth, 1986; Bencze *et al.*, 1988). Whether or not emotional stress precipitates epileptic seizures has not been firmly established. Certainly individuals complain that this occurs, and reports have occasionally appeared in the literature (Moffett & Scott, 1984; Feldman & Paul, 1976).

STATUS EPILEPTICUS

Status epilepticus is a clinical condition in which convulsive or nonconvulsive seizure states persist beyond 30 min (Celesia, 1976). Convulsive status can be divided into several subtypes depending on the seizures observed. Tonic–clonic status, which consists of generalized motor seizures, may have breaks in convulsive seizures without return to consciousness. Myoclonic status is rare but seen in certain epileptic syndromes, most typically with progressive myoclonic epilepsy or in metabolic states such as cerebral anoxia. Tonic status is also rare but can be seen mostly typically in Lennox–Gastaut syndrome. Focal motor status, also known as epilepsia partialis continuum, is a special situation since it is frequently associated with focal cerebral pathology (Thomas, Reagan, & Klass, 1977; Verhagen, Renier, Terleak, Jasper, & Gabreals, 1988). Status epilepticus may be the presenting finding in convulsive epilepsy or may present in the course of epileptic management (Celesia, 1976; Delgado-Escueta, Wasterlain, Treiman, & Porter, 1983).

Nonconvulsive status is of two generalized types, namely, absence status (Anderman & Robb, 1972) and partial complex status (Ballenger, King, & Gallagher, 1983), which are differentiated by EEG findings. Absence status is associated with generalized, usually 3/sec, spike–wave activity, whereas partial complex status is associated with more focal continuous cerebral discharges (Ballenger *et al.*, 1983). Both of these disorders can lead to a stuporous or confusional state that can be clinically confused with a variety of nonepileptogenic etiologies (Delgado-Escueta *et al.*, 1983).

CONFUSIONAL STATES AND EPILEPSY

Ictal events of either the absence status or partial complex status variety may produce confusion, altered consciousness, or disordered behavior (Delgado-Escueta *et al.*, 1983). Nonictal but epilepsy-related etiologies may also produce a confusional state in epileptic populations.

Of these nonictal etiologies the most common is the postictal confusional state, usually seen after generalized motor seizures or prolonged partial complex seizures, with or without secondary generalization of prolonged duration or repetitive occurrence. Individuals present most typically in an agitated delirium but may also show a persistent mild confusion. Occasionally, however, more complex confusional states and disordered behaviors are seen in the postictal time period, although the frequency of this occurrence is controversial. The so-called epileptic psychosis (Wells, 1975) may very well represent partial complex status in most cases, although a more chronic and less dramatic psychosis has been seen on occasion in epileptics with temporal lobe pathology as a postictal or nonictal phenomena. Differentiation of ictal and nonictal states can be accomplished with EEG techniques including ambulatory monitoring (Bridges, 1988). Epileptic medication intoxication may also produce encephalopathy with delirium. The presence of intoxication can be determined by clinical signs and confirmed by finding serum anticonvulsant levels in the toxic range. Typical symptoms and signs of intoxication to specific medications are discussed further in Chapter 9.

Nonepileptic confusional states should also be mentioned briefly. These include various intoxications (including alcohol, sedative hypnotics, and hallucinogens), metabolic states (including hypoglycemia, hypoxemia, and various organ failure states), head trauma, encephalopathy related to migraine, transient global amnesia, and conversion or dissociative emotional states. Some of these disorders are discussed further in the section dealing with differential diagnosis in paroxysmal disorders.

CLINICAL EVALUATION OF EPILEPSY

The initial clinical approach most appropriate for epilepsy diagnosis and treatment determinations is confirmation of electrocerebral discharges as responsible for paroxysmal behavioral or convulsive phenomena. This is accomplished by a variety of EEG methods. Usually a sleep study is more likely to show epileptogenic discharges than a routine awake EEG. Maximizing the productivity of this study with hyperventilation, photic stimulation, special leads, and more specific trigger techniques may also be appropriate. Usually hyperventilation, photic stimulation, and both awake and sleep studies are combined for a routine epilepsy EEG. A discussion of various electrode montages that are helpful for diagnostic confirmation in epilepsy is beyond the scope of this text and therefore is not discussed here. Ambulatory and telemetry monitoring at times combined with video recordings can also be quite useful, since each allows for prolonged observations of EEG activity and correlation with recorded or observed clinical phenomenon. When the confirmation of electro-cerebral activity in association with seizures is established, the focal versus gener-alized aspects of observed electrocerebral discharges are usually also demonstrated.

Adjunctive studies that may be complementary to the evaluation of a person with epilepsy address possible secondary etiologies such as infections, vascular disorders, immune disorders, toxic exposures, and metabolic abnormalities. Figure 2.1 outlines the clinical and imaging studies applicable to the evaluation of new-onset seizures in an adult.

Brain-imaging techniques are appropriate to establish focal pathology where focal discharges are seen. These studies include computerized tomography (CT), magnetic resonance imaging (MRI), and positron emission tomography (PET). The CT demonstrates variations in brain density and, when coupled with contrast enhancement, also helps visualize vascular patterns. Magnetic resonance imaging provides a more anatomically accurate image of the brain structure that is not determined by density but rather by electrochemical characteristics (Jabbari, Gunder-son, Wippold, Citrin, Sherman, Bartoszek, Daigh, & Mitchell, 1986). Positron emission tomography shows localization of brain metabolic activity. An epilepto-genic focus will usually show an area of altered metabolic activity and is being used currently for purposes of localization in seizure surgery evaluations.

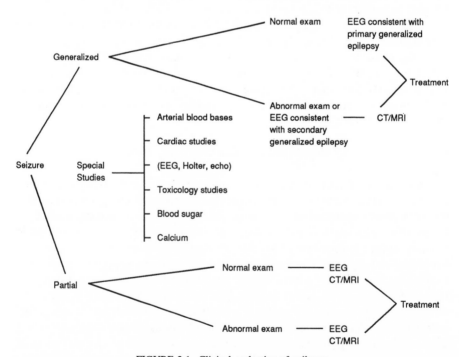

FIGURE 2.1. Clinical evaluation of epilepsy.

DIFFERENTIAL DIAGNOSIS OF EPILEPSY

A variety of disorders associated with altered behavior or consciousness are included in the differential diagnosis of epilepsy. Syncope is loss of consciousness secondary to a decrease in cerebral perfusion. Metabolic and toxic states may alter consciousness or behavior. Migraine is a common neurological disorder that may mimic seizures or at times be associated with seizures. One of the major diagnostic dilemmas in clinical epileptology is the phenomenon of psychogenic or pseudoseizures.

Syncopal Disorders

With transient decreases in cerebral perfusion that may be secondary to cardiac abnormality or autonomic (vasovagal) reactions, loss of consciousness is usually preceded by a vague fade-out sensation or visual dimming. Cough syncope and micturition syncope typify conditions in which autonomic responses initiated by specific inciting factors produce a drop in perfusion pressure followed by syncope.

Syncope of cardiogenic origin is a more clinically serious condition that is likely to lead to major medical complications or even death. The prolonged-QT-interval syndrome may produce alterations in consciousness or syncope or may mimic idiopathic epilepsy (Pignata, Farina, Andria, DelBiudise, Striano, & Adinoffi, 1983) by producing a drop in cerebral perfusion pressure. Various forms of heart block and valvular heart disease may also induce syncope.

Toxic and Metabolic Disorders

Toxic and metabolic problems may transiently alter consciousness with and without associated seizure activity. This is especially true for episodes of hypoxia, as can be seen after pulmonary embolism or with severe bronchospasm. Therefore, clinical and laboratory evaluation for hypoxia and its causation should be considered if clinically warranted. Episodes of transient cerebral ischemia of a focal nature may also significantly alter consciousness and can be confused with partial epilepsy. At times the differential diagnosis of an event of brain dysfunction with or without convulsive accompaniment can be challenging or even unresolvable. Cataplectic attacks in narcolepsy may mimic atonic seizures, and sleep attacks in narcolepsy can be confused with postictal lethargy but usually not convulsive or partial seizures. Sleep apnea may be confused with nocturnal seizures and also induce hypoxic seizures. In most of the abovementioned disorders, clinical features, EEG, or other specific studies aid in the differentiation.

Migraine

In order to cover adequately the relationship of migraine to epilepsy, we would need a format well beyond the scope of this chapter. Transient focal cerebral symptoms may be seen with migraine either with or without associated headache.

Certain epileptic syndromes, notably benign occipital epilepsy and benign rolandic epilepsy, are associated with migraine headaches. The differentiation here may be difficult because the EEG often shows focal, even epileptoform, abnormalities in migraine even without associated seizures but with focal cerebral symptoms. Basilar artery migraine with associated visual and brainstem symptoms is especially known to produce loss of consciousness and possibly also convulsive activity (Bickerstaff, 1961). Partial complex seizures may be followed at times by postictal vascular headaches. Various authors have failed to show a general association or hereditary connection between epilepsy and migraine.

Pseudoseizures

Pseudoseizures present a complex problem for differential diagnosis, especially since a large percentage of individuals with pseudoseizures have an underlying epileptic disorder. Caution should always be exercised when making a diagnosis of conversion-related pseudoseizures or feigned seizures (Krumholz & Niedermeyer, 1983). A recorded episode without electrocerebral discharges may be quite useful in this determination; however, movement artifact can make EEG interpretation difficult. The EEG is more useful when a sequence of normal awake activity followed by movement artifact with no postictal slowing is demonstrated. The actual differentiation process with coexisting pseudoseizures and electrocerebral seizures may be quite tricky. Our practice is to continue therapeutic doses of anticonvulsant medication if clinical or EEG evidence of coexisting epilepsy and pseudoseizures are thought to be present. Openness with the patient and the family is essential. Feigned seizures are usually easier to differentiate, as they are most often motor in nature and clinically obvious depending on the skill of the imitation and the experience of the observer. Tongue biting, lip biting, and incontinence may occur with any pseudoseizure.

SUMMARY

The preceding discussion has reviewed most of the major concepts basic to the understanding of epilepsy, including etiology, localization, classification, evaluation, and differential diagnosis. Mechanisms of epileptogenesis as related to etiology, localization, and type of epileptic seizure are clinically important in the selection of medical therapy with anticonvulsants, surgical therapy, and adjunctive therapies. Basic science research continues to explore the basic mechanisms of epileptogenesis and to promote development of more definitive therapies.

REFERENCES

Ajmone-Marsan, C., & Goldhammer, L. (1973). Clinical ictal patterns and electrographic data in cases of partial seizures of fronto–central–parietal origin. In M. A. B. Brazier (Ed.), *Epilepsy: Its phenomena in man* (pp. 236–260). New York: Academic Press.

Anderman, F., & Robb, J. P. (1972). Absence status: A reapraisal following review of thirty-eight patients. *Epilepsia, 13*, 177–178.

Anderman, K., Berman, S., Cooke, P. M., Dickson, J., Gastaut, H., Kennedy, A., Margerison, J., Pond, D. A., Tizard, J. P. M., & Walsh, E. G. (1962). Self-induced epilepsy. *Archives of Neurology, 6*, 63–79.

Ballenger, C. E. III, King, D. W., & Gallagher, B. B. (1983). Partial complex status epilepticus. *Neurology, 33*, 1545–1552.

Bencze, K. S., Troupin, A., & Prockop, L. D. (1988). Reflex absence epilepsy. *Epilepsia, 29*, 48–51.

Berger, H. (1929). Uber das Elektroenzephalogronom des Menschen. *Archiv fur Psychiatrie und Nervenkrankheiten, 87*, 527–570.

Berkovic, S. T., Andermann, F., Carpenter, S., & Wolfe, L. S. (1986). Progressive myoclonus epilepsies: Specific causes and diagnosis. *New England Journal of Medicine, 315*, 296–303.

Berman, I. W. (1981). Musicogenic epilepsy. *South African Medical Journal, 21*, 49–52.

Bickerstaff, E. R. (1961). Basilar artery migraines. *Lancet, 1*, 15–17.

Bridges, S. L. (1988). Ambulatory cassette electromyography of psychiatric patients. *Archives of Neurology, 45*, 71–75.

Brogna, C. G., Lee, S. I., & Dreifuss, F. E. (1986). Pilanator seizures. *Archives of Neurology, 43*, 1085–1086.

Calderon-Gonzalez, R., Hopkins, I., & McLean, W. T. (1966). Tap seizures. *Journal of the American Medical Association, 198*, 107–109.

Caveness, W. F. (1976). Epilepsy, a product of trauma in our time. *Epilepsia, 17*, 207–215.

Caveness, W. F. (1977). Incidence of craniocerebral trauma in the united states 1970–1975. *Annals of Neurology, 1*, 507–510.

Celesia, G. G. (1976). Modern concepts of status epilepticus. *Journal of the American Medical Association, 235*, 1571–1574.

Cirignotta, I., Zucconi, M., Mondini, S., & Lugaresi, E. (1986). Writing epilepsy. *Clinical Electroencephalography, 17*, 21–23.

Currie, S., Heathfield, K. W. G., Henson, R. A., & Scott, D. F. (1971). clinical course and prognosis of temporal lobe epilepsy. *Brain, 94*, 173–190.

Daube, J. R. (1966). Sensory precipitated seizures: A review. *Journal of Nervous and Mental Disease, 141*, 524–539.

Delgado-Escueta, A. V., Wasterlain, C. G., Treiman, D. M., & Porter, R. J. (1983). *Advances in neurology, Volume 34, Status epilepticus.* New York: Raven Press.

Delgado-Escueta, A. V., Ferrendelli, J. A., & Prince, D. A. (Eds.). (1984). Basic mechanisms of the epilepsies: Proceedings of a workshop at the Kroc Foundation Headquarters. *Annals of Neurology, 16*(5), 1–158.

Delgado-Escueta, A. V., Ward, A. A., Woodburg, P. M., & Porter, R. J. (Eds.). (1986a). Basic mechanisms of the epilepsies. *Advances in Neurology, 44.*

Delgado-Escueta, A. V., Ward, A. A., Woodburg, P. M., & Porter, R. J. (1986b). New wave of research in the epilepsies. *Advances in Neurology, 44*, 3–55.

DeMarco, P., & Miottello, P. (1981). Eye closure epilepsy. *Clinical Electroencephalography, 12*, 66–68.

Devi, T. K. M., & Iyer, G. V. (1985). Pattern of triggering among patients with epilepsy from kerala. *Journal of the Association of Physicians of India, 33*, 513–515.

Dreifuss, F. E., Bancand, J., Henriksen, O., Rubio-Donnadieu, F., Seino, M., & Penry, J. K. (1981). Commission on classification and terminology of the international league against epilepsy. Proposal for revised clinical and electroencephalographic classification of epileptic seizures. *Epilepsia, 22*, 489–501.

Dreifuss, F. E., Martinez-Lage, M., Roger, J., Seino, M., Wolf, P., & Dam, M. (1985). Commission on Classification and Terminology of the International League Against Epilepsy. Proposal for the classification of the epilepsies and epileptic syndromes. *Epilepsia, 26*, 268–278.

Epilepsy Foundation of America. (1975). *Basic Statistics on the Epilepsies.* Philadelphia: F. A. Davis.

Fariello, R. G., Booker, H. E., Chun, R. W. M., & Orrison, W. W. (1983). Reenactment of the triggering situation for the diagnosis of epilepsy. *Neurology, 33*, 878–884.

Faught, E., Falgout, J., Nidiffer, I. O., & Dreifuss, F. E. (1986). Self induced photosensitive absence seizures with ictal pleasure. *Archives of Neurology, 43*, 408–409.

Feldman, R. G., & Paul, N. L. (1976). Identity of emotional triggers in epilepsy. *Journal of Nervous and Mental Disease*, *162*, 345–353.

Gastaut, H., Roger, J., Saulayrol, R., Tassinar, C. A., Regis, H., & Dravet, C. (1966). Childhood epileptic encephalopathy with diffuse slow spike–waves (otherwise known as "petit-mal variant") or Lennox syndrome. *Epilepsia*, *7*, 139–179.

Gibbs, F. A., Davis, H., & Lennox, W. G. (1936). The electroencephalogram in diagnosis and in localization of epileptic seizures. *Archives of Neuropsychiatry*, *36*, 1225–1535.

Goetz, C. G. (1987). Charcot at the Salpetriere: Ambulatory automatisms. *Neurology*, *37*, 1084–1088.

Goldensohn, E. S., & Purpura, D. P. (1963). Intracellular potentials of cortical neurons during focal epileptogenic discharges. *Science*, *139*, 840–842.

Gowers, W. R. (1964). Epilepsy and other chronic convulsive disorders 1885. *American Academy of Neurology Reprint Series*, New York: Dover Publications. Original work published 1885.

Green, J. B. (1969). Photosensitive epilepsy. *Archives of Neurology*, *20*, 191–198.

Holmes, G. L., Blair, S., Eisenberg, E., Scheebaum, R., Margraf, J., & Zimmerman, A. W. (1982). Toothbrushing induced epilepsy. *Epilepsia*, *23*, 657–661.

Ingvar, D. H., & Nyman, G. E. (1962). Epilepsia arthmetries. *Neurology*, *12*, 282–287.

Iwato, T., Itoh, I., Mikami, T., & Anano, K. (1980). Focal epileptiform discharges triggered by opening the eyes. *Folia Psychiatrica et Neurologica Japonica*, *34*, 325–326.

Jabbari, B., Gunderson, C. H., Wippold, F., Citrin, C., Sherman, J., Bartoszek, D., Daigh, J. D., & Mitchell, M. H. (1986). Magnetic resonance imaging in partial complex epilepsy. *Archives of Neurology*, *43*, 869–872.

Keranen, T., Sillanpaa, M., & Riekkinen, P. J. (1988). Distribution of seizure types in an epileptic population. *Epilepsia*, *29*, 1–7.

Krumholz, A., & Neidermeyer, E. (1983). Psychogenic seizures: A clinical study with followup data. *Neurology*, *33*, 498–502.

Lance, J. W., & Adams, R. D. (1963). The syndrome of intention or action myoclonus as a sequel to hypoxic encephalopathy. *Brain*, *86*, 111–136.

Lishman, W. A., Symonds, C. P., Whitly, C. W. M., & Willison, R. G. (1962). Seizures induced by movement. *Brain*, *85*, 93–108.

Lombroso, C. T. (1983). A prospective study of infantile spasms: Clinical and therapeutic correlations. *Epilepsia*, *24*, 135–158.

Ludwig, B. I., & Ajmone-Marsan, C. (1975). Clinical ictal patterns in epileptic patients with occipital electroencephalographic foci. *Neurology*, *25*, 463–471.

Macdonald, R. L., & McLean, M. J. (1986). Anticonvulsant drugs: Mechanisms of action. *Advances in Neurology*, *44*, 713–736.

McNamara, J. O. (1984). Kindling: An animal model of complex partial epilepsy. *Annals of Neurology, 16*, S72–S76.

Mesri, J. C., & Pagano, M. A. (1987). Reading epilepsy. *Epilepsia*, *28*, 301–304.

Moffett, A., & Scott, D. F. (1984). Stress and epilepsy: The value of a benzodiazepine—Lorazepam. *Journal of Neurology, Neurosurgery and Psychiatry*, *47*, 165–167.

Newark, M. E., & Penry, J. D. (1979). *Photosensitivity and epilepsy: A review*. New York: Raven Press.

Niedermeyer, E. (1972). *The generalized epilepsies*. Springfield, IL: Charles C. Thomas.

Penfield, W., & Jasper, H. H. (1954). *Epilepsy and the functional anatomy of the human brain*. Boston: Little, Brown.

Penfield, W., & Kristiansen, K. (1951). *Epileptic seizure patterns*. Springfield, IL: Charles C. Thomas.

Perlstein, M. A., & Gibbs, F. A. (1949). Clinical significance of electroencephalography in cases of cerebral paralysis. *Archives of Neurology and Psychiatry*, *62*, 682–685.

Pignata, C., Farina, V., Andria, G., DelGiudice, E., Striano, S., & Adinaffi, L. (1983). Prolonged Q–T interval syndrome presenting as idiopathic epilepsy. *Neuropediatrics*, *14*, 235–236.

Prince, D. A., & Conners, B. W. (1984). Mechanisms of epileptogenesis in cortical structures. *Annals of Neurology*, *16*, S59–S64.

Prince, D. A., & Conners, B. W. (1986). Mechanisms of interictal epileptogenesis. *Advances in Neurology*, *44*, 275–299.

Rafal, R. D., Laxer, K. D., & Janowsky, J. S. (1986). Seizures triggered by blinking in a non-photosensitive epileptic. *Journal of Neurology Neurosurgery, and Psychiatry*, *49*, 445–447.

Riikonen, R. (1983). Infantile spasms: Some new theorectical aspects. *Epilepsia*, *24*, 159–168.

Roberts, E. (1984). GABA-related phenomena, models of nervous system function and seizures. *Annals of Neurology*, *16*, S77–S89.

Rodin, E. (1987). An assessment of current views of epilepsy. *Epilepsia*, *28*, 267–271.

Sands, H. (1982). *Epilepsy: A handbook for the mental health professional*. New York: Brunner/Mazel.

Satishchandra, P., Shivaramakrishana, A., Kaliaperumal, V. G., & Schoenberg, B. S. (1988). Hot water epilepsy. *Epilepsia*, *29*, 52–56.

Schmidt, R., & Wilder, B. J. (1968). *Epilepsy. Contemporary neurology series*. Philadelphia: F. A. Davis.

Servitz, Z., Kristof, M., & Stejckova, A. (1981). Activating effect of nasal and oral hyperventilation of epileptic electrographic phenomena: Reflex mechanisms of nasal origin. *Epilepsia*, *22*, 321–329.

Stensman, R., & Ursing, B. (1971). Epilepsy precipitated by hot water immersion. *Neurology*, *21*, 559–562.

Stevens, H. (1957). Reading epilepsy. *New England Journal of Medicine*, *257*, 165–170.

Taylor, J. (Ed.). (1958). *Selected writings of John Hughlings Jackson, I. On epilepsy and epileptiform convulsions*. New York: Basic Books.

Thomas, J. E., Reagan, T. J., & Klass, D. W. (1977). Epilepsia partialis continua. A review of 32 cases. *Archives of Neurology*, *34*, 266–275.

Verhagen, W. M., Renier, W. O., Terleak, H., Jaspar, H. H. J., & Gabreals, J. M. (1988). Anomalies of the cerebral cortex in a case of epilepsia partialis continua. *Epilepsia*, *29*, 57–62.

Vieth, J. (1986). Vigilance, sleep and epilepsy. *European Neurology*, *25*, 128–133.

Weiss, G. H., Salazar, A. M., Vance, S. L., Grafman, J. H., & Jabbari, B. (1986). Predicting post-traumatic epilepsy in penetrating head injury. *Archives of Neurology*, *43*, 771–773.

Wells, C. E. (1975). Transient ictal psychosis. *Archives of General Psychiatry*, *32*, 1201–1203.

West, W. J. (1841). On a peculiar form of infantile convulsions. *Lancet*, *1*, 724.

Wilkins, A. J., Darby, C. E., & Binnie, C. D. (1979). Neurophysiological aspects of pattern sensitive epilepsy. *Brain*, *102*, 1–25.

Zuckerman, E. G., & Glaser, G. H. (1972). Urea-Induced myoclonic seizures. *Archives of Neurology*, *27*, 14–28.

3

A Multietiological Model of Psychological and Social Dysfunction in Epilepsy

BRUCE P. HERMANN, STEVE WHITMAN,
and MICHAEL ANTON

One of the fascinations, and part of the frustration, inherent in epilepsy research is the multiplicity of forces that impinge on people with epilepsy. Although many of these factors are of conceptual or theoretical interest to those of us involved in epilepsy research, they are often a more immediate and brutal reality to people with epilepsy. For instance, consider an individual, perhaps a 22-year-old man with a high school education, who presents with the following: a history of a significant neurological insult (e.g., perinatal stroke), extremely overprotective parents, associated neuropsychological deficits, poor academic achievement, less than optimal medical management characterized by polytherapy and the use of barbiturate anticonvulsant medications, poor seizure control, and (as a child) a history of considerable teasing and abuse by his peers because of his seizure disorder. What are the important etiological variables, and where should intervention be aimed if the patient is profoundly depressed? If he is unemployed, what are the likely causes of his joblessness, and how should rehabilitation and intervention proceed? Are the biological factors (etiology, seizure control, neuropsychological deficits) the primary determinants of his psychopathology? Perhaps the social factors we have outlined are among the key causes of his difficulties, and it is likely that pharmacological variables play some role as well.

BRUCE P. HERMANN and MICHAEL ANTON • Epi-Care Center, Baptist Memorial Hospital, and Semmes-Murphey Clinic, Departments of Neurosurgery and Psychiatry, University of Tennessee-Memphis, Memphis, Tennessee 38103.   STEVE WHITMAN • Center for Urban Affairs and Policy Research, Northwestern University, Evanston, Illinois 60201.

The Neuropsychology of Epilepsy, edited by Thomas L. Bennett. Plenum Press, New York, 1992.

Complexities such as these have led us to attempt to develop a conceptual model of psychological and social dysfunction in epilepsy (Hermann & Whitman, 1984, 1986). This model was initially stimulated by our own limitations in understanding the causes of psychosocial problems in epilepsy. At the time, a large and diverse array of potential risk factors had been identified or suggested for a number of psychosocial problems. With only a few exceptions (e.g., Reynolds, 1981), however, there was little in the way of conceptual theorizing that united these variables into a schema of clinical utility or suggested directions for future research.

In the material that follows we first present a proposed model of psychosocial functioning in epilepsy. Following presentation of the model, we survey the findings from two investigations of the experimental utility of this model. In the first data set we examine the model in regard to understanding the determinants of depression in adults with epilepsy, and in the second data set we examine the predictors of social competence in children with epilepsy.

MAJOR CATEGORIES OF RISK FACTORS

Of importance is some organization of the many potential risk factors for psychological and social problems in epilepsy. As reflected in the individual case study just described, a diverse spectrum of potentially important variables may exist in any given case. Several reviews of the literature have specified the diversity of potential risk factors that may be involved, and, overall, a very heterogeneous group of variables have been identified or suggested (Fenwick, 1987; Hermann & Whitman, 1984; Stevens, 1975; Trimble & Bolwig, 1986). We initially proposed that these identified or suggested risk factors could be grouped into three conceptual categories: neurobiological, psychosocial, and treatment or medication related (Table 3.1). We review these categories and identify examples of variables to be considered under each.

TABLE 3.1.   Potential Multietiological Risk Factors

Neurobiological	Psychosocial	Medication
Age at onset	Locus of control	Monotherapy versus polytherapy
Duration of disorder	Fear of seizures	Presence/absence of barbiturate
Seizure type	Adjustment to epilepsy	medications
Degree of seizure control	Parental overprotection	Folate deficiency
Ictal/interictal EEG characteristics	Perceived stigma	Hormonal/endocrine effects
Presence/absence of structural	Perceived discrimination	Medication-induced alterations in
damage	Stressful life events	monoamine metabolism
Phenomenological aspects of the	Financial stress	Medication-induced alterations in
seizures	Employment status	cerebral metabolism
Neuropsychological function	Social support	
Efficiency of cerebral metabolism		
Alterations in neurotransmitter		
systems		

Neurobiological Factors

Many neurobiological and neurophysiological variables define the characteristics of an individual's epilepsy (Table 3.1). For instance, in an attempt to understand a patient's epilepsy, one must consider the etiology, the age at onset of the epilepsy, the number of years that the patient has had the disorder, the specific classification of the patient's seizure type or types, and the degree of seizure control that has been achieved over the years. Information is also needed about the interictal and ictal EEG characteristics, results of imaging studies (MRI and CT scans), phenomenological characteristics of the seizures, and the neuropsychological correlates of the epilepsy. Additional potentially important but perhaps less discussed factors include disruptions and alterations in the efficiency of cerebral metabolism (as revealed by PET scan), alterations in neurotransmitter systems, and disruptions in other basic neurobiological mechanisms. As noted, these and other variables constitute the so-called neurobiological spectrum of epilepsy. A considerable amount of research to date has centered around the relationship between particular psychosocial problems (e.g., psychopathology) and select subsets of these neurobiological factors, the hope being that the results would yield information pertaining to the organic precursors of psychopathology.

Psychosocial Factors

Psychosocial factors constitute a particularly salient dimension of epilepsy (Table 3.1). Although the term "psychosocial" is widely utilized, it is relatively generic and somewhat uninformative. For the purposes of this discussion we will present these risk factors in terms of what we believe to be their intrapersonal versus extrapersonal origins. Even this preliminary dichotomy is somewhat flawed, as the careful reader will discern that intrapersonal factors ultimately depend on the patient's interaction with others. Nevertheless, through this classification we are attempting to emphasize the difference between risk factors related to dysfunctional interpersonal relationships (e.g., stigma, discrimination, overprotection), and those intrapersonal risk factors that derive from how the patient perceives his or her epilepsy and how this in turn affects the nature of his or her interaction with, and perception of, society at large.

Intrapersonal Factors

Several factors can be considered to constitute the intrapersonal spectrum of psychosocial variables. To begin, epilepsy, like some other chronic disorders with episodic manifestations (e.g., asthma), can lead to special stresses. Specifically, seizures can occur anywhere, anytime, with little or no warning. Further, the seizures can be associated with significant embarrassment and loss of personal dignity. This unpredictability associated with the disorder has been hypothesized to alter the patient's perceived locus of control, i.e., the belief that powerful others, chance, or fate (external locus of control) determines important events in life rather than the patient himself or herself (internal locus of control) (Arnston, Droge, Norton, & Murray, 1986; Matthews & Barabas, 1986; Ziegler, 1981). Since an external locus of control has been found to be associated with an increased risk of psychopathology, this appears to be a relevant risk factor, particularly since patients with epilepsy have been found to manifest a more external locus of control than do healthy control subjects and those in other patient groups (e.g., diabetics) (Matthews & Barabas, 1986).

Another intrapersonal factor relates to the individual's perception and understanding of his or her disorder. Mittan (1986) has demonstrated that some adults harbor significant misperceptions of their epilepsy (e.g., that there is a high probability that they may die during a seizure). Perhaps most distressing, some patients act on these misperceptions in ways that are either self-defeating (e.g., avoidance of any and all stress with virtual retirement to the home) or dangerous (e.g., self-medication or self-initiated alterations in anticonvulsant medication usage), either of which would be expected to affect adversely the quality of their lives. Mittan (1986) has argued that fear of seizures is a potent predictor of maladjustment in adults with epilepsy.

In a somewhat similar vein it is a common clinical observation that patients vary enormously in their resources and strength in coping with epilepsy. Some individuals are able to proceed through life relatively unencumbered by their epilepsy, even if it is moderate to marked in severity. Other patients feel resentful, believe that their lives have been ruined by epilepsy, and continually dread the occurrence of a seizure. Further, some patients resent their need for medication, hide the disorder, and in general exhibit what may be best characterized as a poor adjustment to epilepsy. It has been hypothesized that these characteristics are associated with the adequacy of emotional and social adjustment.

Extrapersonal Factors

Particularly troublesome is the fact that individuals with epilepsy may be treated quite differently by friends, family, and society in general merely because of their condition. This differential treatment may be well-meaning in some cases, hostile in others, but may be expected to alter the patient's adjustment in either instance. For example, well-meaning parents may be extremely overprotective of their children with epilepsy. Their expectations for the child may be lowered and patterns of familial interaction altered (Long & Moore, 1979; Ritchie, 1981). At school the child may be teased, harassed, and socially excluded, and the seizures may be feared by the teacher. We have encountered numerous intellectually intact young adults who had been excluded from the regular school system as children because of their seizures and the disruption that they allegedly had caused. These alterations in development surely constitute potential risk factors for poor adjustment.

Perhaps the stigma and discrimination directed against individuals with epilepsy are the most obvious of the extrapersonal psychosocial risk factors, but even here there are subtle considerations. On the one hand, there is often clear abject social exclusion of the individual with epilepsy, reluctance or refusal of an employer to hire an individual with epilepsy, difficulty gaining entrance to various occupations, and discrimination in various other areas (housing, transportation) (Dell, 1986; Schneider & Conrad, 1980, 1983). On the other hand, some individuals will report perceived discrimination and/or stigma yet will be unable to provide specific instances of explicit discriminatory behavior (Ryan, Kempner, & Emlen, 1986). Sociologists have begun to discuss stigma/discrimination in terms of "real versus perceived," which may represent a mixture of explicit versus subtle stigma/discrimination or, in some cases, real versus imagined stigma (Schneider & Conrad, 1980, 1983).

Finally, given all that has been said to this point, it would seem that individuals with epilepsy may be at increased risk for a greater number of stressful life events—a factor of known importance in the susceptibility to psychopathology (Sarason, Johnson, & Siegel, 1978). Additionally, given the financial stresses of this chronic medical condition and the increased probability of employment difficulties, financial stress would clearly seem to be an added risk factor (Fraser, 1980; National Commission for the Control of Epilepsy and Its Consequences, 1978).

In summary, epilepsy contains not only a significant neurobiological dimension, but also an important psychosocial dimension composed of intra- and extrapersonal risk factors that need to be considered in models of adjustment in epilepsy. We now turn to the third major consideration.

Pharmacological Factors

The treatment of epilepsy rests primarily on the administration of anticonvulsant medications. Significant advances have resulted in the development of new such medications that are especially effective for particular seizure types and that produce fewer adverse side effects. These medications, as well as some of the older, well-established drugs, clearly improve seizure control in a majority of patients. Some characteristics of these medications, however, are relevant to our discussion of risk factors for psychosocial problems (Table 3.1).

From our own clinical standpoint, perhaps the most common problem is the inappropriate use of anticonvulsants. We unfortunately see a number of individuals who have been placed on three, four, and sometimes five medications, occasionally in conjunction with a stimulant medication that has been prescribed to counter the sedating effect of the anticonvulsants. This practice of polytherapy is counter to the prevailing suggested modern medical practice of monotherapy whenever possible, utilizing the most efficacious drug (with the fewest side effects) for the patient's particular seizure type (Porter, 1985).

In addition to the number of medications that are used, specific consideration needs to be given to the particular anticonvulsant that is prescribed. Some very effective, safe, and well-established drugs can predispose some individuals to significant psychological and social problems. Perhaps the best-known example concerns the drug phenobarbital. This barbiturate anticonvulsant may cause paradoxical hyperactivity in children while predisposing susceptible individuals to significant depression (Reynolds, 1981; Trimble & Reynolds, 1976).

A recent report indicates that the use of phenobarbital in children with epilepsy is associated with depression in cases in which there is a familial history of psychopathology (Brendt, Crumrine, Varma, Allan, & Allman, 1987).

The effects of the anticonvulsant medications can be somewhat insidious. Theodore and colleagues (Theodore, Bairamian, Newmark, Chiro, Porter, Larson, & Fishbein, 1986a; Theodore, Chiro, Margolin, Fishbein, Porter, & Brooks, 1986b) at the National Institutes of Health have reported interesting findings concerning the effects of drug withdrawal on cerebral metabolism as measured by positron emission tomography. When phenobarbital administration was discontinued cerebral metabolism increased by 37%. When phenytoin (Dilantin®) was removed, there was a rise of about 14%, and when carbamazepine (Tegretol®) was removed, there was a rise of about 10%. Therefore, anticonvulsant drugs clearly affect cerebral metabolism, and this can be noted on PET studies. At present it is not clear exactly what the effects of a global rise in cerebral metabolism are, but it is reasonable to suggest that such improvements in brain function may be associated with improvements in psychological function.

An extended discussion of the mechanisms whereby anticonvulsant medications affect behavioral and social function is beyond the scope of this chapter. It should be noted, however, that Reynolds (1971, 1981, 1982) and his colleagues have suggested that anticonvulsants can adversely affect mental functioning by (1) causing neuropathological changes in the central nervous system, (2) inducing folate deficiency, (3) altering monoamine metabolism, and/or (4) affecting hormonal or endocrine functioning.

Comment

In summary, a large number of potential risk factors for salient problems in living are found among patients with epilepsy. Each patient presents with his or her own unique combination of potential risk factors, and, on clinical grounds alone, it appears difficult to identify those variables that actually represent causal factors. We have here suggested that in order to begin to gain some experimental control over this clinical situation we first categorize each known or suspected risk factor into one of three conceptual groupings (neurobiological, psychosocial, medication), each of which reflects a major dimension of epilepsy.

Such a grouping might then reasonably lead to some systematic investigations. For instance, if these various factors were measured in a substantial number of patients, which variables would be most predictive of, for example, depression or unemployment or psychosis? Conversely, which would be predictive of successful life performance? Is there a shifting of risk factors for specific psychological and social problems? Does the relative importance of neurobiological, psychosocial, and/ or medication variables shift as a function of the problem under investigating; e.g., are neurobiological factors more important in determining academic underachievement whereas psychosocial factors are particularly predictive of depression? Clearly, such studies would need to use statistical procedures to control for the intercorrelation that surely exists among the variables within each of the three domains (as well as across the domains), so that truly independent, nonredundant risk factors would be identified.

We will now turn to a brief presentation of two empirical efforts to determine the utility of this model in identifying the predictors of psychopathology in patients with epilepsy. The first example reviews a previous study involving depression in adults (Hermann & Whitman, 1989) adults with epilepsy, and the second example reviews a previous study of children with epilepsy (Hermann, Whitman, Hughes, Melyn, & Dell, 1988).

DEPRESSION IN ADULTS WITH EPILEPSY

Among the interictal behavioral problems that have been investigated among adults with epilepsy, it now appears that depression is one of the most common (Robertson, Trimble, & Townsend, 1987). This is also reflected in the rate of suicide, which, although very low, is elevated in those with epilepsy relative to the general population (Matthews & Barabas, 1986; Zielinski, 1974). A relevant question is, therefore, what factors predict the development of significant interictal depression? Several investigations have attempted to identify causal factors; interestingly, most have focused on neurobiological risk factors, including seizure type, lateralization and localization of the epileptogenic lesion, duration of the disorder, degree of seizure control, and the presence or absence of a structural lesion (Kogeorgos, Fonagy, & Scott, 1982; Robertson & Trimble, 1983; Robertson et al., 1987; Trimble & Perez, 1980).

In general, the results have been disappointing in that most studies have failed to identify neurobiological correlates of depression. One American group has reported increased depression among patients with complex partial seizures originating from the left temporal lobe (Mendez, Cummings, & Benson, 1986), but this work awaits confirmation. Although the possibility exists that other, as yet uninvestigated, biological variables are predictive of depression, we have hypothesized that psychosocial considerations are particularly promising factors (Hermann & Whitman, 1986). After all, given the social ramifications of epilepsy, it would not be surprising if some of these factors were predictive of interictal depression. The purpose of this study was, therefore, to investigate the utility of our model in investigating depression in epilepsy in general and inquiring into its psychosocial determinants in particular.

Method

Subjects

The subject pool consists of referrals to the inpatient monitoring units of the Baptist Memorial Hospital Epilepsy Center. Patients are referred to the Center for assessment of suitability for focal resection of their epileptogenic lesion, for further diagnostic evaluation because of an unacceptable degree of seizure control, or for reasons concerning differential diagnosis.

The specific sample investigated here consisted of 102 patients with epilepsy, whose diagnosis was confirmed by continuous (24-hr) closed-circuit TV and EEG monitoring with scalp and/or sphenoidal and/or subdural strip electrodes. Monitoring was typically carried out until several spontaneous seizures had been recorded. The sample comprised a consecutive series of individuals undergoing inpatient evaluation, excluding patients who were mentally retarded (WAIS-R Full-Scale IQ less than 70) or who had a significant reading disability (below the fifth percentile on the Reading Scale on the Wide-Range Achievement Test–Revised). Table 3.2 provides characteristics of the final sample.

Since a primary aim of the present study was to determine the multietiological correlates of depression, three sets of predictor variables were investigated (Table 3.3): neurobiological, psychosocial, and medication variables. These factors are reviewed below.

TABLE 3.2.   Subject Characteristics

Average ages (years)	31.2 (9.3)[a]
Average education (years)	12.7 (2.3)
Average IQ	89.9 (10.97)
Gender	45 males
	57 females
Seizure type	Patial (*n* = 97)
	8 simple partial
	90 complex partial
	57 secondarily generalized
	Generalized (*n* = 5)
	2 absence
	4 tonic–clonic
	4 other
Average age at onset (years)	14.9 (11.1)
Average duration (years)	16.3 (10.6)
Number of seizure types	1, 40
	2, 59
	3, 3
Secondarily generalized seizures in addition to simple and/or complex partial seizures?	Yes 55
	No 42
	Unknown, 5
Structural abnormality underlying the epilepsy?	Yes 15
	No 87
Medication	55 monotherapy
	46 polytherapy
	1 none
Taking barbiturate medications?	Yes 14
	No 88

[a]Standard deviation in parentheses.

TABLE 3.3. Multietiological Predictor Variables

Neurobiological	Psychosocial	Medication
Age at onset	Perceived stigma	Monotherapy versus polytherapy
Duration of epilepsy	Perceived limitations	Presence/absence of barbiturate
Laterality of seizure onset	Adjustment to seizures	medications
Seizure type	Vocational adjustment	
Etiology	Financial status	
Presence/absence of secondarily	Life event changes	
generalized seizures	Social support	
Number of different seizure types	Locus of control	

Neurobiological Variables

Several neurobiological variables that are among those commonly considered to play some role in the etiology of psychopathology in epilepsy were included for evaluation. These seven variables were coded from patient charts by a board-certified neurosurgeon with special expertise in epilepsy while blinded to all the behavioral and psychological data. These predictor variables included (1) age at onset of recurrent seizures, (2) duration of disorder, (3) lateralization of unilateral temporal lobe seizure onset using scalp and/or sphenoidal or subdural strip electrodes, (4) seizure type [partial seizures (simple, complex and/or secondarily generalized) versus primary generalized seizures], (5) presence versus absence of a structural lesion believed to underlie the patient's epilepsy (e.g., tumor, cyst), (6) presence or absence of secondarily generalized seizures in addition to simple and/or complex partial seizures, and (7) the number of different seizure types experienced by the patient. We did not analyze the frequency of seizures. Most patients presented to our Center because of an unacceptable degree of seizure control, and the distribution of this variable was therefore relatively truncated. We sought to index the severity of the patients' epilepsy through other variables (e.g., number of different seizure types, presence/absence of secondarily generalized seizures).

Psychosocial Variables

As reviewed above, a wide variety of social and psychological constructs have been hypothesized to be among the determinants of psychopathology in epilepsy. Variables selected for inclusion in this study were those that could be assessed with self-report instruments of adequate reliability and validity and/or measured via questionnaires specifically designed to assess psychosocial problems in patients with epilepsy. The following eight variables were included for evaluation.

(1, 2) *Perceived stigma and perceived limitations.* These variables were assessed by two scales developed by factor analysis of the responses of 445 adults with epilepsy to a 21-item questionnaire inquiring about their attitudes and experiences with epilepsy (Ryan *et al.*, 1980). Factor analyses were performed on the total group of 445 subjects as well as on several subgroups of subjects, and the same factors consistently emerged from the analyses.

The Perceived Stigma scale consists of six items to which subjects respond on a four-point scale reflecting their degree of agreement. The scale specifically assesses the extent to which people with epilepsy feel that they are victims of prejudice because of their epilepsy. The coefficient of internal reliability was high ($\alpha = .75$).

The Perceived Limitation scale consists of five items that are the statements or expressions of constraints that may be imposed by the disorder. Their underlying theme is the sense of vulnerability to the physical consequences of the disorder. The coefficient of internal reliability was again high ($\alpha = .80$).

(3–5) *Adjustment to seizures, vocational adjustment, and financial status*. These three areas of psychosocial concern were assessed by the Washington Psychosocial Seizure Inventory (WPSI) (Dodrill, Batzel, Queisser, & Temkin, 1980).

The Adjustment to Seizures scale of the WPSI consists of 15 items that inquire into whether the person resents having epilepsy, feels less worthwhile because of the epilepsy, and is embarrassed about the diagnosis and/or seizures, and whether or not he or she feels accepted by others.

The Vocational Adjustment scale of the WPSI consists of 13 items that assess whether epilepsy is interfering with the person's ability to obtain a job, degree of satisfaction with current vocational situation, and whether or not there appears to be a need for vocational counseling services.

The Financial Status scale of the WPSI consists of seven items that assess whether the individual has significant financial problems and whether he or she worries a great deal about financial difficulties.

For each scale, increasing scores reflect increasing seriousness of impairment and concern.

(6) *Life event changes*. Assessment of the number of stressful life events occurring during the past 6 months was carried out via the Life Experiences Survey (LES) (Sarason *et al.*, 1978). The LES consists of 47 life event changes, which can be rated on a six-point Likert scale according to their desirability or undesirability. The LES items were originally chosen to represent life changes frequently experienced by individuals in the general population. An acceptable degree of test–retest reliability has been demonstrated, as has the fact that the LES scores are not associated with measures of social desirability (Sarason *et al.*, 1978). For this investigation we used the absolute number of life event changes that had occurred during the past year as the predictor index from the LES.

(7) *Social support*. The Social Support Questionnaire (SSQ) (Sarason, Levine, Basham, & Sarason, 1983) is a 27-item survey that assesses two major aspects of social support, the amount of social support available to the individual and his or her satisfaction with the available support. Items ask the subject to list the people whom he or she can turn to and rely on in a variety of situations and the satisfaction with the support rendered.

Factor analyses of the SSQ have supported the notion of two social support indices (number, satisfaction). Coefficients of internal reliability are uniformly high

($\alpha > .95$), and scores do not correlate with measures of social desirability (Sarason *et al.*, 1983).

For the purposes of this investigation, we utilized the number of individuals available to provide social support (SSN) as the measure of interest derived from the SSQ. The higher the score, the more social support available to the patient.

(8) *Locus of control.* In order to assess each patient's locus of control, we utilized Rotter's (1966) Internal/External Control of Reinforcement scale. Although this scale has been widely utilized, some concerns have been raised regarding its factor structure, scale format, and correlation with social desirability measures. Based on Ashkanasy's (1985) findings (i.e., the scale most likely taps a unitary construct, no significant correlation between social desirability and total score on Rotter's scale), we relied on the scoring procedures originally described by Rotter, with higher scores indicating a more external locus of control.

Medication Factors

Only two medication variables were utilized because at the time of CCTV–EEG monitoring the patients were receiving markedly reduced levels of their anticonvulsant medications, or the medications were withdrawn altogether. Therefore, we examined the patient's most recent (preadmission) medication schedule and determined (1) whether the patient was on a program of monotherapy or polytherapy and (2) whether his or her anticonvulsant program included any barbiturate medications.

Dependent Measure

In order to assess each patient's level of self-reported depression, we utilized the Center for Epidemiological Studies in Depression scale (CES–D). This is a self-report measure of depression with demonstrated reliability and validity (Radloff, 1977).

Data Analyses

First, Pearson correlation coefficients were computed between each of the neurobiological, psychosocial, and medication variables and the total CES–D score. A subsequent intercorrelation matrix of the predictor variables revealed that there was substantial intercorrelation. Therefore, in order to identify independent (nonredundant) predictors of psychopathology, those variables that showed a significant correlation ($p < .05$) with the CES–D score were subsequently entered into a stepwise multiple regression analysis.

Results

Table 3.4 shows the eight predictor variables that exhibited a significant relationship with the CES–D results and their Pearson correlation coefficients and

TABLE 3.4. Statistically Significant Associations
between Depression and Potential Predictor Variables[a]

Variable	r	p
Increased perceived stigma	.32	<.001
Amount of social support	−.21	.014
Increased number of stressful life events	.22	.014
Poor adjustment to epilepsy	.46	<.001
Poor vocational adjustment	.21	.015
Less adequate financial status	.36	<.001
External locus of control	.28	.002

[a]The effect of gender was analyzed via t-test, and females reported significantly increased depression ($t = 3.7$, $p < .001$).

significance levels. Increased depression scores were associated with increased perceived stigma, less social support, an increased number of stressful life events in the past 6 months, poor adjustment to seizures, vocational difficulties, financial stress, an external locus of control, and female gender.

Four of the seven variables remained statistically significant when entered into a stepwise multiple regression analysis (Table 3.5). Specifically, increased depression was associated with an increased number of stressful life events during the past 6 months ($p = .013$), poor adjustment to seizures ($p = .0002$), financial stress ($p = .007$), and female gender ($p = .003$). The multiple correlation ($R = .58$) indicated that these four variables accounted for about 34% of the variance in the CES–D scores. Two remaining variables just missed reaching conventional levels of statistical significance, in the regression model: lower social support ($p = .06$) and an external locus of control ($p = .07$).

Comment

This investigation demonstrated increased self-reported depression in epilepsy to be correlated with several specific risk factors, most of which are psychosocial. Consistent with the bulk of the existing literature, we did not find neurobiological

TABLE 3.5. Significant Independent Predictors of
Depression as Determined by Stepwise Regression Analysis

Predictor variable	p
Increased number of stressful life events	.013
Poor adjustment to epilepsy	.0002
Less adequate financial status	.007
Female gender	.003

factors to be associated with increased depression, and we were not able to confirm previous reports of an association between complex partial seizures of left temporal lobe origin and increased depression.

As we would predict, several of the individual risk factors found to be associated with depression were intercorrelated, and the use of procedures that control for this reduced the initial list of seven variables to four independent risk factors. Specifically, increased depression was found to be associated with an increased number of stressful life events during the past 6 months, poor adjustment to epilepsy, financial stress, and female gender.

Because our procedures were correlational in nature, we cannot, of course, infer causation, but a research agenda is suggested. It is interesting that existing prospective longitudinal investigations of depression in the general population have identified some of these same variables (financial stress, stressful life events, female gender) as bearing a causal relationship to the development of a depressive disorder (Kaplan, Roberts, Camacho, & Coyne, 1987; Lewinsohn, Hoberman, & Rosenbaum, 1988). Whether this is the case for epilepsy remains to be seen.

SOCIAL COMPETENCE IN CHILDREN WITH EPILEPSY

We now turn to an investigation of children with epilepsy (ages 6–16) and attempt to identify the predictors of a different area of behavioral function, social competence. Most research in the area has attempted to identify the correlates of behavioral and social deficiencies, but here we attempt to use our model to predict behavioral and social competence in the pediatric population. The main results of this study have been published elsewhere (Hermann, Whitman, Hughes, Melyn, & Dell, 1988). We briefly present this study so that we can later contrast it with the study of depression presented above.

Method

Subjects

The subject pool consisted of children with epilepsy between the ages of 6 and 16 who were attending a special Epilepsy Clinic at the University of Illinois Medical Center. Children excluded from the regular school system because of mental handicap (i.e., placed in educationally mentally handicapped or trainable mentally handicapped settings) were excluded from consideration for this investigation. Children attending alternative schools because of behavioral dysfunction were included in the subject pool, as were children who attended special learning disorder classes as part of their regular educational programming.

The final sample consisted of 183 consecutively referred children with epilepsy, excluding families who were Spanish-speaking only.

Predictor Variables

The variables identified in Table 3.6 represent the potential predictor variables of interest for this study. Previous publications from our group allow the interested reader to obtain more detailed information about the methodology and operational definitions of each potential predictor variable (Hermann *et al.*, 1988). Table 3.7 provides summary information regarding the characteristics of our sample and their distribution on each of the predictor variables.

Dependent Measure

The behavior and social competence of each child was assessed by means of an interview with the child's mother or guardian using the Child Behavior Checklist (CBCL) (Achenbach & Edelbrock, 1981, 1983). This behavioral assessment inventory was designed to record, in a standardized format, the behavioral problems and social competence of children aged 6–16 years. The CBCL consists of 20 social competence and 118 behavioral problem items.

For the purposes of this investigation we utilized the CBCL measure of Total Social Competence. This represents a composite measure reflecting the amount and quality of the child's participation in sports, hobbies, games, activities, organizations, and friendships as well as school performance and social interaction. Raw scores are converted to standardized T-scores ($x = 50$, S.D. $= 10$). Higher scores indicate increasing social competence, and lower scores indicate less adequate social competence (Achenbach & Edelbrock, 1983).

Data Analysis

Data analysis was similar to that described above. First, simple Pearson correlation coefficients were computed between each of the predictor variables and the measure of social competence. Because there is intercorrelation among the potential predictor variables, those factors showing a significant relationship with social competence were then entered into a stepwise multiple regression analysis so that independent (nonredundant) predictors of social competence could be identified.

TABLE 3.6.   Multietiological Predictor Variables

Neurobiological	Psychosocial	Medication
Age at onset	Parents' marital status	Monotherapy versus polytherapy
Duration of disorder	Family income	Drug type
Seizure type		Number of drug categories
EEG pattern		
Degree of seizure control		
Etiology		

TABLE 3.7.   Average Values or Proportions for the
Independent Variables, Grouped by Hypothesis ($n = 183$)

Biological variables	
Average age at onset	6.3 years
Average duration of disorder	5.1 years
Seizure type	
Partial	53%
Primary generalized	40%
Partial and primary generalized (mixed)	7%
EEG pattern	
Corticoreticular	33%
Focal	43%
Mixed	12%
Other	12%
Seizure control	
Good	30%
Fair	30%
Poor	40%
Etiology	
Symptomatic	21%
Idiopathic	68%
Unknown	11%
Psychosocial variables	
Parents' marital status	
Married	57%
Divorced or separated	34%
Other	8%
Average median family income	$17,835
Medication variables	
Number	
Monotherapy	49%
Polytherapy	37%
None	14%
Drug class[a]	
Barbiturates	53%
Succinamides	14%
Hydantoin	43%
Valproic acid	18%
Carbamazepine	12%
Other	14%
Number of drug categories	
0	14%
1	49%
2	26%
3	8%
4	3%

[a]Percentages are based on the number of children receiving medication ($n = 157$) and add to more than 100% since several children were taking more than one type of medication.

Results

Table 3.8 presents the six variables that were significantly associated with social competence, their Pearson correlation coefficients, and the levels of statistical significance. As can be seen, increased social competence was associated with an intact parental marriage, good seizure control, higher family income, later age at onset of epilepsy, a shorter duration of epilepsy, and the absence of multiple seizure types. Interestingly, monotherapy ($p = .087$) was positively associated, and polytherapy ($p = .051$) was negatively associated with increasing social competence, but these relationships did not reach conventional levels of statistical significance. It is also worth noting that of those variables that did reach statistical significance, the correlations were not high and explained relatively small proportions of the variance.

Because there was intercorrelation among the identified significant predictor variables, they were subsequently entered into a stepwise multiple regression analysis, and the resultant multiple R was .39, indicating that 15% of the variance was accounted for by the predictor variables. Four significant ($p < .05$) variables were identified: good seizure control, an intact parental marriage, shorter duration of epilepsy, and higher family income were associated with increased social competence.

Comment

The results of this investigation demonstrate that it is possible to identify multietiological predictors of social competence in children with epilepsy. Biological (good seizure control and shorter duration of epilepsy) and psychosocial (intact parental marriage and higher family income) variables were associated with increased social competence in children with epilepsy. These findings are intuitively appealing. They suggest that a multidisciplinary approach to children with epilepsy is indicated, stressing both up-to-date, modern medical management in order to bring seizures under the best control possible, and attention to the intactness of the family unit and adequate financial arrangements.

TABLE 3.8. Statistically Significant Pearson
Correlations between Social Competence
and Potential Predictor Variables

Variable	r	p
Intact parental marriage	.20	.004
Multiple seizure types	−.12	.049
Good seizure control	.21	.003
Higher family income	.18	.007
Later age at onset of epilepsy	.17	.013
Shorter duration of epilepsy	.17	.012

CONCLUSION

As we discussed at the beginning of this chapter, the prevailing paradigm in this field, up to now, has been one of pursuing neurobiological predictors of psychopathology in people with epilepsy, almost to the total exclusion of social and medication variables (Whitman & Hermann, 1989). This chapter, and the model on which it is based, should be seen as a response to this paradigm, as an initial step in searching for a more comprehensive way of viewing treatment for and research about psychopathology in epilepsy.

By way of conclusion, let us first analyze the findings in a manner consistent with the model and then suggest implications for future treatment and research in this area.

A large number of predictor variables were examined in the two studies reported on. Of these, eight variables (four in each study) emerged as being statistically significant in stepwise multiple regression analyses. These were good seizure control, shorter duration of epilepsy, intact parental marriage, higher income (twice), an increased number of stressful life events, poor adjustment to epilepsy, and the female gender. If we group these eight variables into the categories of risk factors that have been employed in this chapter, we see that one is demographic, two are neurobiological, and five are psychosocial. Of these five, one is generally seen as being "psychological" (poor adjustment to epilepsy), whereas the other four are generally seen as being "social" (number of stressful life events, an intact parental marriage, and income—twice). This is, to our knowledge, one of the few times that a multietiological model has been tested, and the results clearly suggest the appropriateness of such a model.

We do not believe that the details of this model are yet essential issues. We have tried to establish a comprehensive model in terms of both concept and detail, but much is lacking at this early stage of model building. For example, we have not been able to include many variables that have been hypothesized to be relevant in this area of study. This is particularly the case for variables related to antiepilepsy drugs. Additionally, our grouping of variables may not be optimal, and/or there may be other groupings that should be added.

Nonetheless, it seems apparent to us that this type of multietiological model offers an avenue for investigation in this field. For example, it suggests that attention must not only be paid to biological issues but to issues of medication and to psychosocial concerns. This is, of course, an obvious formulation, and yet the general paradigm in this field has been so strong as to urge us away from this perspective in terms of both research and treatment. This is a trend that should be reversed.

The past 40 years or so, at least since Gibbs's work in the 1940s (Gibbs, Gibbs, & Fuster, 1948), have been spent in studying, refining, and rerefining the hypothesized particularity of complex partial seizures to psychopathology. Few variables have turned up that are consistently related to psychopathology, and they explain relatively little of the variance in the process that we must begin to understand. It seems time for at least some researchers in this area to turn their attention to psychosocial precursors of psychopathology in people with epilepsy. We hope that this model and the associated results will facilitate such a pursuit.

REFERENCES

Achenbach, T. M., & Edelbrock, C. S. (1981). Behavioral problems and social competencies reported by parents of normal and disturbed children aged four through sixteen. *Monographs of the Society for Research in Child Development, 46*, 1–82.

Achenbach, T. M., & Edelbrock, C. S. (1983). *Manual for the Child Behavior Checklist and Revised Child Behavior Checklist.* Burlington: University of Vermont.

Arnston, P., Droge, D., Norton, R., & Murray, E. (1986). The perceived psychosocial consequences of having epilepsy. In S. Whitman & B. P. Hermann (Eds.), *Psychopathology in epilepsy: Social dimensions* (pp. 143–161). New York: Oxford University Press.

Ashkanasy, N. M. (1985). Rotter's Internal–External Scale: Confirmatory factor analysis and correlation with social desirability for alternative scale formats. *Journal of Personality and Social Psychology, 48*, 1328–1341.

Brendt, D. A., Crumrine, P. K., Varma, R. R., Allan, M., & Allman, C. (1987). Phenobarbital treatment and major depressive disorder in children with epilepsy. *Pediatrics, 80*, 909–917.

Dell, J. L. (1986). Social dimensions of epilepsy: Stigma and response. In S. Whitman & B. P. Hermann (Eds.), *Psychopathology in epilepsy: Social dimensions* (pp. 185–210). New York: Oxford University Press.

Dodrill, C. B., Batzel, L. W., Queisser, H. R., & Temkin, N. R. (1980). An objective method for the assessment of psychological and social difficulties among epileptics. *Epilepsia, 21*, 123–135.

Fenwick, P. (1987). Epilepsy and psychiatric disorders. In A. Hopkins (Ed.), *Epilepsy* (pp. 511–552). New York: Demos Publications.

Fraser, R. T. (1980). Vocational aspects of epilepsy. In B. P. Hermann (Ed.), *A multidisciplinary handbook of epilepsy* (pp. 74–105). Springfield, Ill.: Charles C. Thomas.

Gibbs, F. A., Gibbs, E. L., & Fuster, B. (1948). Psychomotor epilepsy. *Archives of Neurology and Psychiatry, 60*, 331–339.

Hermann, B. P., & Whitman, S. (1984). Behavioral and personality correlates of epilepsy: A review, methodological critique and conceptual model. *Psychological Bulletin, 95*, 451–497.

Hermann, B. P., & Whitman, S. (1986). Psychopathology in epilepsy. A multietiologic model. In S. Whitman & B. P. Hermann (Eds.), *Psychopathology in epilepsy: Social dimensions* (pp. 5–37). New York: Oxford University Press.

Hermann, B. P., & Whitman, S. (1989). Psychosocial predictors of depression in epilepsy. *Journal of Epilepsy, 2*, 231–237.

Hermann, B. P., Whitman, S., Hughes, J. R., Melyn, M., & Dell, J. (1988). Multietiological determinants of psychopathology and social competence in children with epilepsy. *Epilepsy Research, 2*, 51–60.

Kaplan, G. A., Roberts, R. E., Camacho, T. C., & Coyne, J. C. (1987). Psychosocial predictors of depression. *American Journal of Epidemiology, 125*, 206–220.

Kogeorgos, J., Fonagy, P., & Scott, D. F. (1982). Psychiatric symptom profiles of chronic epileptics attending a neurologic clinic: A controlled investigation. *British Journal of Psychiatry, 140*, 236–243.

Lewinsohn, P. M., Hoberman, H. M., & Rosenbaum, M. (1988). A prospective study of risk factors for unipolar depression. *Journal of Abnormal Psychology, 97*, 251–264.

Long, C. G., & Moore, J. L. (1979). Parental expectations for their epileptic children. *Journal of Child Psychology and Psychiatry, 20*, 299–312.

Matthews, W., & Barabas, G. (1986). Perceptions of control among children with epilepsy. In S. Whitman & B. P. Hermann (Eds.), *Psychopathology in epilepsy: Social dimensions* (pp. 162–182). New York: Oxford University Press.

Mendez, M. F., Cummings, J. L., & Benson, D. F. (1986). Depression in epilepsy: Significance and phenomenology. *Archives of Neurology, 43*, 766–770.

Mittan, R. J. (1982). Fear of seizures. In S. Whitman & B. P. Hermann (Eds.), *Psychopathology in epilepsy: Social dimensions* (pp. 90–121). New York: Oxford University Press.

National Commission for the Control of Epilepsy and Its Consequences. (1978). *Plan for nationwide action on epilepsy. DHEW Publication No. NIH78–276.* Washington, D.C.: NIH.

Porter, R. J. (1985). *Epilepsy: 100 Elementary Principles.* Philadelphia: W. B. Saunders.

Radloff, L. S. (1977). The CES–D scale: A self-report depression scale for research in the general population. *Applied Psychological Measurement, 1*, 388–401.

Reynolds, E. H. (1971). Anticonvulsant drugs, folic acid metabolism, fit frequency and psychiatric illness. *Psychiatria, Neurologia, Neurochirurgia, 74*, 167–174.

Reynolds, E. H. (1981). Biological factors in psychological disorders associated with epilepsy. In E. H. Reynolds & M. R. Trimble (Eds.), *Psychiatry and epilepsy* (pp. 264–290). Edinburgh: Churchill-Livingstone.

Reynolds, E. H. (1982). Anticonvulsants and mental symptoms. In M. Sandler (Ed.), *Psychopharmacology of anticonvulsants.* New York: Oxford University Press.

Ritchie, K. (1981). Research note: Interaction in the families of epileptic children. *Journal of Child Psychology and Psychiatry, 22*, 68–71.

Robertson, M., & Trimble, M. R. (1983). Depressive illness in patients with epilepsy: A review. *Epilepsia, 24* (Suppl. 2), S109–S116.

Robertson, M. M., Trimble, M. R., & Townsend, H. R. A. (1987). Phenomenology of depression in epilepsy. *Epilepsia, 28*, 364–372.

Rotter, J. B. (1966). Generalized expectancies for internal versus external control of reinforcement. *Psychological Monographs, 80*, whole No. 609.

Ryan, R., Kempner, K., & Emlen, A. C. (1980). The stigma of epilepsy as a self-concept. *Epilepsia, 21*, 433–444.

Sarason, I. G., Johnson, J. H., & Siegel, J. M. (1978). Assessing the impact of life changes: Development of the Life Experience Survey. *Journal of Consulting and Clinical Psychology, 46*, 932–946.

Sarason, I. G., Levine, H. M., Basham, R. B., & Sarason, B. R. (1983). Assessing social support: The Social Support Questionnaire. *Journal of Personality and Social Psychology, 44*, 127–139.

Schneider, J. W., & Conrad, P. (1980). In the closet with epilepsy: Epilepsy stigma potential and information control. *Social Problems, 28*, 32–44.

Schneider, J. W., & Conrad, P. (1983). *Having epilepsy: The experience and control of illness.* Philadelphia: Temple University Press.

Stevens, J. R. (1975). Interictal clinical manifestations of complex partial seizures. In J. K. Penry & D. D. Daly (Eds.), *Advances in Neurology*, Vol. 11 (pp. 85–112). New York: Raven Press.

Theodore, W. H., Bairamian, D., Newmark, M. E., Chiro, G. D., Porter, R. J., Larson, S., & Fishbein, D. (1986a). Effects of phenytoin on human cerebral glucose metabolism. *Journal of Cerebral Blood Flow and Metabolism, 6*, 315–320.

Theodore, W. H., Chiro, G. D., Margolin, R., Fishbein, D., Porter, R. J., & Brooks, R. A. (1986b). Barbituates reduce human cerebral glucose metabolism. *Neurology, 36*, 60–64.

Trimble, M. R., & Reynolds, M. R. (1976). Anticonvulsant drugs and mental symptoms. *Psychological Medicine, 6*, 169–178.

Trimble, M. R., & Perez, M. M. (1980). Quantification of psychopathology in adult patients with epilepsy. In B. Kulig, H. Meinardi, & G. Stores (Eds.), *Epilepsy and behavior '79.* Lisse, Holland: Swets & Zeitlinger.

Trimble, M. R., & Bolwig, T. G. (Eds.). (1986). *Aspects of epilepsy and psychiatry.* Chichester: John Wiley & Sons.

Whitman, S., & Hermann, B. P. (1989). The architecture of research in the epilepsy/psychopathology literature: A review. *Epilepsy Research, 3*, 93–99.

Ziegler, R. G. (1981). Impairments of control and competence in epileptic children and their families. *Epilepsia, 22*, 339–346.

Zielinski, J. J. (1974). Epilepsy and mortality and causes of death. *Epilepsia, 15*, 191–201.

4

Neuropsychological Assessment in the Diagnosis of Nonepileptic Seizures

BRUCE P. HERMANN and BRYAN E. CONNELL

The diagnosis of epilepsy is often a rather straightforward matter. The clinical episodes are classic, the EEG is confirmatory, and the response to medications is positive. At other times the picture is murky. The spells are of an uncharacteristic type, EEG findings of uncertain clinical significance are obtained, and the neurologist subsequently struggles with issues of differential diagnosis, for example, are the spells caused by cardiac disease, cerebrovascular disease, migraine, or some other neurological or systemic process? Often, but not always, the etiology underlying these nonepileptic phenomena is identified and treated, and the patient subsequently improves. In both of these scenarios, the neurologist does not question the organic nature of the attacks, and consultation from the psychology service is neither mandatory nor asked for.

However, if the diagnostic process continues without success and the results of numerous tests and procedures are negative or equivocal, the specter of a psychiatric etiology may be raised. At these times, the patient often is referred for psychological or neuropsychological evaluation. The psychologist generally is asked to provide an opinion as to the probability of an organic versus functional etiology. In other words, "Does the patient have epilepsy or pseudoseizures [nonepileptic seizures (NES) in the current terminology]?"

The clinical situation described above, although a simplification of the realities

BRUCE P. HERMANN • Epi-Care Center, Baptist Memorial Hospital and Semmes-Murphey Clinic, Departments of Neurosurgery and Psychiatry, University of Tennessee-Memphis, Memphis, Tennessee 38103.   BRYAN E. CONNELL • Carolinas Epilepsy Center, Carolinas Medical Center, Charlotte, North Carolina 28232.

The Neuropsychology of Epilepsy, edited by Thomas L. Bennett. Plenum Press, New York, 1992.

involved (Rowan & Gates, in press), probably accurately reflects the position in which the neuropsychologist is placed and the logic that may be imposed. For instance, in an ideal case of NES, the patient would be completely neuropsychologically intact and would show significant psychopathology, particularly of a type suggesting conversion symptomatology. Such a conceptualization would consider it unlikely for patients with unequivocal epilepsy to be cognitively intact or to exhibit the types of psychopathology expected in patients with NES. Similarly, this idea suggests that NES patients seldom demonstrate neuropsychological impairment. It also assumes that epilepsy and NES are mutually exclusive diagnoses, that NES is to be understood only in terms of conversion disorder, and, therefore, that other explanations (e.g., modeling) are unnecessary. Further, it suggests that the traditional methods used by the neurologist to diagnose epilepsy are sufficiently robust not to "miss" cases of unusual but real epilepsy and that the methods of the psychologist are sufficiently powerful to discriminate epilepsy from NES.

As might be inferred from the development of this straw man, the diagnosis of NES versus epileptic seizures (ES), in fact, can be a very difficult venture. Patients with suspected NES constitute a surprisingly frequent and difficult diagnostic problem, even in experienced epilepsy centers. What is not exaggerated is the difficult position in which the psychologist is placed. If they have not had the opportunity to see the wide-ranging gamut of unselected epilepsy patients with their concomitant variability in neuropsychological and emotional functioning, it can be difficult to relate the findings in a case of suspected NES to those with known epilepsy. Further, epilepsy can reveal itself in unusual and frankly bizarre attacks, the epileptogenic lesion can be beyond the sensitivity of interictal and even ictal scalp recordings, and imaging studies can be normal. In this context, the psychologist often is asked to give a judgment as to "organic" versus "functional."

Using this common clinical dilemma as a model, we review the literature concerning the neuropsychological assessment in the diagnosis of NES. First, the literature pertaining to the neuropsychological status of patients with NES is reviewed. An attempt is made to determine whether the neuropsychological (including intellectual) functioning in patients with NES differs from that of ES patients. If differences were found to exist, then such findings might be of clinical utility in the evaluation of patients with suspected NES.

Second, the literature examining personality characteristics of NES patients is discussed. Most of the data on this subject (particularly those emanating from the United States) have utilized the MMPI; therefore, the following discussion focuses on work conducted with this instrument. Interest in this area has stemmed from reports that scores on a subscale (Matthews, Shaw, & Klove, 1966; Shaw, 1966; Shaw & Matthews, 1965), presence of a conversion profile (Matthews et al., 1966; Ramani, Quesney, Olson, & Gumnit, 1980; Wurzman & Matthews, 1982), and the results of decision rules (Henrichs, Tucker, Farha, & Novelly, 1988; Vanderzant, Giordani, Berent, Dreifuss, & Sackellares, 1986; Wilkus, Dodrill, & Thompson, 1984; Wilkus & Dodrill, 1989) discriminate NES from ES patients. The success with which the MMPI captures the distinction between ES and NES patients is reviewed.

REVIEW OF THE NEUROPSYCHOLOGICAL LITERATURE

There has been only limited formal inquiry into the neuropsychological characteristics of NES (Sackellares, Giordani, Berent, Seidenberg, Dreifuss, Vanderzant, &
Boll, 1985; Wilkus *et al.*, 1984; Wilkus & Dodrill, 1989). Variability in several
characteristics, including intelligence, has been reported among patients with NES.
Further, signs of significant compromise of higher cognitive functions in patients with
NES have been reported (Ramani & Gumnit, 1982). However, the number of well-
controlled investigations examining the neuropsychological status of NES versus ES
patients is very small. The pertinent studies are reviewed below.

University of Virginia Study

Sackellares and colleagues (1985) examined patients admitted to the Diagnostic,
Treatment, and Research Unit of the Comprehensive Epilepsy Program at the
University of Virginia and the University of Michigan Epilepsy Laboratory. Using a
strict set of inclusion and exclusion criteria, they obtained three groups of subjects: (1)
patients with NES only ($n = 19$); (2) patients with ES plus NES ($n = 18$); and (3)
patients with documented generalized ES who were randomly selected during the
same period ($n = 20$). The patient groups were administered the Halstead–Reitan
Neuropsychology Test Battery and Allied Procedures and the Wechsler Adult Intelligence Scale (WAIS).

The authors found that patients with only NES had significantly higher mean
WAIS IQ scores (FSIQ = 102, VIQ = 103, PIQ = 100) than both the mixed group
(FSIQ = 90, VIQ = 90, PIQ = 90) and the generalized ES group (FSIQ = 86, VIQ
= 90, PIQ = 83), although the latter two groups did not differ from one another. The
Halstead–Reitan Impairment Index (II) of the NES group (II = 0.45) was significantly lower in comparison to the generalized ES group (II = 0.71) and marginally
lower ($p = .08$) than the mixed group (II = 0.62), the latter two groups again not
differing from one another. Results of specific tests in the Halstead–Reitan Battery
indicated that the NES group performed significantly better than the generalizes ES
group on the TPT test (total time, memory, and location), Category test, Seashore
Rhythm test, and Speech Sounds Perception test. Compared to the mixed group, the
NES patients performed significantly better on the TPT test (total time, memory,
location) and Seashore Rhythm test and marginally better ($p = .08$) on the Speech
Sounds Perception test. Again, there were no significant differences between the
mixed and generalized ES groups.

Although at first glance these results suggested that patients with NES had
relatively intact neuropsychological function, the authors pointed out that the performance of NES patients on the neuropsychological tests was less than that expected for
"normal" individuals of similar intelligence. Their mean Impairment Index was in
the range generally considered borderline between normal and impaired brain
function. Interestingly, the authors raised the hypothesis that neurological impairment
may play a role in the pathogenesis of NES.

University of Washington Investigations

Wilkus *et al.* (1984), in a comprehensive study of NES, also evaluated the intellectual and neuropsychological status of the patients (as well as personality functioning, to be discussed later in this chapter). Twenty-five patients with documented NES were compared to 25 patients with ES who were comparable in age, sex, and level of education. The two groups were compared on the WAIS and Dodrill's Neuropsychological Battery for Epilepsy (NBE). The results were relatively straightforward. There were no differences between the groups on any of the WAIS subtests or IQ values, nor on any of the 16 measures from the NBE. Finally, there was no difference between the groups in the proportion of scores on the NBE that were outside of normal limits. Both groups demonstrated relatively elevated scores (poorer performances). The NES group had 46% of their scores outside normal limits compared to 51% of the scores for ES patients.

The authors concluded that both groups exhibited evidence of brain damage or impairment of brain function. Citing this evidence, together with a high incidence of events suspicious for exacting CNS insult in the NES group (e.g., history of trauma, disease), the authors again raised the possibility that organic factors may, in some cases, contribute to the appearance of NES. Although the results of Wilkus *et al.* (1984) appear to differ from those of Sackellares *et al.* (1985) in that their findings suggested better cognitive function in NES patients compared to ES patients, both investigations reported very comparable impairment indices (i.e., the proportion of test scores outside of normal limits) of 46% and 45%, respectively.

In a later investigation, Wilkus and Dodrill (1989) investigated differences in the neuropsychological findings reported in their previous investigation relative to those of others. Specifically, they evaluated in detail the reasons for the different neuropsychological findings reported by Sackellares *et al.* (1985) and Wilkus *et al.* (1984) (MMPI findings from the investigation also are reviewed later in this chapter).

Wilkus and Dodrill (1989) pointed out that their previous investigation (Wilkus *et al.*, 1984) utilized groups of patients with ES and NES that were matched for age, sex, and education. As reviewed above, they did not find differences in neuropsychological functioning between the two groups. However, the study by Sackellares *et al.* (1985) did not match their ES and NES groups on these characteristics, and their generalized ES group had 2 years less education, a significant difference. Wilkus and Dodrill (1989) speculated that the lack of matching in regard to education was responsible for differences in the results of the two studies.

Four groups formed the basis for comparison in their second study: (1) the 25 NES patients from their earlier study and three additional groups of 25 patients each randomly selected from the neuropsychology lab files, including (2) patients with partial ES, (3) patients with generalized ES matched to the NES patients in terms of age, sex, and education, and (4) patients with generalized ES who were matched to the NES patients in terms of age and sex but not education (similar to Sackellares *et al.*, 1985). The groups were compared on the WAIS and Dodrill's NBE.

Comparing the age-, sex-, and education-matched groups of patients with NES, partial ES, and generalized ES revealed very few differences. These results reportedly were similar to the findings in the original study by Wilkus *et al.* (1984). Only two of 22 comparisons reached statistical significance, and no discernible pattern was noted in the findings. On the other hand, when the NES patients were compared to the group of patients with generalized ES who were not matched on education, there were significant differences between the groups on 11 measures (three IQ measures and eight measures from the NBE). The NES groups performed in a less-impaired direction on all 11 measures. It should be remembered, however, that their overall performance was not within normal limits.

Summary

These few controlled investigations suggest that it is not uncommon for patients with NES to exhibit signs of compromised brain function. Although there may or may not be differences between ES and NES patients on standardized measures of neuropsychological status (presumably because of the adequacy of matching), there is some consensus that groups of NES patients do not exhibit normal brain function. In some cases, NES patients show indices of impairment comparable to patients with verified epilepsy.

These group data are of interest; however, they are of unknown utility to the clinician dealing with individuals. Although they suggest that the presence of "organicity" on neuropsychological examination does not rule out the possibility of NES, they do not provide information about the proportion of patients with NES that exhibit normal versus impaired neuropsychological performance or the factors underlying such differential performance. It also is not entirely clear what proportion of patients with simple or complex partial ES exhibit completely normal neuropsychological function. In other words, the degree of success with which neuropsychological assessment ascertains the presence of NES versus ES remains unclear. This task is confounded by the use of anticonvulsant medications in NES patients, the history of CNS insult in a sizable proportion of NES patients, and other complicating factors such as personality functioning.

REVIEW OF THE MMPI LITERATURE

The evaluation of the MMPI literature is difficult for three major reasons. First, until recently, interpretations (e.g., Nicholl, 1981; Ramani *et al.*, 1980) rather than quantifications of the MMPI profiles were often reported in research articles. Second, the number of subjects included in many studies is quite low (studies of <10 subjects are not uncommon), limiting the generalizability of the findings. Third, inclusion and matching criteria for determining what constitute appropriate NES patients and controls have differed over studies. These differences limit the ability to know the criteria by which the interpretation of conversion was made, the parameters (means and variability) of the results, and the comparability of experimental groups in order to make comparisons across studies.

In general, MMPI studies may be categorized into three major types according to the use of the instrument. These types include work with the Pseudo-Neurologic (Pn) scale, conversion profiles, and decision rules. The development and utility of the findings in each of these three areas are reviewed.

Pn Scale

The first MMPI index reported to separate NES and ES patients was the Pseudo-Neurologic (Pn) scale (Shaw & Matthews, 1965). The Pn scale was developed to differentiate neurologically impaired patients from patients with symptomatology suggestive of CNS dysfunction but without positive findings on neurological examination. The Pn scale consisted of 17 MMPI items derived from scales 1, 3, and 4. Patients scoring at seven or more items in the expected direction were considered to have a nonneurological disorder. In the initial and subsequent validation studies, this cutoff correctly identified 81% and 67% of pseudoneurological patients while misclassifying 25% and 22% of the patients with neurological disease.

Shaw (1966) later used the Pn scale to discriminate 15 NES patients (a subgroup of all pseudoneurological patients) from 15 ES patients matched for age and sex. It is notable that 13 NES subjects in this study were identified as "pseudoseizures with concurrent epilepsy," while only two NES subjects were labeled as "pseudoseizures without concurrent epilepsy." Discriminating patients with ES from those with ES and NES is a most difficult diagnostic challenge, and, indeed, most current research excludes patients with both ES and NES. Nevertheless, Shaw correctly differentiated 73% (11/15) of NES from ES patients using the seven or more criterion; only 7% (1/15) of ES patients were misclassified, a significant difference.

Twenty-two years later, Henrichs *et al*. (1988) reexamined the utility of the Pn scale in discriminating NES patients from ES patients. Their results indicated that the Pn scale correctly identified 68% of NES patients but only 37% of patients with generalized ES. They concluded that the Pn scale was not a particularly helpful clinical tool with which to differentiate NES from ES patients.

To examine why the Pn scale was considered unsuccessful at capturing the NES–ES distinction, the rules provided by decision theory should be examined. According to the decision theory matrix, dichotomous decisions fall into the four categories of true positives, false positives, true negatives, and false negatives. Overall, these categorizations label not only how well a measure correctly identifies what it purports to identify but how often it appropriately excludes as well. True positives and true negatives are correct classifications known as "hits," whereas false positives and false negatives are incorrect classifications known as "misses." These categorizations are depicted in Table 4.1.

Table 4.2 depicts the results of the Henrichs *et al*. (1988) evaluation of the MMPI Pn Scale according to this decision theory matrix. Here, the Pn scale yielded correct

TABLE 4.1. Categorizations of
Dichotomous Decisions
According to Decision Theory

	1	2	Total
A	1A Hit n 1A	2A Miss n 2A	*Total A*
B	1B Miss n 1B	2B Hit n 2B	*Total B*
	Total 1	*Total 2*	

Hit rate X = hits/(hits + misses)
Hit rate for 1 = 1A/(1A + 1B)
Hit rate for 2 = 2A/(2A + 2B)
Hit rate for A = 1A/(1A + 2A)
Hit rate for B = 2B/(2B + 1B)

classifications or "hits" [hit rate = hits/(hits plus misses)] for 68% [21/(21 + 10)] of NES and 37% [10/(10 + 17)] of ES patients, respectively. Thus, incorrect classifications or "misses" occurred for 32% of NES patients and 63% of ES patients, respectively. Using the concept of hit rate for each index, Henrichs *et al.* (1988) calculated that the hit rate was 55% [21/(21 + 17)] when predicting NES (by the seven-or-more cutoff rule) and 50% [10/(10 + 10)] when predicting ES (not-NES by a less-than-seven cutoff rule). Therefore, while the correct identification of 68% of NES patients is relatively high and actually quite close to the 73% identification rate originally found by Shaw (1966), the hit rate for the index is basically at chance levels.

Conversion Profiles

Studies of MMPI results in NES patients have often examined the mean profiles for signs of neurotic or conversion symptomatology. The classic conversion profile includes a denial of psychological distress and simultaneous focus on somatic symptoms without evidence of significant depression or other psychopathology. Typically, this profile has been quantified by significant elevations ($T > 70$) on scales 1 (Hypochondriasis, Hs) and 3 (Hysteria, Hy), with both of these scales at least 10 T higher than scale 2 (Depression, D), and no significant elevations on any other scales (Marks & Seeman, 1963).

Matthews *et al.* (1966) found significant mean scale elevations on scale 3 but not on scale 1 in patients with pseudoneurological symptoms including (but not limited to) NES patients relative to patients with unequivocal brain damage. Wurzman and Matthews (1982) found higher mean scales 1, 3, and 2 in NES patients compared to ES patients. Wilkus *et al.* (1984) reported prominent elevations on scales 1 and 3 and

TABLE 4.2. Results of the Henrichs et al.
(1988) Evaluation of the MMPI Pn Scale
According to the Decision Theory Matrix

	ES ($n = 27$)	NES ($n = 31$)	Total
<7	ES/< 7 Hit 10	NES/< 7 Miss 10	20
≥7	ES/≥ 7 Miss 17	NES/≥ 7 Hit 21	38
Total	27	31	

Hit rate X = hits/(hits + misses)
Hit rate for ES patients = 73% [10/(10 + 17)]
Hit rate for NES patients = 68% [21/(21 + 10)]
Hit rate for <7 cutoff rule = 50% [10/(10 + 10)]
Hit rate for ≥7 cutoff rule = 55% [21/(21 + 17)]

less substantial but nonetheless significant elevations on scales 4 (Psychopathic
Deviate, Pd) and 8 (Schizophrenia, Sc) in their NES patients relative to ES patients.
They suggest that their NES profiles demonstrated MMPI patterns "seen in the
conversion form of hysteria," although their mean scale 2 was only 2–4 T-scores
lower than scales 1 and 3.

Wilkus and Dodrill (1989) attempted to refine NES evaluations by classifying
patients into subgroups based on their "seizure" behavior. This classification system
dichotomized patients into independent subgroups based on (1) extent of *motor
behavior*, including (a) limited motor psychogenic seizures—the seizures resemble
partial motor seizures with mild localized movements—or (b) mostly motor psychogenic seizures—resembling generalized convulsive attacks with "vigorous, diffuse,
tonic, and/or clonic motor activity," often with ictal unresponsiveness—and (2)
extent of *affectual behavior*, including (a) prominently affectual psychogenic
seizures—behaviors include crying, choking, panic, and fear, among others—or (b)
limited no affectual psychogenic seizures—little affectual expression observed.

Wilkus and Dodrill (1989) reported that when classified by this system, the
MMPI profiles of NES patients differed with respect to their "seizure" behavior.
Specifically, they reported that the limited motor subgroup had significant elevations
on scales 1, 3, and 8, and the prominently affectual subgroup revealed elevations on
scales 1, 3, 7 (Psychasthenia, Pt), and 8 in comparison to ES patients with partial
seizures. In contrast, the mostly motor and limited/no affectual subgroups did not
differ from ES patients with generalized seizures.

These findings suggest that MMPI differences may be found in some NES
patients. However, they do not appear to support suppositions that hysteria or

conversion disorder is a specific form of psychopathology that consistently earmarks NES patients as a group, at least from the standpoint of the classical MMPI conversion profile.

Decision Rules

In 1984, Wilkus *et al.* reported the development of a set of MMPI-based decision rules for discriminating patients with NES from those with ES. These rules were defined empirically based on comparisons between groups of NES and ES patients ($n = 15$ per group) matched for age, sex, and education. The rules are as follows:

1. Scale 1 or 3 is 70 or higher and is one of the two highest points disregarding scales 5 and 0.
2. Scale 1 or 3 is 80 or higher, even though not one of the two highest points.
3. Scales 1 and 3 are both higher than 59, and both are at least 10 points higher than scale 2.

Patients meeting rule 1 or rule 2 or rule 3 were called NES.

Wilkus *et al.* (1984) reported hit rates for discriminating groups by these decision rules of 92% [11/(11 + 1)] when predicting NES and 78% [14/(14 + 4)] when predicting ES. The authors then used these decision rules to distinguish two additional groups of NES and ES patients ($n = 10$ per group). Results of the cross-validation study indicated hit rates of 82% [9/(9 + 2)] when predicting NES and 89% [8/(8 + 1)] when predicting ES by these rules. When the results of both groups of NES and ES patients were combined, the hit rates were 81% [22/(22 + 5)] when predicting NES and 87% [20/(20 + 3)] when predicting ES. These results suggest that this system misclassified 19% of the time when predicting NES and 13% of the time when predicting ES.

When dealing with group data, these results appear quite promising. However, the level of misidentification of individuals still may be too high to warrant clinical use at the present time, especially considering the consequences of misclassification for ES patients. For example, misclassification of a true ES patient as an NES patient may entail cessation of anticonvulsant medication(s) with the attendant associated dangers. According to Wilkus *et al.* (1984), nearly 20% of MMPIs predicting NES would misclassify patients with actual seizures. Of course, misclassification of NES patients as having true seizures also carries its own caveats in terms of treatment initiation and maintenance.

Vanderzant *et al.* (1986) undertook a replication of the Wilkus *et al.* (1984) study with one major exception: their NES and epilepsy patients were not matched demographically (e.g., according to age, sex, and education). These researchers found only a mildly elevated Scale 8 in their NES group (mean T score = 71.2) and no statistically significant difference between the groups on any MMPI scale. There was no striking difference in the mean number of scales elevated between the groups (NES = 3.4, ES = 2.4). Further, and similar to Wurzman and Matthews (1982), they reported that Scale 2 elevations were almost as numerous in the NES group as Scale 1 elevations, and five of their 18 NES patients had elevated Scale 2 with "normal" (30 < T-score < 70) scales 1 and 3. They reported that only 37% (7/19) of NES patients were correctly classified by the Wilkus et al. (1984) decision rules, while 10% (2/20) of ES patients were misclassified as having NES. From these data, index hit rates for their study are 78% [7/(7 + 2)] when predicting NES and 60% [18/(18 + 12)] when predicting ES. Therefore, similar to Wilkus et al. (1984), 22% of the NES predictions in this study misclassified patients with actual seizures as having NES. Further, another 40% of ES predictions incorrectly considered NES patients to have actual seizures.

Henrichs et al. (1988) also attempted to replicate the findings of Wilkus et al. (1984) using the MMPI decision rules. This study included a sample of 144 subjects including 59 ES with left temporal foci, 27 ES with right temporal foci, 27 ES with primary generalized ES, and 31 NES. Subjects were matched for age, education, age at onset of recurrent seizures, and duration of recurrent seizures (Some gender differences were evident). Results indicated that 68% of NES patients and 73% of ES patients were classified correctly (27% of ES patients were misclassified) by this system. Further, their index hit rates were only 41% [21/(21 + 30)] when predicting NES, although they were 89% [83/(83 + 10)] when predicting ES. By these results, 59% of predictions would misclassify patients with actual seizures as having NES.

Across these studies, 19–59% of predictions by the Wilkus et al. (1984) decision rules misclassified patients with verified epilepsy as having NES. These findings suggest that the decision rules carry a sizable risk of misclassification.

Wilkus and Dodrill's (1989) results from subtyping NES patients suggest that refinement in the application of the decision rules may enhance their hit rates. For example, they argued that Vanderzant et al. (1986) failed to find MMPI differences in their NES patients because of differences in their samples other than those derived from failure to match on demographics. They emphasized that Vanderzant et al. (1986) evaluated only NES and ES patients with major motor displays in their "seizures," comparisons that also failed to yield significant findings in their own investigations, whereas their significant results stemmed from comparisons of NES and ES patients with prominent affectual and limited motor behavior. They also suggest that the NES patients in the Vanderzant et al. (1986) study probably closely resemble their own mostly motor NES subgroup. However, Wilkus and Dodrill (1989) did not include data regarding hits and misses in this second study, leaving the power of this technique to improve classification rates unknown.

Summary

These findings suggest that use of the MMPI to discriminate NES patients from ES patients is a tenuous and risky business at best. There is considerable disagreement regarding the MMPI's utility. Its proper use, if it has one, may be limited to discriminating NES patients who exhibit specific behaviors during "seizures." Clearly, the hit rates for correct MMPI classification are not high enough to warrant its use as a basis for deriving clinical decisions. The risks of misclassification appear substantial, particularly for the actual patient with epilepsy. Therefore, although the MMPI may be quite helpful as a general clinical instrument, the findings to date suggest that use of the MMPI to discriminate NES and ES patients should be carried out with extreme caution.

CONCLUSIONS

What should be evident from this review is that the neuropsychological discrimination of NES from ES can be extremely difficult. Part of the difficulty may be that the traditional approach to the problem has been too narrow-minded. Perhaps, as originally suggested by Wilkus and Dodrill (1989), patients with NES are a heterogeneous group that may be characterized by a spectrum of identifiable neuropsychological and personality types, types that might differ either qualitatively or quantitatively from patients with epilepsy. In perhaps one of the more creative approaches to the problem, neuropsychologists at the University of Minnesota Epilepsy Center have gathered a large number of patients with "nonepileptic events" and have cluster-analyzed their neuropsychological and MMPI data. The preliminary findings, as yet unpublished except in abstract form (Barrash, Gates, Heck, & Berriak, 1989), have demonstrated that patients with NES are a heterogeneous group indeed, characterized by a variety of MMPI and neuropsychological profile types. This information, in conjunction with an understanding of the distribution of similar profile types among patients with actual epilepsy, may allow for more accurate probability statements regarding the presence of either epilepsy or NES. Unfortunately, it probably will be some time until that level of sophistication is available. Until then, ongoing collaborative efforts with neurological and psychiatric colleagues will help to reduce the error inherent in this difficult diagnostic task.

REFERENCES

Barrash, J., Gates, J. R., Heck, D. G., & Berriak, T. E. (1989). MMPI subtypes among patients with nonepileptic events. *Epilepsia*, *30*, 730.

Henrichs, T. F., Tucker, D. M., Farha, J., & Novelly, R. A. (1988). MMPI indices in the identification of patients evidencing pseudoseizures. *Epilepsia*, *29*, 184–187.

Marks, P. A., & Seeman, W. (1963). *The actuarial description of abnormal personality.* Baltimore: Williams & Wilkins.

Matthews, C. G., Shaw, D. J., & Klove, H. (1966). Psychological test performances in neurologic and "pseudo-neurologic" subjects. *Cortex*, *2*, 244–253.

Nicholl, J. S. (1981). Pseudoseizures: A neuropsychiatric diagnostic dilemma. *Psychosomatics*, *22*, 451–454.

Ramani, S. V., & Gumnit, R. J. (1982). Management of hysterical seizures in epileptic patients. *Archives of Neurology*, *39*, 78–81.

Ramani, S. V., Quesney, L. F., Olson, D., & Gumnit, R. J. (1980). Diagnosis of hysterical seizures in epileptic patients. *American Journal of Psychiatry*, *137*, 705–709.

Rowan, A. J., & Gates, J. (Eds.). *Nonepileptic seizures: Causation, diagnosis, classification, and treatment* (in press). New York: Demos.

Sackellares, J. C., Giordani, B., Berent, S., Seidenberg, M., Dreifuss, F., Vanderzant, C. W., & Boll, T. J. (1985). Patients with pseudoseizures: Intellectual and cognitive performance. *Neurology, 35,* 116–119.

Shaw, D. J. (1966). Differential MMPI performance in pseudoseizure epileptic and pseudo-neurologic groups. *Journal of Clinical Psychology, 22,* 271–275.

Shaw, D. J., & Matthews, C. G. (1965). Differential MMPI performance of brain-damages vs. pseudo-neurologic groups. *Journal of Clinical Psychology, 21,* 405–408.

Vanderzant, C. W., Giordani, B., Berent, S., Dreifuss, F. E., & Sackellares, J. C. (1986). Personality of patients with pseudoseizures. *Neurology, 36,* 664–668.

Wilkus, R. J., & Dodrill, C. B. (1989). Factors affecting the outcome of MMPI and neuropsychological assessments of psychogenic and epileptic seizure patients. *Epilepsia, 30,* 339–347.

Wilkus, R. J., Dodrill, C. B., & Thompson, P. M. (1984). Intensive EEG monitoring and psychological studies of patients with pseudoepileptic seizures. *Epilepsia, 25,* 100–107.

Wurzman, L. P., & Matthews, C. G. (February, 1982). The borderlands of epilepsy: Explorations with the MMPI. Paper presented at International Neuropsychological Society, Pittsburgh.

II

Cognitive and Emotional
Consequences of Epilepsy

5

Cognitive Effects of Epilepsy and Anticonvulsant Medications

THOMAS L. BENNETT

The apparent association between cognitive impairment and epilepsy has been observed for at least several centuries. For example, in his 17th century Oxford Lectures, Thomas Willis remarked: "It often happens that epileptic patients, during their paroxysm and afterwards, suffer a severe loss of memory, intellect, and phantasy. . ." (Dewhurst, 1980). This view of epilepsy pervaded the thinking of physicians through the 19th century, and it was based entirely on clinical impressions. This approach continued into the early 20th century as clinicians continued to note a high frequency of cognitive impairment in patients with epilepsy (for example, Turner, 1907).

A significant limitation of the early observations was that they were typically confined to investigating patients in institutions. Thus, even when IQ began to be used as an index of intellectual ability (for example, Fox, 1924), the results were biased by sampling error. Since the 1950s, the trend has been to sample the population more generally and to investigate intellectual functions in noninstitutionalized individuals. As these latter studies were published, it soon became quite evident that epilepsy and cognitive impairment are not highly correlated. Lack of cognitive impairment began to be stressed (for example, Keating, 1960; Lennox & Lennox, 1960). In a study of 1,905 individuals with epilepsy, Lennox and Lennox concluded that fully two-thirds of their patients were intellectually normal, and only one-seventh were clearly impaired.

Many problems were encountered in the early studies of cognitive impairment in epilepsy. Major factors known to affect cognitive processes in patients with epilepsy were not controlled, and indeed, this remains a major problem for research conducted

THOMAS L. BENNETT • Department of Psychology, Colorado State University, Fort Collins, Colorado 80523.

The Neuropsychology of Epilepsy, edited by Thomas L. Bennett. Plenum Press, New York, 1992.

on this topic today. These factors include age of onset and duration of the seizure disorder, seizure type, seizure frequency, medication variables, and whether the seizures are idiopathic or symptomatic. These variables are discussed later in this chapter.

A second major problem deals with the assessment of epilepsy. Early studies that employed objective measures used IQ testing. However, although IQ testing is in general a good measure of a person's biological level of adaptive functioning, it is nevertheless highly dependent on achievement. Furthermore, having not been developed originally to evaluate cerebral dysfunction, IQ tests are not particularly sensitive to the types of cognitive problems that people with brain injury experience. Neuropsychologists use IQ scores along with other information to estimate premorbid functioning in brain-injured individuals because of the IQ's resistance to brain injury.

Rather than using IQ as a measure of cognitive functions, recent research has used a process approach in evaluating cognitive abilities in epileptic populations. The cognitive processes investigated have included sensory processes, attention and sustained concentration, learning and memory, language skills, perceptual abilities, conceptualization and reasoning, and motor abilities. The majority of studies do not investigate all of these processes, and within a given process such as attention, one is struck by the fact that few investigators use the same task. Another problem is that a test may not evaluate what it purports to evaluate. Thus, a test of memory may actually be a test of attention, or it might be failed becaused of impaired attention, language, or conceptualization processes.

This latter difficulty can potentially be circumvented by utilizing a battery approach in assessment, an example of which is the Halstead–Reitan Neuropsychological Test Battery (Reitan & Wolfson, 1985). Reitan (1974) believed that this approach would be sensitive to the aggregate of cognitive impairments that might characterize a particular type of epilepsy under investigation.

Although generally in agreement with Reitan's view, Carl Dodrill has further refined the battery approach in the assessment of individuals with epilepsy (for example, Dodrill, 1978, 1981). He has modified and/or extended the Halstead–Reitan Battery to optimally assess the cognitive deficits associated with epilepsy. His battery used 16 measures of performance. Eleven of these were from the Halstead–Reitan Battery (Category test; Tactual Performance test; total time, memory, and localization scores; Seashore Rhythm test; Tapping, total; Trails B; Aphasia Screening test errors; Constructional Dyspraxia; Sensory/Perceptual exam; and Name Writing, total (letter/ second). He added the following: Seashore Tonal Memory; Stroop test, Part I and II – Part I; and the logical and visual reproduction portions of the Wechsler Memory Scale. Norms that reliably distinguished performance of patients with epilepsy from that of closely matched control subjects were established. The two groups were matched according to sex, age, education, occupational status, and race.

The sensitivity to cognitive deficits associated with epilepsy that Dodrill attempted to achieve was apparently realized as illustrated in a study by Dodrill and Troupin (1977). This study investigated the effects of phenytoin and carbamazepine on cognitive function. Use of the standardized Halstead–Reitan Battery yielded no statistically significant findings. However, several important differences emerged when Dodrill's Epilepsy Battery was employed.

The application of neuropsychological test batteries to evaluate the cognitive effects of epilepsy and Dodrill's development of a battery specific to epilepsy represent major advances in the relationship between cognition and epilepsy. Unfortunately, the most common approach still remains narrow, and the majority of inquiries on this topic have continued to focus on a single, or only a few, cognitive abilities.

Three major topics are discussed in this chapter. The first is the effects of epilepsy on cognitive processes such as attention, memory, and reasoning ability. That section is introduced by a model of the brain's functions in neuropsychological processes. Neural factors underlying cognitive deficits are discussed next. These include such factors as the age of onset and duration of the seizure disorder, seizure type, seizure frequency, and whether the seizures are idiopathic or symptomatic. Finally, the influence of anticonvulsant medications on cognitive processes is considered.

EPILEPSY AND COGNITIVE PROCESSES

This section of the chapter discusses the effects of epilepsy on cognitive processes. I discuss this against a model of neuropsychological function, which is described next.

Neuropsychological Model of Brain Functioning

To appreciate fully the effects of epilepsy on cognitive processes, it is helpful to consider these processes within a theoretical or conceptual model of the behavioral correlates of brain functioning. In my own conceptualization, I have found it helpful to expand on and modify the model presented by Reitan and Wolfson (1985); their model denotes six categories of brain–behavior relationships. I have expanded the number of categories to seven to separate attention from memory and to emphasize the dependence of memory on attention and concentration. I have expanded on their level of logical analysis and renamed it "executive functions." Note that this is a process model and not an anatomic model. With the exceptions of language skills and visual–spatial, visuoconstructive, and manipulospatial skills, which are more represented, respectively in the left and right hemispheres, these processes are bilaterally represented. This model is diagrammed in Fig. 5.1 (from Bennett, 1988b).

According to this model, the first level of neuropsychological processing is input to the brain via one of the sensory systems. It should be remembered that input could also arise endogenously from within the brain. The input must be attended to or concentrated on for information processing to occur and for the significance of the input to be ascertained (second level). Determining the significance of the stimulus or remembering it for later reference requires involvement of the memory system (level 3).

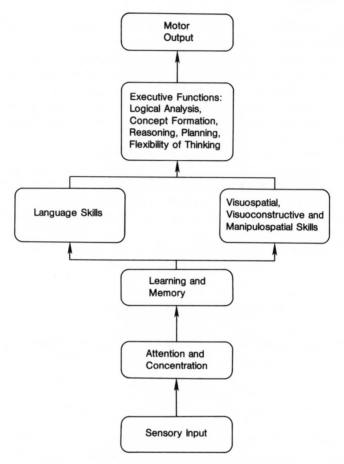

FIGURE 5.1. Conceptual model of the behavioral correlates of brain functioning. (After Reitan and Wolfson, 1985; from Bennett, 1988b).

The interdependence of attention and memory illustrates the fact that this neural system is dynamic, with activity flowing in both directions. In general, if information is to be remembered, it must be attended to, although, on the other hand, attention is no guarantee for memory. Similarly, attention is dependent on memory in terms of attentional processes being involved in such activities as habituation and filtering or gating out nonrelevant information.

Input material that is verbal in nature requires the processing activities of a fourth neuropsychological category, language skills. Nonverbal material similarly requires processing mechanisms of a fifth category, visuospatial, visuoconstructive, and manipulospatial skills.

Executive functions represent the highest level of information processing. These activities are involved in logical analysis, conceptualization, planning, self-monitoring, and flexibility of thinking. Poor performance on tests of executive functions can result from a primary deficit to those functions themselves, or it can result from a primary deficit to one of the lower levels of processing on which executive functions depend. Executive functions quickly become quite impaired in the person who is distractable, forgetful, language-impaired, or who cannot perform higher-level perceptual processes.

Motor functions are the basis for responding and represent the final common path of the neuropsychological processes. They reflect the output capabilities of the system. This is the rationale for placing motor output at the top of the diagram. With this neuropsychological model as a backdrop, the effects of epilepsy on specific cognitive processes can be discussed.

Effects of Epilepsy on Specific Cognitive Processes

Sensory Input

Both impairment and exaggeration of sensory input can be said to result from seizures. Absence or petit mal attacks are generalized nonconvulsive seizures that occur particularly in children. They are characterized by brief episodes of loss of consciousness lasting approximately 5–15 s. During these episodes, the child seems to be unaware of his or her surroundings and stares with a vacant expression. Sensory input occuring during these periods is neither attended to nor registered.

Complex partial seizures, on the other hand, may be manifested as sensory misperceptions and/or hallucinations. Misperceptions are often visual and complex. They typically involve distortions in depth perception or size. Size misperceptions can result in objects being perceived as much smaller (micropsia) or larger (macropsia) than they are. Visual misperceptions reflect a posterior temporal lobe seizure focus. For example, they were observed to occur in a patient prior to discovery of a right temporal lobe astrocytoma, and they diminished following its removal.

Misperception of voices results from a focal discharge of the anterior temporal lobe neocortex, especially from the left hemisphere. Voices will be perceived as too high or too low in pitch or as being too loud or too soft. The patient might complain that the voices around him or her sound as if they are coming out of a tunnel.

Hallucinations or auras that are experienced by complex partial seizure patients are typically simple. In general, olfactory–gustatory sensations, which are often quite displeasing, result from a focal discharge in the uncus of the hippocampus. My patients who experience these auras most typically report salty or bitter taste sensations and/or olfactory sensations best described as burning flesh or putrid. One patient, whose seizures were particularly refractory to anticonvulsant therapy and who experienced secondary generalized seizures correlated with menstruation, was anosmic except when she experienced olfactory auras just prior to and during menstruation each month.

Abdominal and epigastric sensations typically arise from an amygdala focus. Simple auditory phenomena, such as buzzing, ringing, and hissing sounds, are produced by focal activity on the surface of the temporal lobe, especially the primary auditory reception area. Complex visual hallucinations, although uncommon, arise from the temporo–parieto–occipital junction (Rodin, 1984).

Cephalgic auras reflect discharge originating in the central regions of the temporal lobes. They consist of severe, sharp, stabbing, knife-like head pains that are often associated with the head feeling too big, too small, or off the body. Cephalgic auras will occasionally be misdiagnosed as migraine headaches and subsequently incorrectly medicated.

An important feature of auras is that they are passive experiences. The patient feels like an observer to those ictal (seizure) events, dissociated from the actual experience. This is different from the schizophrenic, who firmly believes his or her hallucinations are "real" experiences. The ictal events are unrelated to the environment except for rare seizures triggered by specific stimuli (e.g., musicogenic seizures, sexual seizures). I once had a patient whose seizures were reliably triggered whenever he played the arcade game *Foosball!* More typically for the complex partial seizure patient, the ictal events begin spontaneously with an arrest of all activity, and the aura and/or psychomotor responses follow. Finally, although attention is usually paid to the most salient attribute of the epileptic patient's aura, the dream-like quality of the epileptic aura will often encompass many experiences. For example, a patient of mine regularly experienced a series of events including epigastric sensations, time distortion, detachment from her surroundings, and olfactory sensations as components of her seizure episodes.

Attention and Concentration

Impairment of attention and concentration, in the absence of overt clinical seizures, has been documented by several writers. For example, Holdsworth and Whitmore (1974) reported that 42% of their population of children with epilepsy were rated by their teachers as being markedly inattentive, and other writers have noted the detrimental effects of epilepsy-associated inattention on school success (for example, Stores, 1973). In adults, Mirsky and Van Buren (1965) noted that the presence of epileptic spike waves was associated with decreased attention and concentration that was particularly apparent just prior to onset of and following spike–wave activity.

Attention difficulties in epilepsy are related to seizure type. Patients with generalized seizures are more impaired on measures of sustained attention than are patients with focal seizures (Lansdell & Mirsky, 1964; Mirsky, Primoc, Marsan, Rosvold, & Stevens, 1960). Mirsky and his colleagues argue that this occurs because generalized seizures are more likely than focal seizures to affect central subcortical structures that are responsible for maintaining attention.

In contrast, it appears that patients with focal seizures are more impaired on selective attention than are patients with generalized seizures (Loiseu, Signoret, & Strube, 1984; Stores, 1973). Loiseu *et al.* demonstrated that individuals with focal seizures and persons with generalized seizures performed significantly worse on tests of selective attention than nonepileptic individuals. The worst performance was seen in the group with focal seizures. Stores explains this phenomenon by indicating that although subcortical structures may be important in the maintenance of attention, cortical structures are important in determining what to pay attention to (selective attention). Focal seizures in the cortex thus produce inattentiveness by disrupting selective attention.

Learning and Memory

Memory deficits in association with epilepsy have been documented for over 100 years. Evidence has accumulated associating these deficits with temporal lobe epileptic foci. In an early study that compared cognitive abilities in patients with generalized seizures versus those with focal complex partial seizures of temporal lobe origin, Quadfasel and Pruyser (1955) found that memory impairment was significant only in the focal group.

It should be noted, however, that most studies have been based on investigations of patients who were surgical candidates for intractable epilepsy. Little attention has been directed toward patients with complex partial seizures who were not candidates for surgical intervention. In addition, the findings from existing studies have not been entirely consistent.

When present, the memory deficit seen in individuals with complex partial seizures can exist in isolation. For example, when a complex partial seizure patient was initially evaluated using the Halstead–Reitan Battery, he showed a severe memory deficit that was more pronounced when he attempted to learn verbal material than when he attempted to learn nonverbal material (patterns). His Full-Scale WAIS-R IQ score was in the high average range, and his performance on all of the tests of the Halstead–Reitan Battery was within the normal range. Unfortunately, he showed a more global disruption of cognitive ability when tested a year later. Although his overall intellectual ability, as evaluated by the WAIS-R, had not significantly changed, he showed, in addition to his memory deficits, impairments in word-finding (dysnomia), psychomotor speed, and attention and sustained concentration. His conceptualization and logical analysis abilities remained unimpaired, but his memory deficits were even more pronounced than they had been in the initial evaluation.

The pattern of the neuropsychological deficits may prove to be an aid in determining the laterality of a temporal lobe focus, just as it is in determining the laterality of dysfunction after brain damage. One discrepancy worth noting is a difference in the severity of a deficit in processing, consolidating, and recalling verbal versus nonverbal information. It is well established that left temporal lobe dysfunction yields relatively greater verbal than nonverbal deficit, and the opposite pattern is obtained with right temporal lobe dysfunction (Jarvis & Barth, 1984; Milner, 1975). An analogous phenomenon occurs in patients with left versus right temporal lobe foci. For example, the patient I described who had a greater deficit in verbal memory than he did in nonverbal apparently had a left temporal lobe focus, as indicated by his EEG evaluations.

Although clinical evidence that memory disorders exist in complex partial seizures is longstanding, few carefully designed experiments on this topic have been carried out, and verbal memory has been studied more often than nonverbal memory. Studies of verbal memory in complex partial seizure patients indicate that those individuals with a left temporal lobe focus perform worse on tests of verbal memory than those with a right temporal lobe focus (Masui, Niwa, Anzai, Kameyama, Saitoh, & Rymar, 1984; Mayeux, Brandt, Rosen, & Benson, 1980).

Fedio and Mirsky (1969) studied verbal and nonverbal memory in children with right versus left seizure foci. Although no differences on short-term memory were found, recall of verbal material after a 5-min delay was significantly poorer in the left-focus group. In contrast, delayed recall of nonverbal material was significantly poorer in the right-focus children. Glowinski (1973) confirmed the direction of these laterality differences in adults, but the magnitude of these differences was not significant.

Since these initial studies were conducted, methodology for categorizing and matching patients has been improved, and the basic findings have been confirmed, with long-term memory more significantly affected than short-term memory. For example, Lavadas, Umilta, and Provinciali (1979) investigated patients with epileptic foci in either the left or right temporal lobe who had no evidence of structural lesions on their CT scans. Short- and long-term memory was assessed. No difference in short-term memory was observed. On the other hand, patients with a left temporal lobe focus were more impaired on verbal long-term memory tasks, and right-temporal-lobe patients were more impaired on nonverbal memory tasks. Delaney, Rosen, Mattson, and Novelly (1980) reported similar findings in right- and left-temporal-lobe-focus patients matched for age of onset, duration of epilepsy, and seizure frequency.

Taken together, these studies suggest a significant impairment of memory functions in patients with complex partial seizures of temporal lobe origin. A word of caution comes from the work of Mayeux et al. (1980), who have published findings that indicate that dysnomia contributes greatly to the interictal memory impairment seen in complex-partial-seizure patients. Impairment on memory testing was highly correlated with deficits on the Boston Naming Test. They wrote that ". . .the relative anomia demonstrated in temporal lobe epilepsy patients may have been interpreted by these patients and their relatives as poor memory" (p. 123). The authors further suggested that the verbosity and circumstantiality observed in some patients with complex partial seizures (for example, Bear and Fedio, 1977; Bennett, 1987) may be the expression of a compensatory mechanism for dysnomia. This research points to the difficulty in attempting to evaluate deficits in specific cognitive processes for patients with epilepsy.

Language Skills

Both experimental inquiry and clinical observation indicate that epilepsy may adversely affect language skills. As indicated earlier, Mayeux et al. (1980) demonstrated that dysnomia was prominent in their complex-partial-seizure patients who had a left temporal lobe focus. This deficit was indexed by scores on the Boston Naming Test. They also suggested that dysnomia contributed to the verbosity and circumstantial speech that is often observed in these individuals.

Circumstantiality is seen in both their spoken and written communication. Their communications are often overinclusive and include excessive background detailing, precise times, clarifications, qualifications, and other nonessentials (Bear, Freeman, & Greenberg, 1984). A simple question may elicit a lengthy and circuitous discussion before an answer is finally given. Their verbosity can prevent a conversation from reaching a normal end. This interpersonal communication style can lead to such patients being shunned.

Hypergraphia is also often seen in patients with complex partial seizures. Hypergraphia refers to a tendency toward excessive and compulsive writing, and it was first well documented in these patients by Waxman and Geschwind (1980). It is often characterized by verbosity and circumstantiality, but perhaps it facilitated the writing of the complex partial seizure victim and legendary author Feodor Dostoievsky (Geschwind, 1984).

Impaired language skills as a consequence of epilepsy are also suggested by studies indicating that children with epilepsy have difficulty learning to read. Tizard, Rutter, and Whitmore (1969), for example, reported that 25% of their sample of children with epilepsy who were 9 to 12 years old were more than 28 months behind in reading and comprehension compared to only 4% of the general population. In their Isle of Wight study, Rutter and his colleagues found that children with epilepsy showed a 12-month lag in reading ability compared to their chronological age (Rutter, Graham, & Uyle, 1970). Bagley (1971) and Long and Moore (1979) have published similar findings.

Perceptual–Motor Skills

There has not been a great deal of research investigating the effects of epilepsy on perceptual–motor skills, but the following has been reported. As was noted earlier, Dodrill (1978, 1981) found that total time, memory, and localization scores from the Tactual Performance test were sensitive measures of the effects of epilepsy on cognitive processes. The total time score is a measure of perceptual–motor (manipulospatial) ability. A deficit in spatial memory can be evaluated via the localization score if a significant discrepancy exists between the localization score and the memory score from this task.

Several studies using the Bender Gestalt test have indicated that children with epilepsy perform more poorly than control subjects (for example, Schwartz & Dennerll, 1970; Tymchuk, 1974). Tymchuk found that a score that combined errors with reproduction time reliably distinguished between children with epilepsy and children with school/behavior problems and borderline to mildly retarded children without epilepsy. No attempt was made to distinguish differential effects according to seizure type in these studies. Regarding this latter factor, Morgan and Groh (1980) reported greater impairment on the Frostig Test of Developmental Visual Perception in children with focal seizures than in those with generalized seizures.

Executive Functions

Because of their dependence on lower-level neuropsychological functions, executive functions of the brain involved in such processes as conceptualization, logical analysis, reasoning, planning, sequential thinking, flexibility of thinking, and self-monitoring are especially sensitive to cerebral dysfunction, including that associated with epilepsy. As indicated earlier in this chapter, executive functions will typically be impaired in the person who is distractable, has a poor memory, is language impaired, or who has difficulty with perceptual–motor skills. In a general sense, executive functions are the basis for a person's ability to effectively meet the expectations of others and the demands of his or her environment. Although these impairments may be easily overlooked, they are commonly seen in individuals with epilepsy as indicated by performance on such tests as the Trail Making Tests, the Wisconsin Card-Sorting Test, and the Category Test. Trails B and the Category Test from the Halstead–Reitan Battery are components of Dodrill's Epilepsy Battery, and both Reitan (1974) and Dodrill (1981) stress the use of tests of executive functions in evaluating cognitive functions in patients with epilepsy.

An interesting study by Hermann, Wyler, and Richey (1988) investigated Wisconsin Card-Sorting Test performance (a test of frontal lobe functions) in patients with complex partial seizures of temporal lobe origin. Performance was studied in individuals whose seizures arose from the dominant versus nondominant temporal lobe as well as in an epilepsy control group comprised mainly of patients with primary generalized seizures. Thirty-seven percent of the dominant-hemisphere-focus group and 79% of nondominant-temporal-lobe groups were impaired on this task, suggesting frontal lobe involvement. Only 17% of the epilepsy controls were impaired. It was suggested that these findings reflected dysfunction of the frontal lobes because of epileptic discharge ("neural noise") being propagated from a temporal lobe/hippocampal epileptic focus. Pathways that could transmit such temporal–frontal discharges are well known. After partial resection of the epilepto-genic temporal lobe, Wisconsin Card-Sorting Test performance improved, presumably because of a significant diminution of the neural noise. A similar explanation was used to account for the finding by Novelly, Augustine, Mattson, Glaser, Williamson, Spencer, and Spencer (1984) that patients who underwent unilateral temporal lobectomy experienced a postoperative improvement in material-specific memory mediated by the hemisphere contralateral to the resection (Novelly *et al.*, 1984).

Motor Output

Decreased reaction time and psychomotor speed are common difficulties for individuals with epilepsy. Thus, McGuckin (1980) proposed that lack of speed is one of four main barriers to competitive employment faced by individuals with epilepsy. Using subjects with absence seizures, Goode, Penry, and Dreifuss (1970) reported that the presence of spike–wave activity was accompanied by disruption of attention, increased reaction time, and impaired movement on tasks of motor performance, thereby producing more errors. Errors further increased when spike–waves were present for more than 3 s. Bruhn and Parsons (1977) also showed that slowed reaction time was common in patients with epilepsy.

NEURAL FACTORS UNDERLYING COGNITIVE DEFICITS

This part of the chapter briefly considers some of the neural variables that must be considered in evaluating the effects of epilepsy on cognitive processes. The following factors are discussed: etiology of the seizure disorder, seizure type and frequency, age of onset, and duration of the seizures. Relevant information that is more restricted to epilepsy in children is found in another chapter by the author (Bennett and Krein, 1989).

Etiology of the Seizure Disorder

Of the intellectual correlates associated with epilepsy and the variables that alter them, the most predictable is that of etiology and its relationship to IQ. In his review of research concerned with intellectual and adaptive functioning in epilepsy, Tarter (1972) summarized studies in which etiological factors were considered. The IQ scores of individuals whose seizures were idiopathic ranged from 4 to 11 points higher than scores attained by patients whose seizures were secondary to known pathology (symptomatic). These differences were observed in both institutionalized and non-institutionalized children and adults.

The same relationship between severity of IQ impairment in known versus unknown etiology has been found to occur on measures of neuropsychological functions as well. In one of a series of investigations, Klove and Matthews (1966) found that although adult patients with idiopathic seizures demonstrated neuropsychological impairment as measured by the Halstead battery when compared to nonepileptic controls, the greatest degree of impairment was noted in patients whose seizures were symptomatic.

As noted by Dotten (1988), etiology can significantly confound attempts to study neuropsychological processes in persons with epilepsy. For example, Fowler, Richards, Berent, and Boll (1987) conducted a study, utilizing a modified Halstead–Reitan Neuropsychological Test Battery, to assess cognitive impairments in persons with epilepsy and to investigate correlations between deficits on these tests and EEG indices of focus localization. They were able to demonstrate cognitive impairments on most of the measures employed and, where applicable, correlate these findings with EEG localization. For example, persons scoring low on tests of verbal comprehension usually had a left temporal lobe focus. However, approximately half of the subjects in this study knew the origin of their seizure disorder. Etiologies listed included head injury, infectious disease (e.g., encephalitis), intracranial tumors, and cerebral vascular disease (e.g., stroke). Because brain damage alone can severely impair cognitive functioning and the Halstead–Reitan Neuropsychological Test Battery is highly sensitive to the effects of these conditions, it would seem impossible to sort the cognitive impairments caused by epilepsy from those caused by the disorder underlying the epilepsy in this inquiry.

Dikmen and Reitan's (1978) results support this view. They have demonstrated that, when coupled with head injury with or without persistent focal cortical signs, persons with posttraumatic epilepsy demonstrate impaired performance on the Halstead–Reitan Neuropsychological Test Battery. It is not surprising that such impairments are seen in persons with persistent focal cortical signs, since there are obvious signs of brain pathology. It is their contention that it is not possible to tell if the impairments seen in persons without persistent cortical signs are caused by the epilepsy or by the effects of the head injury. They argue, however, that they are most likely the result of the residual effects of the head injury picked up by a neuropsychological test sensitive to these effects.

Based on these and other findings, Sandra Dotten, for her Master's thesis, took great care to rule out prior history of head injury or neurological disease in her study of the cognitive effects of epilepsy in adults with clear evidence of focal left versus focal right temporal lobe seizures (Haynes & Bennett, 1991). Subjects with epilepsy were closely matched to a normal group on sex, age, IQ, and education. The test battery administered included the Weschsler Adult Intelligence Scale–Revised, lateral dominance exam, Seashore Rhythm test, Speech Sounds Perception test, Seashore Tonal Memory test, Ray–Osterreith Figure Memory test, Story Memory test, Boston Naming test, Trail Making tests, Category test, Finger Oscillation test, and the Grooved Pegboard test.

The number of experimental subjects was small (four in each group), but in the absence of prior head injury or neurological disease, there were no lateralized deficits observed. The only trend that appeared was that the subjects with epilepsy as a group exhibited generalized deficits in the areas of psychomotor speed, selective attention, and reasoning ability. This study emphasizes the importance of ruling out underlying cerebral pathology caused by head injury or other neurological disease in studying cognitive processes in persons with epilepsy.

Seizure Type and Frequency

In addition to etiological factors, type and frequency of seizures constitute important variables influencing the nature and extent of intellectual and cognitive dysfunction. A number of studies have shown generalized tonic–clonic seizures to be associated with greater intellectual and cognitive impairment than other types of seizures. An early study by Zimmerman, Burgemeister, and Putnam (1951) investigated intellectual ability in children and adults using the Stanford–Binet, Weschsler–

Bellevue, and Merrill–Palmer Performance Tests. Mean IQ measured in children and adults with idiopathic absence seizures ranged from 10 to 14 points higher than that in patients with tonic–clonic seizures. Using the Weschsler Adult Intelligence Scale and the Halstead–Reitan Battery, Matthews and Klove (1967) found that adult patients who experienced generalized tonic–clonic seizures demonstrated greater overall intellectual–cognitive impairment than patients with other types of seizures regardless of whether the seizures were idiopathic or symptomatic. Wilkus and Dodrill (1976) also observed poorer performance by adults with EEG evidence of generalized discharge compared to a focal seizure group. In addition, they noted that more frequent seizures were associated with greater deficits. This negative correlation between cognitive ability and frequency of seizures was also reported by Dikman and Matthews (1977) in a study of 72 adults with tonic–clonic seizures of known and unknown etiology.

A similar relationship between seizure frequency and intellectual–cognitive impairment has been reported in children. In an early study, Keith, Ewart, Green, and Gage (1955) reviewed medical records of 296 children and found a regular increasing progression in percentage of retarded children as frequency of seizures increased. This relationship was consistent across all seizure types considered. Also, cases in which the seizures were symptomatic showed a greater incidence of retardation (73%) than those in which the cause of seizures could not be attributed to organic abnormality (22.2%).

More recently, Farwell, Dodrill, and Batzel (1985) evaluated a large group of children whose ages ranged from 6 to 15 years. Within each seizure type studied, lower seizure frequency was associated with higher scores on the WISC–R. In addition, seizure type was found to be a discriminating factor when both IQ and neuropsychological functions were evaluated. The minor motor and atypical absence groups showed statistically significant lower IQ scores than all other groups. However, children with partial or generalized tonic–clonic seizures demonstrated proportions of Full-Scale IQ scores comparable to those observed in the control group. When considered together, children with epilepsy showed significantly greater neuropsychological impairment than controls as measured by the age-appropriate Halstead–Reitan battery. Overall neuropsychological impairment was found to differentiate between seizure types with greater sensitivity than did Full-Scale IQ (WISC–R). Children with minor motor or atypical absence seizures showed mild impairment. The majority of children who experienced only classical absence seizures demonstrated no detectable neuropsychological impairment, but when seizure types were mixed (classic absence plus generalized tonic–clonic), impairment was again evident.

Seizure type has been found to affect selected cognitive functions differentially: Quadfasel and Pruyser (1955) compared cognitive abilities in adult male patients with generalized seizures versus complex partial seizures and found that memory was impaired only in the partial-seizure group. Fedio and Mirsky (1969) assessed the performance of outpatient groups of children (6 to 14 years old) who had left temporal lobe epileptic focus, right temporal lobe focus, or centrencephalic epilepsy (generalized seizures). Children were evaluated using measures of attention, verbal and nonverbal learning and memory, and IQ. Regardless of seizure type, the performance of children with epilepsy was below that of the nonepileptic control group. Of greater interest, however, was the pattern of deficits observed between seizure types and within the temporal lobe seizure groups. Children with left temporal lobe seizure focus showed learning and memory deficits on measures that required delayed recall of verbal material, whereas children with right temporal lobe focus had greater difficulty with recall tasks involving visuospatial abilities. Significant differences between performance on measures of short-term memory were not evident between groups. Further, children whose seizures were centrencephalic in nature performed at a significantly lower level on tasks of sustained attention than did the temporal lobe groups, but they did not demonstrate either short-term or long-term memory impairment.

Patterns of intellectual performance on the Weschsler Intelligence Scales (WAIS or WISC–R) that varied with seizure type were observed by Giordani, Berant, Sackellares, Rourke, Seidenberg, O'Leary, Dreifuss, and Boll (1985). Adults and children with partial seizures performed better on Digit Span, Digit Symbol (or Coding), Block Design, and Object Assembly than did patients with either generalized or partial secondarily generalized seizures, although significant differences between groups on Full-Scale IQ scores were not present.

In contrast, some studies have not shown a clear relationship between seizure type and cognitive impairment (Arieff & Yacorzynski, 1942; Scott, Moffett, Matthews, & Ettlinger, 1976) or frequency of seizures and greater intellectual impairment (Delaney et al., 1980; Loiseau, Strube, Brouslet, Battellochi, Gomeni, & Morselli, 1980; Scott et al., 1976). O'Leary, Lovell, Sackellares, Berent, Giordani, Seidenberg, and Boll (1983) found only one variable that showed a significant difference in performance between groups of children with differing seizure disorders. Children with partial seizures performed significantly better on the Tactual Performance test (TPT, total time) than children with generalized seizures. The partial-seizure group in this study, however, was composed of simple partial, complex partial, and partial secondarily generalized seizure types, and this wide variation of seizure types within one group may have accounted for the limited differences seen when groups were compared.

Because seizure classifications and their inclusion criteria have not been consistent, particularly in the earlier studies, and populations tested have not been uniform across investigations (institutionalized versus noninstitutionalized), direct comparisons between studies are not always possible. The study of seizure type and frequency and its effect on intellectual and cognitive function is further complicated by the severity of seizures and the levels of antiepileptic medications necessary to achieve adequate seizure control. It is also possible that in some cases, the association between observed cognitive deficits and frequency of seizures reflects the extent of cerebral damage that is responsible for both. When considered as a whole, however, current studies suggest that the extent of intellectual and cognitive dysfunction in epilepsy varies with type of seizure and increases with greater seizure frequency.

Age at Onset and Duration of Disorder

More than a century ago, Gowers recognized the relationship between early onset of seizure disorder and poor prognosis for mental functioning (Brown & Reynolds, 1981). In general, current research supports this early observation. Studies of intellectual and neuropsychological functions in people with epilepsy, regardless of seizure type, indicate that onset of seizures early in life and a consequently long duration of seizure disorder place individuals at higher risk for cognitive dysfunction. Many studies of the effect of age at seizure onset on cognitive processes have considered only generalized tonic–clonic seizures. Dikman, Matthews, and Harley (1975, 1977) found that adult patients with early onset of major motor seizures (0–5 years of age) obtained significantly lower Verbal, Performance, and Full-Scale IQ scores (WAIS) than a group of patients with later onset of seizures (10–15 years of age). Both seizure groups showed impaired neuropsychological functions (Halstead–Reitan) compared to a nonepileptic control group. However, differences in performance between the early- and late-onset epileptic groups were not significant. On the other hand, Matthews and Klove (1967) found that early onset of tonic–clonic seizures resulted in greater impairment of both intellectual and neuropsychological abilities. This difference was observed in both idiopathic and symptomatic seizures.

More recently, O'Leary *et al.* (1983) studied the effects of early onset of epilepsy in children 9 to 15 years of age with partial versus generalized seizures. Results indicated that both groups of children with early seizure onset performed more poorly on measures of neuropsychological abilities than children whose seizures began when they were older. These findings are consistent with observations of the effect of seizure onset by Farwell *et al.* (1985), who studied a variety of seizure types, and Scarpa and Corassini (1982) in their study of children with partial seizures.

As in studies of seizure frequency, investigation of the effects of age at onset is complicated by anticonvulsant medications. Anticonvulsants have been found to affect cognitive performance in both children and adults, as discussed next. In cases of early seizure onset, the effects of anticonvulsant drugs on the developing brain become an important consideration, as well as does the subsequent long-term drug therapy that must follow.

COGNITIVE EFFECTS OF ANTICONVULSANT MEDICATIONS

Intellectual and cognitive impairments in people with epilepsy, especially memory deficits, were observed and noted in the literature over 100 years ago, long before anticonvulsant drugs that are used today were available (Trimble & Thompson, 1984). Unfortunately, there is increasing evidence that many, if not most, anticonvulsants themselves adversely affect cognitive ability. As a result, anticonvulsants may compound the cognitive difficulties and behavioral problems seen in persons with epilepsy (Bellur & Hermann, 1984; Blumer & Benson, 1982; Committee on Drugs, 1985; Corbett, Trimble, & Nichol, 1985; Himmelhock, 1984; Reynolds & Trimble, 1985; Walker & Blumer, 1984; Wilson, Petty, Perry, & Rose, 1983).

For most anticonvulsants, favorable reports, usually based on subjective impressions, have been noted immediately after they have been introduced for general use. With more widespread use and experimental inquiry into their neuropsychological influence, adverse effects soon emerged for most anticonvulsants. Toxic doses of virtually all anticonvulsant medications will affect cognitive functioning. It is, however, the possibility of cognitive impairment resulting from serum concentrations of antiepileptic medications within the therapeutic range that is of most concern in the long-term treatment of epilepsy.

For example, Reynolds and Travers (1974) studied a group of 57 outpatients who were, or were not, experiencing intellectual deterioration, psychiatric illness, personality change, or psychomotor slowing. Those that were experiencing these difficulties had significantly higher blood levels of phenytoin or phenobarbital than those without such changes, even though these individuals all had blood levels of these drugs that were within the optimum or therapeutic range. Patients with overt drug toxicity, detectable cerebral lesions, or psychiatric illness that preceded the onset of epilepsy had been excluded from the study. These observations were also not simply related to seizure frequency. Similar findings were reported by Trimble and Corbett (1980) is a study of 312 children in a residential hospital school. Children who experienced a decline in IQ of between 10 and 40 points over a 1-year interval had significantly higher levels of phenytoin and primidone, with a similar trend for phenobarbital, than those who did not. Again, blood levels of these anticonvulsants were within the therapeutic range.

The nature and extent of these deficits vary with the drug or combination of drugs administered to the patient. As would be expected, polytherapy (administration of more than one anticonvulsant) has been found to result in greater deficits than monotherapy (MacLeod, Dekaban, & Hunt, 1978; Shorwon & Reynolds, 1979; Thompson & Trimble, 1983). Shorwon and Reynolds were able to reduce polytherapy to monotherapy in 29 of 40 outpatients studied. In over half of the patients reduced to monotherapy, an improvement of alertness, concentration, drive, mood, and sociability was observed. This was especially noted in association with withdrawal of phenobarbital or primidone. Similarly, Fischbacher (1982) reported that reduction of at least one anticonvulsant in institutionalized patients improved alertness, psychomotor performance, and behavior. The cognitive effects produced by commonly prescribed anticonvulsants are described in the following sections.

Barbiturates

Early studies investigating the cognitive effects of phenobarbital led to the conclusion that despite its sedative properties, phenobarbital had no adverse effects on cognitive ability (Grinker, 1929; Lennox, 1942). However, with the development of more sensitive neuropsychological tests and the medical technology required to accurately evaluate serum anticonvulsant levels, it soon became apparent that cognitive deficits were produced by this drug. For example, Hutt, Jackson, Belsham, and Higgins (1968) tested phenobarbital on nonepileptic volunteers and found that it impaired psychomotor speed and sustained attention.

Hyperactivity is often a paradoxical side effect of phenobarbital therapy (Wolf & Forsythe, 1978; McGowan, Neville, & Reynolds, 1983). In a comparative study of monotherapy with four major anticonvulsants in previously untreated children with epilepsy, McGowan *et al.* found that 5 of the 10 children assigned to the phenobarbital group developed hyperactivity or aggressive behavior or difficulty coping with school work. This necessitated withdrawal of the drug from the patients and discontinuing its use in the study.

Primidone (Mysoline®) is a barbiturate analogue that is metabolized into phenobarbital and phenylethylmalonamide. There is little direct experimental evidence on the cognitive effects of this medication, but it is generally believed that the effects closely parallel those produced by phenobarbital.

Phenytoin

Phenytoin (Dilantin®), when originally introduced, was thought to improve alertness (Trimble, 1981), but later research indicated that this was an incorrect conclusion. It is now clear that even therapeutic doses of phenytoin can adversely affect psychomotor performance (Idestrom, Schelling, Carlquist, & Sjoquist, 1972; Thompson & Trimble, 1982), concentration (Andrewes, Tomlinson, Elwes, & Reynolds, 1984; Dodrill & Troupin, 1977), memory (Andrewes *et al.*, 1984, Thompson & Trimble, 1982), and problem solving (Dodrill & Troupin, 1977).

A reversible phenytoin-induced encephalopathy, characterized by intellectual impairment and memory deficits, has been reported (Trimble & Reynolds, 1976). This is associated with toxic blood levels of phenytoin, but it is not accompanied by other clear neurological evidence of toxicity such as nystagmus or ataxia. This encephalopathy can occur in adults, but it has been more often observed in children, especially those with preexisting brain damage or mental retardation. It may mistakenly be interpreted as progressive neurological disease rather than as a reversible condition.

Sodium Valproate

Trimble & Thompson (1984) reported minimal adverse cognitive effects associated with administration of sodium valproate (Depakote®) on performance of neuropsychological tests. Barnes and Bower (1975) asserted that administration of this drug actually improved alertness and school performance in children with epilepsy. On the negative side, there have been several reports of a sodium-valproate-induced encephalopathy similar to that described above for phenytoin (Davidson, 1983; Reynolds, 1985).

Carbamazepine

Carbamazepine (Tegretol®), like sodium valproate, appears to produce minimal adverse effects on cognitive processes. Dalby (1975) reported that behavioral alterations associated with complex partial seizures of temporal lobe origin, namely, slowness of information processing, interpersonal viscosity, emotional lability, and increased aggressivity, improved with carbamazepine in approximately 50% of his patients.

An interesting study by Schain, Ward, and Guthrie (1977) evaluated the cognitive consequences of replacing phenobarbital and primidone with carbamazepine treatment in children with tonic–clonic and complex partial seizure disorders. A battery of neuropsychological tests intended to evaluate general intelligence, problem-solving ability, and attention was administered. Substantial improvement in problem-solving measures was noted when carbamazepine was given. In addition, the children appeared to be more alert and attentive than when they were treated with phenobarbital or primidone. Seizures were still adequately controlled. Thompson and Trimble (1982), using adults, similarly found carbamazepine to have a less detrimental effect on cognitive functioning than did phenobarbital or primidone.

Taken together, these studies indicate that some anticonvulsants can have significant negative effects on cognitive functions. These findings allow us to conclude that some of the neuropsychological changes that are observed in people with epilepsy occur as a direct result of anticonvulsant therapy rather than as a consequence of the many variables, reviewed earlier, that can themselves alter cognitive ability in these individuals. This is an important consideration in prescribing these agents. Although these subtle yet significant cognitive effects may easily be overlooked without careful neuropsychological monitoring, they may be a large price to pay for seizure control or, quite commonly, inadequate seizure control. This is especially true for children and others in academic pursuits (Stores, 1981) and for adults whose occupations require psychomotor speed, sustained concentration, and high levels of information processing.

CONCLUSIONS AND RECOMMENDATIONS FOR FUTURE RESEARCH

Two themes emerge in this chapter. First, epilepsy in its own right can produce cognitive difficulties. However, the nature and extent of the deficits depend on seizure type and frequency, age at onset and duration of the disorder, and etiology of the seizure disorder. The major consideration with respect to etiology was whether the seizure disorder was idiopathic or symptomatic. Symptomatic seizures are secondary to known neuropathology. Cognitive impairments associated with symptomatic seizures are typically more reflective of the consequences of underlying pathology (for example, traumatic brain injury) than they are reflective of consequences of epilepsy *per se*. A major failure in research that has investigated cognitive impairments associated with epilepsy has been the lack of good control for prior history of neurological disease or injury. Future research must control for this factor. Once this is adequately accomplished, then the influence of other neurological variables, such as seizure type, frequency, age at onset, and duration of disorder, on cognitive processes can be clarified.

A second theme that has emerged is that many anticonvulsant medications can themselves produce cognitive impairment. This phenomenon has been demonstrated in nonepileptic volunteers and patients with epilepsy. Future research will be needed to further explore this phenomenon and its interaction with polytherapy. The fact that medications themselves produce cognitive disturbances makes it doubly hard to determine the influence on cognitive performance produced by the variables associated with epilepsy itself.

Neuropsychological assessment may not contribute greatly to the actual diagnosis of epilepsy because, although these individuals may often show cognitive impairment, there is probably no consistent neuropsychological profile seen that will reliably distinguish individuals with epilepsy from individuals with other neurological conditions that impair cognitive functioning. It is also apparently not possible to distinguish reliably patients with one category of idiopathic epilepsy from another. On the other hand, knowledge of the cognitive processes impaired in an individual with epilepsy may be useful in devising remedial or cognitive rehabilitation programs that will help the patient overcome or minimize the effects of these deficits (for example, Bennett, 1988a).

Neuropsychological assessment can be used to monitor cognitive changes related to the epilepsy or the drugs administered to treat it. It can be used to detect subtle, but significant, alterations in cognitive processes resulting from anticonvulsant therapy. The most beneficial anticonvulsant regimen for a patient may be one in which a compromise is reached between degree of seizure control and neuropsychological impairment (or benefit) if the patient is carefully monitored from a neuropsychological perspective.

ACKNOWLEDGMENTS.   The author wishes to acknowledge the aid of Linda K. Krein, M.S., R.Ph., and S. D. H. Dotten, Ph.D., for their help in surveying the research on neural factors underlying cognitive deficits in epilepsy.

REFERENCES

Andrewes, D. G., Tomlinson, L., Elwes, R. D., & Reynolds, E. H. (1984). The influence of carbamezepine and phenytoin on memory and other aspects of cognitive function in new referrals with epilepsy. *Acta Neurologica Scandinavica, Supplement, 99,* 23–30.

Arieff, A. J., & Yacorzynski, G. K. (1942). Deterioration of patients with organic epilepsy. *Journal of Nervous and Mental Disease, 96,* 49–55.

Bagley, C. (1971). *The social psychology of the child with epilepsy.* London: Routledge, Kegan and Paul.

Barnes, S. E., & Bower, B. D. (1975). Sodium valproate in the treatment of intractable childhood epilepsy. *Developmental Medicine and Child Neurology, 17,* 175–181.

Bear, D. M., & Fedio, P. (1977). Quantitative analysis of interictal behavior in temporal lobe epilepsy. *Archives of Neurology, 34,* 454–467.

Bear, D. M., Freeman, R., & Greenberg, M. (1984). Behavioral alterations in patients with temporal lobe epilepsy. In D. Blumer (Ed.), *Psychiatric aspects of epilepsy* (pp. 197–227). Washington, DC: American Psychiatric Press.

Bellur, S., & Hermann, B. P. (1984). Emotional and cognitive effects of anticonvulsant medications. *The International Journal of Clinical Neuropsychology*, *6*, 21–23.

Bennett, T. L. (1987). Neuropsychological aspects of complex partial seizures: Diagnostic and treatment issues. *The International Journal of Clinical Neuropsychology*, *9*, 37–45.

Bennett, T. L. (1988a). Neuropsychological rehabilitation in the private practice setting. *Cognitive Rehabilitation*, *6*(1), 12–15.

Bennett, T. L. (1988b). Use of the Halstead–Reitan Neuropsychological Test Battery in the assessment of head injury. *Cognitive Rehabilitation*, *6*(3), 18–24.

Bennett, T. L., & Krien, L. K. (1989). The neuropsychology of epilepsy: Psychological and social impact. In C. R. Reynolds & E. Fletcher-Janzen (Eds.), *Handbook of clinical child neuropsychology* (pp. 419–441). New York: Plenum Press.

Blumer, D., & Benson, D. F. (1982). Psychiatric manifestations of epilepsy. In D. F. Benson & D. Blumer (Eds.), *Psychiatric aspects of neurologic disease*, Volume 2 (pp. 25–48). New York: Grune & Stratton.

Browne, S. W., & Reynolds, E. H. (1981). Cognitive impairment in epileptic patients. In E. H. Reynolds and M. R. Trimble (Eds.), *Epilepsy and psychiatry* (pp. 147–164). London: Churchill Livingstone.

Bruhm, P., & Parsons, O. A. (1977). Reaction time variability in epileptic and brain-damaged patients. *Cortex*, *13*, 373–384.

Committee on Drugs. (1985). Behavioral and cognitive effects of anticonvulsant therapy. *Pediatrics*, *76*, 644–647.

Corbett, J. A., Trimble, M. R., & Nichol, T. C. (1985). Behavioral and cognitive impairments in children with epilepsy: The long term effects of anticonvulsant therapy. *Journal of the American Academy of Child Psychiatry*, *24*, 17–23.

Dalby, M. A. (1975). Behavioral effects of carbamazepine. In J. K. Penry & D. D. Daly (Eds.), *Advances in Neurology*, Volume 11 (pp. 331–343). New York: Raven Press.

Davidson, D. L. W. (1983). A review of the side effects of sodium valproate. *British Journal of Clinical Practice*, *27*(Suppl.), 79–85.

Delaney, R. C., Rosen, A. J., Mattson, R. H., & Novelly, R. A. (1980). Memory function in focal epilepsy: A comparison of non-surgical, unilateral temporal lobe and frontal lobe samples. *Cortex*, *16*, 103–117.

Dewhurst, K. (1980). *Thomas Willis' Oxford lectures*. Oxford: Sanford.

Dikman, S., & Matthews, C. G. (1977). Effect of major motor seizure frequency upon cognitive–intellectual function in adults. *Epilepsia*, *18*, 21–29.

Dikman, S., Matthews, C. G., & Harley, J. P. (1975). The effect of early versus late onset of major motor epilepsy upon cognitive–intellectual performance. *Epilepsia*, *16*, 73–81.

Dikman, S., Matthews, C. G., & Harley, J. P. (1977). Effect of early versus late onset of major motor epilepsy on cognitive–intellectual performance: Further considerations. *Epilepsia*, *18*, 31–36.

Dikmen, S., & Reitan, R. (1978). Neuropsychological performance in posttraumatic epilepsy. *Epilepsia*, *19*, 177–183.

Dodrill, C. B. (1978). A neuropsychological battery for epilepsy. *Epilepsia*, *19*, 611–623.

Dodrill, C. B. (1981). Neuropsychology of epilepsy. In S. B. Filskov & T. J. Boll (Eds.), *Handbook of clinical neuropsychology* (pp. 366–395). New York: John Wiley & Sons.

Dodrill, C. B., & Troupin, A. S. (1977). Psychotropic effects of carbamazepine in epilepsy: A double-blind comparison with phenytoin. *Neurology*, *27*, 1023–1028.

Dotten, S. D. H. (1988). *Cognitive impairments in adults with complex partial seizures*. Unpublished Master's thesis, Colorado State University.

Farwell, J. R., Dodrill, C. B., & Batzel, L. W. (1985). Neuropsychological abilities of children with epilepsy. *Epilepsia*, *26*(5), 395–400.

Fedio, P., & Mirsky, A. F. (1969). Selective intellectual deficits in children with temporal lobe or centrencephalic epilepsy. *Neuropsychologia*, *7*, 287–300.

Fischlacher, E. (1982). Effect of reduction of anticonvulsants on wellbeing. *British Medical Journal, 285*, 425–427.

Fowler, P. C., Richards, H. C., Berent, S., & Boll, T. J. (1987). Epilepsy, neuropsychological deficits and EEG lateralization. *Archives of Clinical Neuropsychology, 2*, 81–92.

Fox, J. T. (1924). Response of epileptic children to mental and educational tests. *British Journal of Medical Psychology, 4*, 235–248.

Geschwind, N. (1984). Dostoievsky's epilepsy. In D. Blumer (Ed.), *Psychiatric aspects of epilepsy* (pp. 325–334). Washington, DC: American Psychiatric Press.

Giordani, B., Berent, S., Sackellares, J. C., Rourke, D., Seidenberg, M., O'Leary, D. S., Dreifuss, F. E., & Boll, T. J. (1985). Intelligence test performance of patients with partial and generalized seizures. *Epilepsia, 26*(1), 37–42.

Glowinski, H. (1973). Cognitive deficits in temporal lobe epilepsy. *The Journal of Nervous and Mental Disorders, 157*, 129–137.

Goode, D. J., Penry, J. K., & Dreifuss, F. E. (1970). Effects of paroxysmal spike wave on continuous visual–motor performance. *Epilepsia, 11*, 241–254.

Grinker, R. R. (1929). The proper use of phenobarbital in the treatment of the epilepsies. *Journal of the American Medical Association, 93*, 1218–1219.

Haynes, S. D., & Bennett, T. L. (1991). Cognitive impairments in adults with complex partial seizures. *The International Journal of Clinical Neuropsychology, 12*, 74–81.

Hermann, B. P., Wyler, A. R., & Richey, E. T. (1988). Wisconsin card sorting test performance in patients with complex partial seizures of temporal-lobe origin. *Journal of Clinical and Experimental Neuropsychology, 10*, 467–476.

Himmelhock, J. M. (1984). Major mood disorders related to epileptic changes. In D. Blumer (Ed.), *Psychiatric aspects of epilepsy* (pp. 271–294). Washington, DC: American Psychiatric Press.

Holdsworth, L., & Whitmore, K. (1974). A study of children with epilepsy attending ordinary schools. I. Their seizure patterns, progress and behavior in school. *Developmental Medicine and Child Neurology, 16*, 746–758.

Hutt, S. J., Jackson, P. M., Belsham, A. B., & Higgins, G. (1968). Perceptual–motor behavior in relation to blood phenobarbitone level. *Developmental Medicine and Child Neurology, 10*, 626–632.

Idestrom, C. M., Schelling, D., Carlquist, V., & Sjoquist, F. (1972). Behavioral and psychophysiological studies: Acute effects of diphenylhydantoin in relation to plasma levels. *Psychological Medicine, 2*, 111–120.

Jarvis, P. E., & Barth, J. T. (1984). *Halstead–Reitan Test Battery: An interpretive guide*. Odessa, Florida: Psychological Assessment Resources.

Keating, L. E. (1960). A review of the literature on the relationship of epilepsy and intelligence in school children. *Journal of Mental Science, 106*, 1042–1059.

Keith, H. M., Ewert, J. C., Green, M. W., & Gage, R. P. (1955). Mental status of children with convulsive disorders. *Neurology, 5*, 419–425.

Klove, H., & Matthews, C. G. (1966). Psychometric and adaptive abilities in epilepsy with differential etiology. *Epilepsia, 7*, 330–338.

Lansdell, H., & Mirsky, A. F. (1964). Attention in focal and centrencephalic epilepsy. *Experimental Neurology, 9*, 463–469.

Lavadas, E., Umilta, C., & Provinciali, L. (1979). Hemisphere dependent cognitive performance in epileptic patients. *Epilepsia, 20*, 493–502.

Lennox, W. G. (1942). Brain injury, drugs and environment as causes of mental decay in epileptics. *American Journal of Psychiatry, 99*, 174–180.

Lennox, W. G., & Lennox, M. A. (1960). *Epilepsy and related disorders*. Boston: Little, Brown.

Loiseau, P., Strube, E., Brouslet, D., Battellochi, S., Gomeni, C., & Morselli, P. L. (1980). Evaluation of memory function in a population of epileptic patients and matched controls. *Acta Neurologica Scandanavica, 62* (Supplement 80), 58–61.

Loiseau, P., Signoret, J. L., & Strube, E. (1984). Attention problems in adult epileptic patients. *Acta Neurologica Scandanavica (Supplement 99), 69*, 31–34.

Long, C. G., & Moore, J. R. (1979). Parental expectations for their epileptic children. *Journal of Child Psychology and Psychiatry, 20*, 313–324.

MacLeod, C. M., Dekaban, A., & Hunt, E. (1978). Memory impairment in epileptic patients: Selective effects of phenobarbital concentration. *Science, 202*, 1102–1104.

Masui, K., Niwa, S., Anzai, N., Kameyama, T., Saitoh, O., & Rymar, K. (1984). Verbal memory disturbances in left temporal lobe epileptics. *Cortex, 20*, 361–368.

Matthews, C. G., & Klove, H. (1967). Differential psychological performances in major motor, psychomotor and mixed seizure classification of known and unknown etiology. *Epilepsia, 8*, 117–128.

Mayeux, R., Brandt, J., Rosen, J., & Benson, F. (1980). Interictal memory and language impairment in temporal lobe epilepsy. *Neurology, 30*, 120–125.

McGowan, M. E. L., Neville, B. G. R., & Reynolds, E. H. (1983). Comparative monotherapy trial in children with epilepsy. *British Journal of Clinical Practice, Symposium Supplement, 27*, 115–118.

McGuckin, H. M. (1980). Changing the world view of those with epilepsy. In R. Canger, F. Angeleri, & J. K. Penry (Eds.), *Advances in epileptology: XIth epilepsy international symposium, 1980* (pp. 205–208). New York: Raven Press.

Milner, B. (1975). Hemispheric specialization: Scope and limits. In B. Milner (Ed.), *Hemispheric specialization and interaction* (pp. 75–89). Cambridge, MA: MIT Press.

Mirsky, A. F., & Van Buren, J. M. (1965). On the nature of the "absence" in centrencephalic epilepsy: A study of some behavioral, electroencephalographic and autonomic factors. *Electroencephalography and Clinical Neurophysiology, 18*, 334–348.

Mirsky, A. F., Primac, D. W., Marson, C. A., Roswold, H. E., & Stevens, J. R. (1960). A comparison of the psychological test performance of patients with focal and non-focal epilepsy. *Experimental Neurology, 2*, 75–89.

Morgan, A., & Groh, C. (1980). Changes in visual perception in children with epilepsy. In B. Kulig, H. Meinardi, & G. Stores (Eds.). *Epilepsy and behavior '79*. Lisse: Swets & Zeitlinger.

Novelly, R., Augustine, E. A., Mattson, R. H., Glaser, G. H., Williamson, P. D., Spencer, D. D., & Spencer, S. S. (1984). Selective memory improvement and impairment in temporal lobectomy for epilepsy. *Annals of Neurology, 15*, 64–67.

O'Leary, D. S., Lovell, M. R., Sackellares, J. C., Berent, S., Giordani, B., Seidenberg, M., & Boll, T. J. (1983). Effects of age of onset of partial and generalized seizures on neuropsychological performance in children. *Journal of Nervous and Mental Disease, 171*(10), 624–629.

Quadfasel, A. F., & Pruyser, P. W. (1955). Cognitive deficits in patients with psychomotor epilepsy. *Epilepsia, 4*, 80–90.

Reitan, R. M. (1974). Psychological testing of epileptic patients. In P. J. Vinken & G. W. Bruyn (Eds.), *A handbook of clinical neurology, Volume 15: The epilepsies* (pp. 559–575). Amsterdam: Elsevier/North-Holland.

Reitan, R. M., & Wolfson, D. (1985). *The Halstead–Reitan Neuropsychological Test Battery: Theory and clinical interpretation*. Tucson, AZ: Neuropsychology Press.

Reynolds, E. H. (1985). Antiepileptic drugs and psychopathology. In M. R. Trimble (Ed.), *The psychopharmacology of epilepsy* (pp. 49–63). New York: John Wiley & Sons.

Reynolds, E. H., & Travers, R. D. (1974). Serum anticonvulsant concentrations in epileptic patients with mental symptoms. *British Journal of Psychiatry, 124*, 440–445.

Reynolds, E. H., & Trimble, M. R. (1985). Adverse neuropsychiatric effects of anticonvulsant drugs. *Drugs, 29*, 570–581.

Rodin, E. (1984). Epileptic and pseudoepileptic seizures: Differential diagnostic considerations. In D. Blumer (Ed.), *Psychiatric aspects of epilepsy* (pp. 179–195). Washington, DC: American Psychiatric Press.

Rutter, M., Graham, P., & Yule, W. (1970). A neuropsychiatric study in childhood. Philadelphia: Lippencott.

Schain, R. J., Ward, J. W., & Guthrie, D. (1977). Carbamazepine as an anticonvulsant in children. *Neurology, 27*, 476–480.

Schwartz, M. L., & Dennerll, R. D. (1970). Neuropsychological assessment of children with and without questionable epileptogenic dysfunction. *Perceptual and Motor Skills, 30*, 111–121.

Scott, D., Moffett, A., Matthews, A., & Ettlinger, G. (1976). Effects of epileptic discharges on learning and memory in patients. *Epilepsia, 8*, 188–194.

Shorvon, S. D., & Reynolds, E. H. (1979). Reduction of polypharmacy for epilepsy. *British Medical Journal, 2*, 1023–1025.

Stores, G. (1973). Studies of attention and seizure disorders. *Developmental Medicine and Child Neurology, 15*, 376–382.

Stores, G. (1981). Problems of learning and behavior in children with epilepsy. In E. H. Reynolds & M. R. Trimble (Eds.), *Epilepsy and psychiatry* (pp. 33–48). Edinburgh: Churchill Lingstone.

Tarter, R. E. (1972). Intellectual and adaptive functioning in epilepsy: A review of 50 years of research. *Diseases of the Nervous System, 33*, 763–770.

Thompson, P. J., & Trimble, M. R. (1982). Anticonvulsant drugs and cognitive functions. *Epilepsia, 23*, 531–544.

Thompson, P. J., & Trimble, M. R. (1983). The effect of anticonvulsant drugs on cognitive function: Relation to serum levels. *Journal of Neurology, Neurosurgery and Psychiatry, 46*, 227–233.

Tizard, J., Rutter, M., & Whitmore, K. (1969). *Education, health and behavior.* London: Longmans.

Trimble, M. (1981). Anticonvulsant drugs, behavior and cognitive abilities. *Current Developments in Psychopharmacology, 6*, 65–91.

Trimble, M. R., & Corbett, J. A. (1980). Behavioral and cognitive disturbances in epileptic children. *Irish Medical Journal, 73*(Supplement), 21–28.

Trimble, M. R., & Reynolds, E. H. (1976). Anticonvulsant drugs and mental symptoms. *Psychological Medicine, 6*, 169–178.

Trimble, M. R., & Thompson, P. J. (1984). Sodium valproate and cognitive function. *Epilepsia, 25*(Supplement 1), 560–564.

Turner, W. A. (1907). *Epilepsy.* London: Macmillan.

Tymchuk, A. J. (1974). Comparison of Bander error and time scores for groups of epileptic, retarded and behavior-problem children. *Perceptual and Motor Skills, 38*, 71–74.

Walker, A. E., & Blumer, D. (1984). Behavioral effects of temporal lobectomy for temporal lobe epilepsy. In D. Blumer (Ed.), *Psychiatric aspects of epilepsy* (pp. 295–323). Washington, DC: American Psychiatric Press.

Wilkus, R. J., & Dodrill, C. B. (1976). Neuropsychological correlates of the EEG in epileptics. I. Topographic distribution and average rate of epileptiform activity. *Epilepsia, 17*, 89–100.

Wilson, A., Petty, R., Perry, A., & Rose, R. C. (1983). Paroxysmal language disturbance in an epileptic treated with clobazan. *Neurology, 33*, 652–654.

Wolf, S. M., & Forsythe, A. (1978). Behavior disturbance, phenobarbital and febrile seizures. *Pediatrics, 61*, 728–731.

Zimmerman, F. T., Burgemeister, B. B., & Putnam, T. J. (1951). Intellectual and emotional makeup of the epileptic. *Archives of Neurology and Psychiatry, 65*, 545–556.

6

Behavioral Alterations in Temporolimbic Epilepsy

PAUL A. SPIERS, DONALD L. SCHOMER, HOWARD W. BLUME, and GAIL S. HOCHANADEL

The study of temporal lobe epilepsy and its relationship to particular psychological phenomena or disorders provides a unique opportunity to investigate the neural and physiological substrates underlying the control of behavior. Historically, epilepsy has been encumbered by myth and superstition. Epilepsy was variously called the "sacred disease" or thought to be evidence of demonic possession because the manifestations of a seizure appeared to onlookers as though the person afflicted had been invaded by some supernatural being. Scientific inquiry and the rise of the medical profession slowly stripped away these misconceptions, however, and what were previously thought to be divine phenomena became the subject of scientific analysis and theoretical speculation. For example, scholars have debated whether the politics of Alexander, the chronicles of Caesar, the faith and epistles of St. Paul, or the writings of Dostoevsky reflect personality alterations resulting from their epilepsy (Geschwind, 1984; Landsborough, 1987). Similarly, it is of interest to speculate whether certain works of art or literature, such as those of Vincent Van Gogh or Lewis Carroll, represent experiences felt during a temporal lobe convulsive state. The association of personality and behavioral disorders with temporal lobe epilepsy has continued to intrigue investigators. This is no longer a matter of speculation and is supported by clinical, experimental, and neuroanatomical evidence.

PAUL A. SPIERS • Clinical Research Center, Massachusetts Institute of Technology, Cambridge, Massachusetts 02142.   DONALD L. SCHOMER • Department of Neurology, Beth Israel Hospital, Boston, Massachusetts 02215.   HOWARD W. BLUME • Department of Surgery, Beth Israel Hospital, Boston, Massachusetts 02215.   GAIL S. HOCHANADEL • Department of Neurology, Lahey Clinic Medical Center, Burlington, Massachusetts 01805.

The Neuropsychology of Epilepsy, edited by Thomas L. Bennett. Plenum Press, New York, 1992.

A consideration of the neuroanatomy and interconnections of the temporal lobe confirms that this region plays a central role within the neural network mediating the control of behavior and emotion. Not only does the temporal lobe encompass neo-cortical areas where complex sensory associations are formed, but it also includes structures such as the amygdala and hippocampus that are pivotal components on the limbic system and have direct access to the hormonal, visceral, and motivational mechanisms of the hypothalamus. The temporal lobe also has widespread reciprocal connections with regions in the frontal, parietal, and occipital lobes as well as with orbitofrontal structures, septal nuclei, the cingulate gyrus, and the basal ganglia (Mesulam, 1985). Because our terminology of necessity reflects the sophistication of our concepts, we have chosen to use the term "temporolimbic" to characterize this network or when referring to partial or complex partial seizures originating in this region (Spiers, Schomer, Blume, & Mesulam, 1987).

In this chapter, the various alterations in behavior that occur in temporolimbic epilepsy are reviewed with special reference to illustrative case examples. This review is divided into two major categories: ictal and interictal behavioral alterations. Although such a gross classification may be artificial and difficult to define, it nonetheless provides a convenient heuristic around which to organize our analysis. We classify behavioral alterations as "ictal" when they (1) have a paroxysmal onset, (2) have a recurrent and, eventually, predictable course, (3) usually resolve gradually, and (4) can ultimately be correlated with appropriate EEG phenomena. Interictal alterations are those changes in behavior that do not share these characteristics but that nonetheless appear to be related to the onset of a seizure disorder and may affect the individual in a variety of contexts. For each type of behavioral alteration, some attempt is made not only to consider the phenomena descriptively but also to discuss the possible mechanisms responsible for the changes observed.

THE IMPORTANCE OF CONNECTIONS

The extensive reciprocal connections that exist between the temporal lobe and the other components of the temporolimbic network frequently make it difficult, if not impossible, to differentiate the manifestations of a seizure that originates in parietal cortex and subsequently incorporates the amygdala or other more anterior, mesial structures from those of a seizure that begins in the hippocampus and then spreads either to overlying temporal cortex or to other synaptically connected regions. These powerful interconnections also bring into question the potentially misleading tendency to consider that patients whose seizure focus has been demonstrated by scalp-surface electrographic recordings to be in some nontemporal area represent a seperate and distinct population from patients with temporal lobe foci. There are two immediately apparent reasons for rejecting such classifications. First, our ability to track the evolution and origin of a seizure discharge on surface electroencephalo-grams (EEG) is extremely limited. Second, no significant electrical event, at least of sufficient magnitude to produce a partial seizure, can occur in isolation in any of the association cortices. The majority of these regions project to primary limbic structures, which, in turn, have direct pathways linking them to the rest of the temporolimbic network. This does not imply that every cortical seizure produces a temporolimbic seizure. Many events remain restricted to a single population of neurons. It is known, however, that when a seizure occurs some discharges may spread (Crowell, 1970). They may be projected forward to neuronal populations in the network to which the seizure focus is connected (orthodromic connections) and, on occasion, may even spread backward to neurons that project to the seizure focus (antidromic connections) (Schwartzkroin, Mutani, & Prince, 1975). The point is that, like 'higher cortical' or cognitive functions, seizures defy simple localization.

The significant interconnections of the temporolimbic network also have important implications for the classification of specific behavioral events such as seizures. Large portions of the temporal lobe are buried within the sylvian fissure. The orbitofrontal and inferotemporal regions are shielded by the base of the skull, and mesial temporal lobe structures are far distant from the scalp. It is not surprising, therefore, that Gloor and colleagues (Gloor, Olivier, Quesney, Andermann, & Horowitz, 1982) at the Montreal Neurological Institute found that nearly half of all the seizures they recorded in a large group of patients who were monitored with depth electrodes had no electrical manifestation at the cortical surface inside the skull. Consequently, the absence of a positive scalp-surface EEG cannot be taken to rule out a seizure disorder. This is true not only when the patient displays stereotyped automatisms but also when atypical behaviors are prominent in the clinical presentation.

A striking example of such a presentation was provided by a 20-year-old male patient who at the age of 12 had begun to experience motor compulsions and obsessions. Most prominent among these was an irresistible urge to gently tap either his own face or objects in the environment repeatedly in an incremental sequence. As a result, he was always touching things with his first two fingers, with a pencil, or by flicking his cigarette in a one–two–three tap sequence. The patient had also displayed more typical obsessions such as requiring an invariant environment or needing additional time to get dressed so that he could examine himself and his clothing in the mirror from every possible angle, this was ". . . to make sure everything looked just right." The patient reported that he was tormented by the motor compulsions in particular, and by the age of 14 he had taken to consuming an average of 6 to 10 beers per day in order to suppress these behaviors. He described them as incessant: "From the time I wake up to the time I go to sleep, it's like someone is in there telling me to do these things!" At the age of 15, he started to use street drugs for symptom control, and within a few months he had to be detoxified from polysubstance abuse. He was subsequently committed to a major psychiatric teaching hospital, where he remained for 4 years. His symptoms were refractory to psychotherapy and behavior therapy interventions as well as to a wide range of antidepressant and antipsychotic medications.

At age 20, this patient was presented to Dr. Norman Geschwind, who referred him for neuropsychological and neurophysiological investigation. Subsequent history obtained from the family indicated that shortly after birth the patient had experienced a transient right hemiparesis, which resolved over 48 h, and blood had been found in the CSF on spinal tap. The patient was the only left-handed child in a multigenerational family of right-handers, had severe reading problems in school, and carried the diagnosis of dyslexia. A CT scan was then obtained and revealed a large parenchymal cyst at the left temporoparietal junction encompassing the angular and supramarginal gyri and the posterior aspect of the superior temporal gyrus. Conventional EEG was unrevealing, but EEG telemetry with sphenoidal electrodes showed almost constant bursts of paroxysmal activity from the left anterior temporal region. Neuropsychological investigation was consistent with an acquired left hemisphere injury with some displacement of function and compensation by the right hemisphere. The patient was placed on anticonvulsants but remained refractory to all major categories and combinations of medications. Telemetry confirmed that the frequency of the patient's motor compulsions appeared linked to increased left temporal discharges, and a surgical approach was considered. Amobarbitol investigation revealed right hemisphere memory control and mixed language dominance with the expressive, motor components of speech interrupted by left hemisphere suppression and comprehension disrupted during right hemisphere injection. Repetition was disturbed during both tests. A surgical approach was subsequently undertaken. Corticography revealed active discharges in the left anterior temporal region, more posteriorly in the vicinity of the parenchymal cyst, as well as from the intraoperative depth electrodes. Stimulation of the left amygdala and anterior hippocampus during surgery elicited several instances of the patient's motor compulsions, with the patient touching his own face and the operating table in the characteristic sequence. Six months after his temporal lobectomy, the patient reported that he was free of compulsions and obsessions; his EEG had shown considerable improvement, and he was discharged from inpatient psychiatric care.

THE BASIS OF BEHAVIORAL ALTERATIONS

Under normal conditions, the affective tone imparted to certain events, stimuli, and even thoughts is related to the individual's past history, present priorities, experience of the environment, current emotional state, and neurogenetic capabilities. In patients with temporolimbic epilepsy, however, this scenario can be disrupted in a number of ways that may produce an incongruent assignment of affect to experience, resulting in both transient and persistent alterations in the patient's behavior. Although it is not always possible to determine the specific mechanisms leading to stereotypic or other behavior alterations in a particular patient with temporolimbic epilepsy, there is considerable evidence to suggest that a variety of physiological and structural changes may be occurring at any time in response to the presence of a discharging seizure focus (Ben-Ari & Krnjevic, 1981; Ben-Ari, Krnjevic, & Reinhard, 1979; Krnjevic, 1983; Delgado-Escueta, 1988; Scwartzkroin, 1983; Goddard, 1983; Morrell, 1988).

Ictal events, for example, may produce sudden, intense alterations in affect that may result in the assignment of an inappropriate emotion to an otherwise neutral experience. Transient epileptiform discharges may prevent the correct association of appropriate affect in certain interpersonal or social situations. Synaptic or membrane alterations and imbalance of the physiological milieu may lead to sensitization of portions of the temporolimbic network resulting in a generalized increase in the intensity of affective tone (Bear, 1979; Jasper & Van Gelder, 1983; Morselli, Lloyd, Loscher, Meldrum, & Reynolds, 1981). Selective neuronal depopulation, a phenomenon observed in animals with discharging seizure foci, may interfere with both emotion and cognition (Schwartzkroin, 1983; Wang & Traub, 1988). These effects are likely to be present not only in the region of maximum epileptogenesis but also at ipsilateral and contralateral sites that are orthodromically and antidromically connected to the seizure focus (Schwartzkroin et al., 1975). Recent research on regional cerebral blood flow (rCBF) in patients with temporal lobe epilepsy, for example, has demonstrated interictal hypoperfusion not only at the site of maximum epileptogenesis but also at distant contralateral and ipsilateral sites (Valmier, Touchon, Daures, Zanca, & Baldy-Moulinier, 1987).

Patients with temporolimbic epilepsy may also have underlying structural lesions that can alter their ability to process certain types of information and influence the consistency with which appropriate or sufficient affective tone will be impaired to certain stimuli or classes of events. These lesions have been well described in the surgical literature and usually take the form of hamartomas, small tumors, and zones of necrosis or sclerosis (Falconer, 1971; Penfield & Jasper, 1954; Purpura, Penry, & Walter, 1975; Rasmussen, 1979). It also seems likely that some patients with temporolimbic epilepsy may have cell migration deficits or neuronal dysplagias of the type described in patients with specific learning disabilities (Galaburda & Kemper, 1970; Galaburda, Sherman, Rosen, Aboitiz, & Geschwind, 1985). Certainly, regions of neuronal loss have been well described, though it is unknown whether this is cause or consequence in relation to the epilepsy (Darn, 1980; Ounsted & Lindsay, 1966; Sagar & Oxbury, 1987). Nevertheless, these structural alterations are presumably related to the source of the epileptogenesis and also may provide the basis for the cognitive deficits, most commonly memory disorders, observed in these patients. These, in turn, affect the manner in which the patients process their environment and may impact significantly on their psychosocial development.

In addition to the seizure disorder itself, patients may experience alterations in their behavior as a result of pharmacological treatment (Delgado-Escueta, Treiman, & Walsh, 1983a,b; Woodbury, Penry, & Peppenger, 1982). These range from such simple, predictable side effects as drowsiness, decreased attention, or interference in learning to potentially less obvious and less likely to be reported changes such as impotence or violent feelings. Finally, patients may experience the effects of various psychological reactions and social–interpersonal variables related to the diagnosis of a seizure disorder. The incidence of depression in particular seems to be elevated in this population and may be accompanied by an important risk of suicide (Barraclough, 1987; Mendez, Cummings, & Benson, 1986). These emotional variables will obviously play a role both in the patient's response to seizures and in determining his or her overall level of adaptation. The relative contributions of each of these sets of variables: physiological, structural, treatment, and psychological, often make it difficult to identify the primary source of a behavioral alteration in a specific patient with temporolimbic epilepsy.

In this chapter, we focus first on what might seem to be the most clear-cut of these categories: those behavioral alterations directly associated with a seizure discharge. It should become apparent, however, that even this source of behavior alteration is mired in significant controversy. Secondly, we examine those changes in behavior and personality that may be more directly attributable to the long-term physiological and structural effects of those seizure discharges. Social, psychological, and treatment variables are addressed in detail elsewhere in this volume, but the reader is reminded that they too influence the patient's behavior, even in the most dramatic cases of seizure-induced behavioral alteration.

ICTAL ALTERATIONS

Ictal events provide the first and most apparent level at which behavior may be altered by temporolimbic epilepsy. Under these circumstances, a sustained pattern of paroxysmal discharges disrupts the normal activity of those structures in which the seizure focus is located and may activate a variety of temporolimbic structures in an unpredictable manner, producing alterations in mood, sensation, perception, or motor behavior and what, to observers, may appear to be abnormal responses to their consensually shared environment. Often the patient's symptoms may mimic the manifestations of psychiatric disorders.

The symptoms produced by ictal discharges often become stereotyped and characteristic in an individual patient. This is probably best understood from a "cell assembly" (Hebb, 1966) perspective, which would argue that the initial facilitation of certain pathways during the ictal discharge results in a preparedness to respond in this same circuit to future occurrences. We now know that this is probably accomplished by the establishment of new synaptic connections that, on repeated stimulation, become relatively fixed. The tendency of untreated or uncontrolled seizures to evolve and become more elaborate probably represents the progressive spread of these discharges into other cell assemblies that overlap the primary or initially stimulated circuit. This has been well illustrated in kindling experiments, where repeated subthreshold stimulation eventually leads to a partial and, if continued, generalized seizure (Goddard, 1983).

In this context, it also seems likely that environmental events that stimulate these same cell assemblies may alter the potential for a seizure discharge either in an excitatory or inhibitory manner. Clinically, it has been our observation, and many patients report, that seizures can be triggered by stressful situations or stimulating activities (e.g., orgasm: Berthier, Starkstein, & Leiguarda, 1987), specific environmental stimuli (e.g., reflex epilepsy: Forster, 1977), particular cognitive activities such as reading (Geschwind & Sherwin, 1967; Newman & Longley, 1984; Ramani, 1983) or mental arithmetic (Wilkins, Zifkin, Andermann, & McGovern, 1982), and even such activities as watching television (Binnie, Darby, & Hindley, 1973), eating (Reder & Wright, 1982), blinking (Terzano, Parrino, Manzoni, & Mancia, 1983), or playing video games (Glista, Frank, & Tracy, 1983). Similarly, patients can often learn strategies for inhibiting or modifying their experience of a seizure, suggesting the possibility of access into certain of the cell assemblies activated by the seizure discharge (Efron, 1956, 1957; Mostofsky & Balashack, 1977). The observation that patients with intractable epilepsy will often stop having seizures on hospital admission for telemetry supports the notion of an interactive neural network that can be influenced by external, environmental stimuli, even in the presence of a frequently discharging seizure focus.

Types of Ictal Events

Certain easily recognized characteristics are widely assumed to be the hallmark manifestations of a temporolimbic ictal event. Typically, these are supposed to involve a dazed or fixated look followed by some interruption or loss of consciousness. This is accompanied by some type of motor automatism, usually lip smacking, a lack of responsiveness to questions, and a tendency to be combative if the patient is touched or restrained. Although this is a representative account of certain complex partial seizures, it unfortunately does not describe the majority of simple partial seizures, which may be extremely elaborate in their manifestations without sharing any of these "telltale" characteristics.

A catalogue of temporolimbic seizure phenomena must, by definition, include a broad spectrum of symptoms and behavioral alterations (Geschwind, 1983; Gloor & Feindel, 1963; Penfield & Jasper, 1954; Spiers et al., 1985; Taylor & Lochery, 1987), and a number of these are listed in Table 6.1. Focal somatic pain, headache, or extremity discomfort, as well as various peripheral sensory changes such as tingling or numbness unaccompanied by any other alteration in behavior, perception, or consciousness may be the sole manifestation of a simple partial seizure (Laplante, St. Hilaire, & Bouvier, 1983; Lesser, Lueders, Conomy, Furlan, & Dinner, 1983; Penfield & Jasper, 1954; Young & Blume, 1983). This may take a very specific form such as pain restricted to a solitary limb, for example, the left thigh (Trevathian & Cascino, 1988), typically in association with a contralateral posterior seizure focus, or may even include such unusual symptoms as scrotal pain accompanied by testicular jerking (Bhaskar, 1987) or unilateral piloerection (Green, 1984). Transient motor paresis, twitching, jerking, posturing, speech arrest, and stuttering are possible motor outcomes of a sustained abnormal electrical discharge (Baratz & Mesulam, 1981; Gilmore & Heilman, 1981; Hamilton & Matthews, 1979; Peled, Harnes, Borovich, & Sharf, 1984; Reilly & Massey, 1980). Aphasia, including neologistic jargon, and even forced singing may occur (Rosenbaum, Siegel, Barr, & Rowan, 1986; Vidailhet, Serdaru, & Agid, 1989; Wilson, Petty, Perry, & Rose, 1983) and may, if accompanied by mood alteration, be misdiagnosed as hysterical or psychiatric

TABLE 6.1. Ictal Manifestations, Often Presenting as Simple Partial Seizures,
Reported by Patients with Temporolimbic Epilepsy and Correlated with Positive EEG

Motor	Sensory	Autonomic
Automatisms	Headache	Flushing
Staring	Focal pain	Apnea
Rapid eye movements	Discomfort	Shortness of breath
Twitching/jerking	Malaise	Dizziness
Head turning	Clumsyness	Vertigo
Grimacing	Paresthesia	Sinus tachycardia
Waxy flexibility	Numbness	Arrhythmia
Paresis	Bugs on skin	Nausea
Stuttering		Abdominal pain
Slurred speech		Vomiting
Jargon aphasia		Piloerection
Speech arrest		
Hallucinatory	Experiential	Emotional/behavioral
Visual	Memory flashbacks	Embarassment
Metamorphosia	Deja vu/vecu	Sadness/depression
Macropsia/micropsia	Jamais vu/vecu	Crying
Auditory	Feeling a presence	Explosive laughter
Gustatory	Feeling possessed	Fear/timor mortis
Olfactory	Feeling dead	Serenity
	Mind–body dissociation	Irritability/anger
	Impending doom	Orgasm/exhibitionism
		Compulsions/obsessions
		Self-mutilation
		Hypomania/confusion

in origin (Plesner, Munk-Andersen, & Luhdorf, 1987). Sudden changes in facial
expression suggesting bewilderment or fear, hand clapping, hugging oneself, kicking
out, drinking water, grunting, and even shouting obscenities have been reported as
well (Remillard, Andermann, & Gloor, 1981; Strauss, Wada, & Kosaka, 1983;
Waterman, Purves, Kosaka, Strauss, & Wada, 1987). Autonomic symptoms such as
flushing, dizziness, and cardiac arrhythmia, sometimes occurring in combination
and mimicking a cardiac disorder or panic attack, have been reported (Devinsky,
Price, & Cohen, 1986; Drake, 1983; Edlund, Swann, & Clothier, 1987; Gilchrist,
1985; Marshall, Westmoreland, & Sharbrough, 1983; Van Buren, 1961; Van Buren &
Ajmone-Marsan, 1960; Wall, Tuchman, & Mielke, 1985; Weilburg, Bear, & Sachs,
1987). These cardiac manifestations of epilepsy may even be life threatening in some
instances (Hirsch & Martin, 1971; Jay & Leetsma, 1981; Keilson, Hauser, Magrill,
& Goldman, 1987; Terrence, Wisotzkey, & Perper, 1975).

   Those ictal events most likely to resemble psychiatric symptoms include visual,
auditory, gustatory, and olfactory hallucinations and illusions (Gloor & Feindel, 1963;
Gloor *et al.*, 1982; Weiser, 1983). Common experiential phenomena include memory
flashbacks, mind–body dissociation, illusions of familiarity or unfamiliarity (*deja*
or *jamais vu*), the illusion of possession, and the feeling of a presence, that is, of

someone nearby or watching (Commission on Classification, 1981; Gloor & Feindel, 1963; Gloor *et al.*, 1982; Mesulam, 1981; Stein & Murray, 1984). Patients may have forced thinking such as obsessions that result in compulsive motor behavior, or forced emotions including embarrassment, sadness, guilt, or fear, often accompanied by epigastric distress (Devinsky, Hafler, & Victor, 1982; Mitchell, Greenwood, & Mersenheimer, 1983; Peppercorn, Herzog, & Dichter, 1978; Robertson & Trimble, 1983; Strauss, Risser, & Jones, 1982; Weiser, 1983; Young & Blume, 1983). Patients who experience combinations of these symptoms may easily be misdiagnosed as suffering from a psychiatric disorder, particularly if there are misleading traumatic life events in their history (Bennett & Curiel, 1988). Sexual ictal manifestations may occur in temporolimbic epilepsy, including but not limited to vaginal sensations, penile erection, spontaneous orgasm, and compulsive masturbation (Jacome & Risko, 1983; Currier, Little, & Suess, 1971; Remillard, Andermann, Tosta, Gloor, Aube, Martin, Feindel, Guberman, & Simpson, 1983). One of our patients, reported elsewhere (Stein & Murray, 1984), suffered from postictal promiscuity, indiscriminately seeking out sexual partners on the street after, or potentially during, her seizure. Seizure-induced Klüver–Bucy syndrome with prominent oral tendencies and hypersexuality has also been reported (Nakada, Lee, Kwee, & Lerner, 1984). We have also observed patients who experienced dissociative personality changes, who were catatonic or unresponsive, who engaged in self-mutilation, or who were confused, hypomanic, and displayed ritualistic or grossly psychotic behaviors. Similar patients have been described by others (Adebimpe, 1977; Drake & Coffey, 1983; Mesulam, 1981; Stein & Murray, 1984), and such patients are often experiencing some form of nonmotor-convulsive status epilepticus (Iivanainen, Bergstrom, Nuitila, & Viukari, 1984; Lim, Yagnik, Schraeder, & Wheeler, 1986). In other instances, psychosis (Logsdail & Toone, 1988) or mania (Rosenbaum & Barry, 1975) has been reported in the post- or interictal period, typically following the acute onset of seizures or after a period of increased seizure frequency.

All of the alterations listed here either have been correlated with ongoing electrographic abnormalities or have responded to anticonvulsant therapy in patients who had interictal EEGs characteristic of temporolimbic epilepsy. Whether the patient experiences only selected symptoms or some combination of these will obviously vary depending on the spread of the seizure within the temporolimbic network and the number of cell assemblies activated. The ictal nature of these symptoms often can only be determined on EEG by the use of sphenoidal electrodes, surgically implanted subdural strip electrodes, or intracerebral depth electrodes because the locus of the abnormality may not be detectable on conventional surface recordings. The sphenoidal electrode is particularly useful in the outpatient setting. It is placed under local anesthetic and passes through the mandibular notch, a natural opening in the jaw joint, toward the foramen ovale, giving more direct access to anterior temporal and inferior, posterior, lateral frontal structures. The electrode can be safely left in place for several days either for inpatient or outpatient monitoring and has frequently led to the demonstration of an ictal electrographic basis for behavioral events that had previously been diagnosed to be psychiatric in origin. In a recent study employing the anterior sphenoidal electrode, Ives (Ives, Schachter, Drislane,

Miles, & Schomer, 1990) showed a 25% improvement in positive EEG correlations between behavior changes and the recording of ictal discharges from patients who had previously had normal scalp telemetry studies during presumed clinical events.

When sophisticated EEG monitoring is not available, the clinician must draw on knowledge of the myriad manifestations of temporolimbic epilepsy and rely on clinical judgment. In some cases, the paroxysmal basis for sudden changes in behavior can be inferred from the patient's clinical presentation by observing the regularity and relatively stereotyped nature of their behavior disturbance. It is important to keep in mind, however, that these symptoms are often experienced in what may appear to be full consciousness and may be as brief as a few seconds in duration, persist for several minutes, or recur with increasing frequency over the course of several days. The relationship of symptoms to certain environments, times of day, activities (e.g., driving: (Allan & Stewart, 1971), and to the menstrual cycle (e.g., catamenial epilepsy: Laidlaw, 1956) may all provide evidence that an inappropriate or maladaptive behavior or emotion is epileptic in origin. The increased frequency of neuroendocrine disorders in male (Herzog, Seibel, Schomer, Vaitukaitis, & Geschwind, 1986b) and female (Herzog, Seibel, Schomer, Vaitukaitis, & Geschwind, 1986a) epileptic patients, and the history, common in our experience, that the onset of seizure symptoms is correlated with puberty, pregnancy, or some other major neuroendocrine event underlines the important interactive and potentially causal role of hormones in temporolimbic epilepsy (Backstrom, Zetterlund, Blom, & Romano, 1984; Herzog, 1989). These findings also may open significant new avenues for the hormonal treatment of seizure disorders (Herzog, 1988). Psychiatric diagnoses should be made cautiously and by inclusion, with good fulfillment of DSM-III-R criteria, and not selected by exclusion on the basis that certain symptoms are too peculiar to be neurological in origin or because a scalp EEG was unrevealing or negative. A careful interview that uncovers a history of birth trauma, learning disability, head injury, or substance abuse, appetite or sexual alterations in relation to the frequency of episodes, or of familial symptoms similar to the patient's, may raise the index of suspicion that certain behaviors are ictal in origin. In this context, a positive EEG is helpful in confirming the diagnosis of temporolimbic epilepsy, but the responsibility of arriving at a diagnosis ultimately rests with the clinician and cannot be abdicated to the electroencephalogram. Signal detection problems notwithstanding, one must question the logic that if the EEG study is negative, the patient is therefore normal. First, one should always be cautious about affirming a null hypothesis. Second, the patient may not have experienced any of the behavioral alterations associated with a discharge in his/her seizure focus during the time when the EEG was being recorded.

Ictal Events and Psychosis

Detailed descriptions of ictal manifestations that mimic symptoms of psychiatric disease date back to early reports of patients with temporolimbic epilepsy and are, in fact, especially prominent in the histories of those patients who were also labeled psychotic (Slater & Beard, 1963; Gibbs, 1951). It is of interest, therefore, that the psychoses of many of these patients were considered to be otherwise atypical. Unlike chronic schizophrenic or paranoid psychotic patients, they frequently had well-preserved affect. Between their episodic hallucinations or delusions, they had no sustained thought disorder and generally failed to show decompensation over time. In addition, these patients had little premorbid disruption of social, interpersonal, or family relationships of the type usually found in psychotic or schizophrenic histories. One explanation for these findings is that many of the symptoms suggestive of a psychiatric disorder in such patients may, in fact, be the manifestations of an ictal event (Flor-Henry, 1969, 1976; Kristensen & Sindrup, 1979; Perez & Trimble, 1980; Sherwin, 1981; Slater & Beard, 1963; Taylor, 1975). Although some patients with temporolimbic epilepsy may remain indistinguishable from psychotics (Kogeorgos, Fonagy, & Scott, 1982), more recent studies have shown that when specific inclusion criteria are scrutinized in psychotic or schizophrenic temporolimbic epilepsy patients, many of these do not meet the necessary conditions for psychiatric diagnosis (Toone, Garralda, & Ron, 1982).

An example of this type of behavioral alteration as result of temporolimbic seizures is provided by the case of a 56-year-old right-handed former lab technician who sustained a closed head injury and had been diagnosed as suffering from paranoid psychosis 3 years later when she first experienced the onset of persecutory visual and auditory hallucinations, recurrent depression, and self-mutilation. These symptoms did not respond to either pharmacological or psychological therapy. The patient had 15 psychiatric hospitalizations over the next 3 years and was admitted to our service for telemetry, now 6 years after the head injury, because her psychosis was atypical and refractory.

By interviewing the patient during her episodes, it was determined that she had only a few distinct hallucinations. The first consisted of a physical form she called "the bloody lady," which she described as the figure of a woman in long, flowing robes whose fingertips dripped blood and who repeatedly told the patient that she was a "bad person." At times the "bloody lady" was accompanied by small weasel-like animals that, the patient complained, were nipping at her fingertips. These symptoms were considered dynamically significant because the patient had been an accomplished amateur pianist who had given up teaching and performances as a result of her illness. The second hallucination was of six soldiers in German World War I uniforms advancing on her and firing their rifles. This had been interpreted to be a representation of physical abuse she had suffered at the hands of her husband, who was formerly in the military. On careful questioning, however, it was found that these hallucinations were restricted solely to the patient's left visual field. When the "bloody lady" was present, the patient often engaged in self-mutilation, scratching her upper torso, always on the left side. She appeared to have no pain sensation on the left and did not respond to visual threat from the left field during the hallucinations. As the episode progressed, she would suddenly become very agitated and fearful and had to be restrained to prevent self-injury or escape. These behaviors notwithstanding, she responded to questions, smiled in reaction to humor, and was able to learn and implement behavioral rehearsal (i.e., repeating "I'm all right. I am not a bad person, and nothing bad can happen to me.") as a means of modifying her response. These attempts at intervention never eliminated or altered the hallucinations, but they did succeed in reducing her combativeness and the frequency of self-injury during these episodes.

The hallucinations lasted from several minutes up to half an hour and occured as frequently as five times per day. The patient was amnestic for some specific episodes but remembered the hallucinations *per se* between occurrences. As an episode began, the patient would scream, and her face would become contorted. There were no automatisms or tonic–clonic components, but she would begin to struggle with her restraints and repeatedly mutter: "Oh no, oh no, it's her again, go away, go away, . . . it's the bloody lady, go away, don't hurt me, . . ." As the episode ended, her face and body would relax, and she would appear as if awakening from a dream, requiring a few moments to become reoriented. Immediately afterwards, she felt sad and frequently expressed a desire to kill herself to put an end to these events and the devastating impact they had on her life. Otherwise, she was appropriately concerned and troubled by her symptoms, family situation, and frequent psychiatric hospitalizations. Neuropsychological testing revealed a memory deficit for nonverbal material and some difficulty with complex constructional tasks. There was no evidence of a thought disorder, she related in a warm and personable manner, and her premorbid history included raising five children, regular employment, and active community involvement.

Telemetry using scalp and sphenoidal electrodes showed a clear correlation between the patient's visual hallucinations and the development of a right posterior temporal seizure discharge. The onset of self-mutilation, agitation, and fear were correlated with spread of the abnormal discharges to the more anterior and mesial portions of the temporal lobe. These behaviors, feelings, and hallucinations all ceased abruptly in conjunction with normalization of the EEG. This correlation of behavioral alteration and seizure discharge was later confirmed by intraoperative electrical stimulation of the cortex at the junction of the posterior temporal and parietal lobes, which elicited her hallucinations. Furthermore, intraoperative cortical and depth recording showed that the self-mutilation and fear occurred only after the seizure had spread forward in the temporal lobe and once a sustained discharge was monitored at the deepest contact point in the anterior hippocampal region. In other words, the emotional components of the event did not manifest themselves until the seizure had incorporated the more specific limbic regions of the temporolimbic network. Previous scarring of the pia and cortex in the posterior temporal and inferior parietal regions presumably from her head injury, was noted at surgery. The etiology of her seizure disorder, therefore, was most likely kindling at the site of a "silent" posttraumatic intracerebral hemorrhage. A similar explanation was offered in another case of delayed-onset "psychosis" after cerebral injury (Levine & Finkelstein, 1982). The "psychotic symptoms," which manifested themselves 3 years later in our patient, meanwhile, have not recurred since her right temporal lobectomy, even though she has continued to have less frequent and more conventional complex partial seizures.

This patient's symptoms provide a dramatic example of the possibilities that exist for the manifestations of temporolimbic epilepsy to mimic psychosis. Nevertheless, the clinical and electrographic evidence that these symptoms were the direct result of a seizure discharge was no less compelling than in patients with more conventional complex partial seizures. In fact, patients who experience continuous focal epileptiform activity during episodes of complex partial status probably will not display stereotyped, nonpurposeful automatisms. They may also vary considerably in their level of responsiveness. Patients may be only mildly confused, continue to respond to commands, and persist in carrying out goal-directed activities, or they may be completely unresponsive and disoriented. Episodes of complex partial status have been reported lasting up to 4 h and a number of patients have been described who became aphasic, severely confused, and displayed such primitive behavior as chanting, muttering, indecent exposure, and even fecal smearing (Adebimpe, 1977; Ballenger, King, & Gallagher, 1983; Drake & Coffey, 1983; Escueta, Buxley, & Stubbs, 1974; Nakada et al., 1984; Shalev & Amir, 1983; Somerville & Bruni, 1983; Stein & Murray, 1984). In addition, patients have been reported who presented with a postictal psychosis, presumeably related to the influence of excessive seizure activity on limbic and frontal structures (Logsdail & Toone, 1988). Similar to earlier observations, however, the psychosis in these patients was atypical, without first-rank symptoms, an appropriate premorbid history, or the usual evolution.

A separate but related issue is whether some patients who, in fact, do fit the diagnostic criteria for psychosis may not suffer from some temporolimbic seizures. In this regard, several studies have attempted to examine electrographic abnormalities in chronic schizophrenic patients. First, it has been demonstrated that between 20% and 30% of these patients have EEG abnormalities such as focal irregular θ and sharp wave activity or θ and δ wave slowing localized over one or both temporal lobes, and in one study more than half of the schizophrenics with abnormal EEGs had frank paroxysmal activity in their records (Abrams & Taylor, 1979; Goon, Robinson, & Levy, 1973; Lifshitz & Gradijan, 1974; Tarrier, Cooke, & Lader, 1978). Schizophrenics have been found to have abnormalities in visually evoked potentials, more over the left than the right hemisphere, and a number of studies have found a correlation between displays of abnormal behavior and certain nonspecific changes in the EEGs of schizophrenics (Roemer, Shagass, Straumanis, & Amaded, 1978). Recently, the EEGs from a carefully defined sample of schizophrenic and control subjects were used to investigate the frequency of occurrence of specific computer-derived, electrophysiological indices (Stevens & Livermore, 1982). These indices had previously been identified in the scalp or dural EEGs of animals that had both surface and implanted electrodes monitored simultaneously, and their occurence in the surface EEG had been shown to coincide with spike activity in subcortical regions recorded from the implanted depth electrodes. In the present study with schizophrenics, these indices were never observed in the records of control human subjects but occurred with significant frequency in sampled portions of the schizophrenics' scalp-surface EEGs. They were also twice as common during periods when the patients were displaying abnormal behaviors such as catatonia, auditory hallucinations, and visual checking.

Although these observations are merely suggestive of a relationship between undetected ictal events and certain manifestations of psychosis in selected schizophrenics, earlier research in which psychotic patients were implanted with depth electrodes confirm such a hypothesis (Monroe, 1982). For example, spike and slow-wave activity was recorded from the septal region during psychotic behaviors, and limbic dysrythmias have been correlated with episodic confusion, often including aggression. One patient who had been diagnosed as a chronic paranoid schizophrenic was monitored from depth electrode contacts during episodes when she was delusional, confused, disoriented, experiencing auditory and visual hallucinations, and, occasionally, while showing intense rage with aggressive and destructive acts. The simultaneous EEG recording showed repeated bursts of paroxysmal, high-amplitude, multiphasic spikes in the hippocampal and septal regions with occasional temporal cortex involvement. These abnormalities were not detected by corresponding scalp leads. Even more striking are those patients in whom a series of stimulations were delivered to the amygdala–hippocampal region in a manner analogous to kindling. These stimulations eventually resulted in the generation of extreme emotional behaviors, such as fear or rage, being directed toward the patients' immediate environment. These emotions occurred suddenly and apparently without any relation to the motive state of the patient just prior to the stimulation.

Although negative results have been reported in attempting to correlate psychotic or aggressive behaviors with EEG changes, and it is widely held that purposeful, directed aggression is not an ictal phenomenon (Delgado-Escueta, Mattson, King, Goldensohn, Spiegel, Madsen, Crandall, Dreyfuss, & Porter, 1981), positive cases may have been missed for a variety of reasons. The EEG findings may be lacking because of the restricted, focal nature of the discharges producing these behavioral alterations or because they are inaccessible to conventional electrodes as a result of localization in mesial temporolimbic structures (Ramani & Gumnit, 1982). These discharges may even be missed by implanted electrodes because they often record from relatively narrow electrical fields. In addition, patients who experience the most severe forms of this type of ictally produced behavioral alteration are probably underrepresented in the epilepsy literature. Telemetry studies capable of detecting changes in mesial temporolimbic or inferior frontal lobe structures are rarely obtained from patients who are frequently aggressive and are even less likely to be obtained during violent outbursts. Such patients are frequently excluded from study in facilities where sophisticated EEG monitoring technology is available by virtue of those same behaviors that are the manifestations of their seizure disorder and that make them difficult to manage clinically (Robb, 1975; Mark, 1982). Consequently, caution should be advised before concluding that certain behaviors are not epileptic in origin, even in those cases where the history may be compatible with a diagnosis of psychosis or antisocial behavior disorder. We have had the opportunity to observe and record a patient whose violence during seizures, which included tearing fixtures off the hospital walls and throwing them at staff members, could easily have been interpreted as purposeful and had led to his arrest in the past. Weiser (1983) reported a patient who attacked a nurse with a knife immediately following a recorded seizure. Cases have also been reported where rage attacks responded to anticonvulsant intervention (Maletzky, 1973; Pellegrini, Lippmann, Crump, & Manshadi, 1984), and aggressive behavior in certain patients has been dramatically reduced by excision of their epileptic focus (Falconer, 1973). The relationship between these behavioral alterations and temporolimbic epilepsy should, therefore, remain open to debate and discussion until more appropriate, relevant studies have been conducted (Mark & Swelt, 1974; Delgado-Escueta *et al.*, 1981; Mark, 1982; Stevens & Hermann, 1981).

Ictal Events and Behavior Disorders

A second important form of behavioral alteration directly related to ictal events can be discerned in patients who experience less dramatic experiential or emotional seizure phenomena but who nonetheless respond directly to the emotional states or sensory perceptions of their seizures rather than to their environment. In this situation, patients may appear appropriately responsive to the environment but project their forced ictal emotions onto external stimuli so that they react to situations or persons in a manner that is not appropriate. The patient's conduct at these times is frequently suggestive of some preserved ability to mediate the expression of the feelings generated by the seizure.

One such patient was a 23-year-old single right-handed athletic female college student who developed "panic attacks" after a series of closed head injuries and a brief period of drug abuse. The attacks were characterized by epigastric distress, tachycardia, left chest, arm, and throat pain, perspiration, and flushing that were typically more pronounced on the left side and a fear that something terrible was about to happen. She was generally oriented and conversational during these episodes but felt she had to run in order to escape whatever danger she felt must be present in the environment, even though she could not identify what this might be. These episodes often occurred without warning under otherwise neutral circumstances and without any apparent provocation. As a result, the patient had developed phobic avoidance to several locations where these symptoms had overwhelmed her, such as certain tennis courts or a particular street near her college. She had been in psychotherapy for 3 years and had also had a trial of behavior therapy for what was believed to be an anxiety disorder. She had once attempted suicide. This was during a time when she was having almost continuous autonomic symptoms, building gradually to attacks of intense fear that were then followed by an hour of feeling relatively asymptomatic but tired. As a result of these episodes she had been unable to complete a teaching internship and was forced to drop out of college. Her sleep was severely disturbed, with frequent nocturnal awakenings, usually in a symptomatic state, and she had begun to avoid sleep by taking a job as a bartender.

During admission for telemetry and observation, this patient frequently would leave her room and use emergency stairways to run away from staff and attempt to escape from the hospital. If interrupted, she could sometimes excercise sufficient control to return to her room, often promising to remain there. Within minutes, however, she would usually try again to escape after making sure that she would not be observed. If she was caught at this point, physical restraint was usually necessary, and she would become argumentative and mildly combative, pleading to be allowed to "go for a walk" or "go for cigarettes." Her initial reaction to the onset of these feelings varied considerably. In some instances she would speak freely of her symptoms and warn staff that she "felt like running." At other times, she was secretive, buried her head in her pillow, and waited for an opportune moment to escape. Regardless of the initial reaction, once the episode had terminated she would return voluntarily to her room. Often, she was still anxious, feeling that something on the ward must have frightened her if she had been trying to run out of the hospital.

Electroencephalographic telemetry with scalp and sphenoidal electrodes and eventually with subdural strip electrodes revealed runs of unsustained bitemporal independent paroxysmal activity with left predominance that increased in association with her behavioral and autonomic manifestations. Recent reports, as well as our own experience from intraoperative depth recording of such patients, suggest that this type of EEG finding probably reflects sustained, ongoing seizure activity in deeper temporolimbic structures. Unlike the patient described earlier, however, this young woman was able to learn adaptive strategies for responding to her autonomic seizures and forced emotions. She was able to use verbal self-instruction with positive coping phrases to reassure herself that the symptoms were transient and "not real feelings." She also learned, when her symptoms were intensifying, to signal that she felt unsafe either to nursing staff in whom she had confidence or to her family. Eventually, she was able to displace herself within the more limited environment of the neurology ward in response to her fear by utilizing the solarium or conference room as an escape area from her own room.

This case provides an example in which a recurrent epileptic event leads to a predictable alteration in behavior but the specific manifestations observed during a particular episode depend on interactions among the immediate environment, the patient's past experience in the surroundings, and the nature of her relationship with those present at the time the seizure occurs. In other words, the ictal behavioral alterations may vary. The core events of the seizure remain constant, autonomic changes and fear, but the patient attempts either to conceal, deny, or report her symptoms and reacts to them in different ways as a function of the context in which they occur. Obviously, such patients challenge the widespread view that seizures are relatively predictable, short-lived, stereotyped occurrences.

Many patients with more stereotypic complex partial seizures report that they experience sudden emotional or behavioral alterations, which they attribute to their epilepsy. Some of these episodes are distinctly abnormal and, with detailed history taking, can often be classified as simple partial seizures. Other emotional states, drives, or compulsions, however, may be more difficult to diagnose as the manifestation of an ictal disturbance, even if the patient has known epilepsy. Nevertheless, it seems likely that patients with temporolimbic epilepsy may experience limited discharges that are sufficient to activate a portion of some cell assembly but do not spread or generalize in such a manner that primary motor or sensory manifestations, interruption of awareness, or automatisms are produced. In some instances these may eventually be correlated with electrophysiological evidence of a seizure discharge, whereas in others such documentation may be impossible.

There is evidence that sudden behavioral or emotional alterations may also occur in patients suffering from other neuropsychiatric conditions (Silberman, Post, Nurnberger, Theodore, & Boulenger, 1985). This has been taken to challenge the formulation that such episodes are "epileptic" in origin. Conversely, however, it raises the question of whether many supposedly nonepileptic psychiatric patients may be experiencing partial seizures either as a correlative manifestation of some neuropathology underlying their behavior disturbance, as an outcome of altered neurotransmitter status, or as the causal factor in the evolution of their psychiatric condition. It will be important to define the parameters of this relationship more closely. Reports already exist concerning abnormal EEG results and temporolimbic seizure symptoms in patients with bipolar mood disorder (Lewis, Feldman, Greene, & Martinez-Mustardo, 1984), obsessive–compulsive disorder (Jenike & Brotman, 1984), and panic disorder (Weilburg et al., 1987). Irrespective of the mechanism, the patient who experiences such events will generally attempt to develop some reasonable explanation for these sudden changes, particularly when they are of an emotional nature. This may be especially difficult if the feelings generated are inappropriate to the patient's mood or activity at the time this alteration occurs. In addition, the unpredictability and intensity of these emotional changes may result in partially distorted perceptions of reality or produce random conditioning of inappropriate stimulus–response relationships. Ultimately, such episodes might lead to more permanent alterations in behavior patterns or in what might be classified as a personality change.

Certainly, it is widely accepted that a single traumatic emotional episode or catastrophic experience may permanently alter an individual's emotional character and future interpersonal transactions. Presumably, the neural representation of such an event involves the formation of new synaptic relationships between previously unrelated cell assemblies paired with a strong discharge arising from limbic structures. If the same process is duplicated by an internally generated episode, such as a partial seizure, why should we be reluctant to consider that such occurrences may significantly affect the individual's overall pattern of behavior. Consider, for example, a report concerned with the behavioral correlates of hippocampal kindling in rats (Mellanby, Strawbridge, Collingridge, George, Rands, Stroud, & Thompson, 1981). Depth electrodes placed in limbic structures were stimulated until the animals developed overt convulsive events and were then discontinued. In association with the onset of seizures, these animals developed alterations in their response to handling, to novel animals placed in their environment, and to the social hierarchy within their groups. Although overt convulsions ceased completely 2 weeks after stimulation was terminated, the behavioral alterations did not improve or disappear. Depth electrode recording from the hippocampus revealed persistent and nearly constant intermittent paroxysmal discharges restricted to this portion of the temporolimbic network. The regular occurrence of transient epileptiform discharges may, therefore, also be responsible for the more persistent, presumably interictal, behavior changes reported in the population of patients with temporolimbic epilepsy.

INTERICTAL ALTERATIONS

At present, the term "interictal" is a problematic one in the field of epilepsy. In cases of temporolimbic epilepsy, in particular, the distinction between ictal and interictal can become extremely blurred. If a patient with known epilepsy has paroxysmal discharges every 5 s in specific limbic structures or shows intermittent bursts of spike-and-wave activity during sleep, what then constitutes their "interictal" behavior? Conversely, consider the patient seen on our service who had a partial seizure consisting of the odor of skunk that sometimes lasted many minutes but did not prevent him for conducting an important business meeting. Later the same day, however, he was unable to perform sexually even though the overt seizure manifestation had disappeared. Was this patient's impotence psychological or interictal? This is an especially difficult question when, in fact, this particular behavioral alteration was reversed and the patient's seizures were brought under excellent control when monthly injections of testosterone were added to his medication regimen.

A different but equally troubling example is provided by an adolescent male surgical candidate on whom we had occasion to perform simultaneous scalp-surface and subdural strip electrode recording, that is, one EEG from electrodes inside the skull resting on the cortical surface and one EEG from corresponding electrodes on the scalp. One of the patient's primary complaints was of constant dysphoric feelings of variable intensity that had been refractory to psychiatric and antidepressant therapies, and he carried the diagnosis of depression. Interestingly, these symptoms had disappeared once, for nearly a week, after he had attempted suicide by phenobarbital overdose. During the simultaneous recording session, the patient was discovered to have constant, periodic bursts of small spike-and-wave, seizure activity from the right posterior temporal region. These electrographic events were observable only in the record from the subdural strip electrodes and were of insufficient amplitude to be detected by the scalp-surface electrodes through the attenuating effect of bone, skin, and muscle tissue. When the patient was administered a single dose of paraldehyde, a potent, short-acting liquid anticonvulsant, these bursts of seizure activity disappeared. The patient then volunteered that his dysphoric mood had lifted. His affect reverted as the paraldehyde dose wore off and the spike-and-wave activity returned. There was no alteration in the signal from the scalp-surface contacts, which had failed to show any abnormal discharges during the test.

The issues raised by such special cases notwithstanding, there are certain stereotyped "interictal" behavioral alterations that have been reported in this population of patients. Although these changes do not appear to be the direct result of a specific ictal discharge, they appear to affect the patient's behavior in a uniform manner across a broad set of circumstances.

The Interictal Behavior Syndrome

In a series of case reports, several of the interictal alterations purported to accompany temporolimbic epilepsy were hypothesized to occur together, forming a cluster that was labeled the interictal behavior syndrome (Waxman & Geschwind, 1975). This term was chosen not only to distinguish these alterations from the ictal or psychotic manifestations associated with temporolimbic epilepsy but also to empha- size that these alterations need not imply psychopathology. This syndrome was believed to be characterized by changes in sexual desire or interest, the appearance of religious, ethical, or moral preoccupations, and hypergraphia, this last being a tendency to voluminous, compulsive, overly detailed writing, frequently concerned with moral issues.

A subsequent report by Bear and Fedio (1977) broadly expanded the limits of the interictal behavior syndrome. First, all of the various clinical observations that had been made in the literature concerning nonpsychotic behavior changes in patients with temporolimbic epilepsy were summarized and sorted into 18 different categories or traits. Second, the authors developed a questionnaire to sample these traits by generating five items, self-statements that the patient endorses or denies, to assess each category of behavioral alteration. Independent ratings could be obtained on two forms of this behavior inventory, one from the patient and one from a spouse, parent, or significant other. The inventories were then administered to patients with "left and right temporal foci," to patients with neuromuscular disorders, and to a group of normal controls. The results indicated that the self-report inventory differentiated the epileptics from the neuromuscular patients and the normals on all 18 traits. When the inventories filled out by the raters were used, 14 of the traits continued to show significant differences between temporolimbic epilepsy and control subjects. Few of the traits, however, significantly differentiated right from left temporal lobe epilep- tics. A factor analysis of the same data yielded two components: the first, labeled *ideative*, consisted of rumination over ethical or philosophical issues, hypergraphia, and paranoia and was more common in left temporal lobe patients; the second, labeled *emotive*, consisted of mood-related behavior changes and was more common in the ratings obtained from right temporal lobe patients. In addition, patients with right hemisphere foci endorsed fewer items in comparison to their independent raters, whereas patients with left hemisphere foci endorsed more items than their raters. These differences in self-perception bias were attributed to the phenomena of denial or minimization frequently noted after right hemisphere injury and of catastrophic reaction reported in certain patients after left hemisphere insult. The findings of this study were considered to validate the concept of an interictal behavior syndrome, and it was concluded that the Behavior Inventory could reliably measure these traits and self-perception biases. Previous studies that had failed to detect these personality changes using conventional psychological tests could therefore be understood as deficient in terms of not sampling the appropriate behaviors or traits.

Since these original case reports and the Bear and Fedio study, the interictal behavior syndrome has been partially confirmed, directly refuted, and declared nonexistent and has developed into a central issue of debate in the field of epilepsy (Master, Toone, & Scott, 1984; Mungas, 1982; Rodin & Schmaltz, 1984; Rodin, Schmaltz, & Twitty, 1984). Attempts to replicate the discriminative power of the Behavior Inventory have met with only limited or mixed success. When more closely matched hospitalized psychiatric control groups have been used, only a few of the original 18 traits have emerged as specific to epilepsy, and only in comparison to certain patient populations (Bear, Levin, Blumer, Chatman, & Reider, 1982). When patients with other forms of seizure disorder have been used as controls, there have been even fewer significant group differences in Behavior Inventory performance (Brandt, Seidman, & Kohl, 1984; Hermann & Riel, 1981). Neverthless, a few traits on the Behavior Inventory consistently seem to be associated with temporolimbic epilepsy. Notably, these include circumstantiality, the tendency to be overly focused on detail in either writing or conversation, significant interest in religious or philosophical matters, humorlessness, and suspiciousness.

In addition to research using the Behavior Inventory, a separate line of investigation has focused exclusively on one feature of the interictal behavior syndrome, hypergraphia. Attempts have been made to measure this trait in a more naturalistic manner by having patients with temporolimbic epilepsy respond to open-ended questions regarding their general health or the history of their seizure disorder. In one such study (Sachdev & Waxman, 1981), where replies were requested by mail, twice as many patients with focal temporal lobe seizure foci responded as patients with nontemporal foci or primary generalized epilepsy. Furthermore, the mean number of words in the responses were 12 times greater for the temporal lobe group, though it is not known whether this result could have been skewed by only a few voluminous replies. Two subsequent studies, using similar control groups, failed to replicate group differences in hypergraphia (Hermann, Whitman, & Arntson, 1983; Hermann, Whitman, Wyler, Richey, & Dell, 1988). In both of these studies, however, the authors did report that the longest written productions were from patients with temporolimbic epilepsy and that they represented approximately 7% of the sample. Unfortunately, when subsequent analyses attempted to relate hypergraphia to other personality traits or to cognitive test results, the pooled group data were used, and there was no focus on what may have been the only important portion of the sample, the minority 7% who were truly hypergraphic. This procedure yielded an inconclusive result.

Methodological Problems

The failure to find clear differences between groups of patients with temporolimbic and other forms of epilepsy, either with regard to a specific behavior trait or on the Behavior Inventory, seems at this time to be more a function of methodological errors and theoretical differences than a statement on the validity of the interictal behavior syndrome. The Behavior Inventory, for example, was clearly an attempt to improve on previous test instruments such as the MMPI. It suffers, however, from numerous design shortcomings of its own and at present remains experimental in structure. For example, self-statements or items reflecting severe psychopathology are grouped under the same trait label as relatively benign and often positive self-attributions. Only five statements sample each trait, and they were neither drawn from statements generated by a population of patients with temporolimbic epilepsy nor determined empirically to differentiate this group from other populations before being organized into *a priori* categories by the investigators (Sorensen, Hansen, Andersen, Hogenhaven, Allerup, & Bolwig, 1989). The statistical methodology of the initial Behavior Inventory study has been questioned, and factors related to the self-report nature of the inventory have not yet been addressed. There is, for example, no internal control for patients answering in an image-enhancing manner, and all responses are scored in the affirmative to increase trait scores. This, obviously, could facilitate the development of an endorsement bias, either positive or negative.

Research concerning the interictal behavior syndrome has also been plagued by a lack of specificity with respect to the subjects under study. Factors such as premorbid intelligence, handedness, memory dysfunction, and learning disabilities, all of which vary considerably in this clinical population, have not been taken into consideration. Length of seizure disorder, seizure frequency, the proximity of data sampling to periods of increased or decreased seizure activity, and the patient's anticonvulsant regimen also represent potential sources of variance that typically remain uncontrolled. These complex subject variables also raise a question as to the general appropriateness of the methodologies and subject groups used to study this topic. First, there may be no appropriate control group for patients with temporo-limbic epilepsy. Given the myriad connections of the temporolimbic region and the representation of cortical association areas in these structures required to mediate emotion and memory, it simply may not be possible to consider that a subject with a parietal or frontal focus has an independent, nontemporal seizure disorder. Recent research demonstrating that interictal psychopathology is more prominent among focal epilepsy patients in general as opposed to those with primary generalized epilepsy reinforces this point of view (Edeh & Toone, 1987). In the study of epilepsy in particular, it would seem naive and potentially dangerous to ignore the current state of knowledge in neuroscience in order to rely on gross, superficial divisions of the cortex when categorizing our subjects. Secondly, it is clear that ictal behavioral alterations cannot be reliably classified as cortical or limbic in origin on the basis of scalp-surface recording.

A final methodological issue in the study of the interictal behavior syndrome concerns the application and relevance of normative statistics in neurologically impaired populations (Shallice, 1979; Spiers, 1981, 1982). These patients do not share common historical antecedents, have a significant variety of premorbid etiological variables, and, in fact, are unlikely to form a homogeneous sample except in regard to very specific, limited data points. There is, in fact, no reason to assume that patients with temporolimbic epilepsy should be evenly distributed either with regard to an interictal behavior syndrome as a whole or in relation to any specific interictal trait or behavioral alteration such as hypergraphia. Rather, the appearance of these behavioral alterations is far more likely to be a function of subject-specific variables such as the presence of a congenital lesion, the frequency of seizure discharges, the involvement of mesial temporal lobe structures in the seizure, or other operant factors that have yet to be identified. These factors may even differ by gender, age at onset of seizure disorder, or manual preference. In summary, groups of "temporal lobe" seizure patients cannot be reliably formed based on current technology, and even if they could, it seems unlikely that any specific behavioral alteration, ictal or interictal, can be represented along a continuum that satisfies the assumptions of normative group statistics. In fact, ictal manifestations are clearly skewed in their distributions, with certain manifestations being consistently associated with specific neuroanatomic sites (e.g., olfactory hallucination and orbitofrontal seizure discharge). Perhaps interictal manifestations are equally specific and should therefore be investigated by a case-study observational approach rather than by a group statistical methodology until the appropriate parameters for grouping subjects have been identified. For the moment, when populations are selected solely by scalp-surface EEG criteria, a compulsion to obsessional, religious writing will probably not be present in every patient or even in a significant proportion of patients who have temporolimbic epilepsy. It may be present in a certain number of these patients, however, and pooling their data with those of subjects who do not show such changes only serves to dilute and conceal the importance of these cases, statistically and theoretically.

Interictal Alterations

That patients exist who display hypergraphia and that this is related to their temporolimbic epilepsy cannot be denied. A left-handed 30-year-old woman in our practice was hypergraphic. Her seizures consisted of irritability, a sense of impending doom, and macropsia limited to the right visual field without impairment of consciousness or motor automatisms. These ictal alterations were correlated on EEG with epileptiform activity in the left temporal–central region. She had experienced these symptoms for over 10 years and had repeatedly sought medical and psychiatric attention without having received the diagnosis of temporolimbic epilepsy. As these episodes persisted, she had become progressively more dependent on her left hand for skilled motor movements, but a dichotic listening test at the time of diagnosis suggested left hemisphere language dominance. Notwithstanding her seizure disorder, she had graduated from an Ivy League college and had been a successful hospital administrator until her seizures became more frequent and she abandoned her career to pursue her writing interests. At the time of our evaluation, she was a published prose translator and was actively writing short stories and poetry. She was aware, however, that her drive and inspiration for writing, and especially for poetry, were related to her seizure frequency. The times when her episodes were most prevalent and intense were also when she felt most compelled to write. Once these were properly identified as seizures, and the option of medications was available to control them, she faced a quandary regarding the desirability of seizure control as opposed to her motivation for writing. Since achieving control on anticonvulsants, she has, for the most part, returned to working in hospital administration.

Consider also the case of a 36-year-old right-handed homosexual male dancer who developed a mixed partial and secondary generalized seizure disorder of temporolimbic origin. There was no lateralized predominance on EEG, and seizures were initially difficult to monitor. Neuropsychological findings, however, clearly implicated compromise in right hemisphere functioning. This patient manifested many of the interpersonal features of the interictal behavior syndrome, including hypergraphia. His writing, however, was largely circumstantial, obsessional, redundant, and highly philosophical. He remained unemployed after the onset of his seizures but pursued his writing vigorously, often spending 8 h a day for several weeks working on a single poem or short story. None of his works had been published, but he nonetheless used his meager income to hire professional typists to prepare his manuscripts. This behavior continued unabated for 3 years until anticonvulsant control was finally achieved through a combination of phenobarbital and carbamazepine. This resulted in a cessation of writing and a return to employment, which lasted 6 months until he could no longer tolerate impotence as an apparent medication side effect and asked to be tapered off all anticonvulsants. His writing compulsion returned as soon as his partial seizures manifested. He left work, applied to college for creative writing, and was successful until an episode of partial and secondary generalized status interrupted his academic year. He resumed a low dose of anticonvulsant therapy but remained uncontrolled with frequent bouts of partial seizures. He continued to pursue his writing, even obtaining a 6-month fellowship to Oxford, and has since been accepted into a graduate literature program.

These two cases illustrate the compulsion to write, and particularly to write poetry, which has been apparent in many of the temporolimbic epilepsy patients we follow. The outcome of this interictal behavioral alteration can often be destructive, but it can also be positive or productive, sometimes in the same patient at different times. Much of the written material produced by these patients is obsessive and circumstantial, but it can also be insightful and amusing, as illustrated by the sample provided in Fig. 6.1. The specific parameters governing the relationship between hypergraphia and temporolimbic epilepsy have yet to be determined. This should not, however, undermine our ability to observe such occurrences in our clinical practice and to design relevant research to further elucidate this phenomenon.

The correlation between temporolimbic epilepsy and some of the other facets of the interictal behavior syndrome appears to be as specific as it is for hypergraphia. The study of these alterations is, therefore, of great importance for understanding the biological basis of behavior. Although the specific cluster of traits constituting an interictal behavior syndrome has yet to be fully outlined and may vary from patient to patient, in our experiences a current list would have to include the following five general categories of behavioral alteration.

First, the patient has an exaggerated level of interest in philosophical, religious, moral, or cosmic concerns and issues. Second, the patient may develop hypergraphia, with a content that usually reflects personal preoccupations, often expressed in poetic

A TLE TRIP TO THE GROCERY STORE OR WHY IT CAN TAKE ALL DAY
(Hypergraphia, Vol. IX)

Maximizing control of a situation is crucial. One way to control a major undertaking like a trip to the grocery store is to break it down into smaller segments which can be coped with once individually organized.

I. MAKING THE LIST

This entails at least 11 trips to the pantry to see what groceries we already have (4 of these trips alone are to check to see if we're out of bread yet), and checking in the refrigerator to see how many eggs are lef (of course, the first few times you look youn can't remember what the answer was when you close the refrigerator door, but evemtually it sinks in). (Hopefully you have already set down your noteboook and pen on the kitchen table so that you can write down each item you need before you forget it, but if you haven't it only takes about 20 minutes to look in all the places you might have put the pen when you first decided to make the list).Think it's simple to make a list? How the hell did I use to spell margarine? And, Chirst, how do you make the letter "E"? Which direction does the letter "S" curve, anyway? Time spent compiling the list varies with the extent of the projected shopping expedition but its a trade-off between one lengthly, complex, potentially terrrifying and humiliating experiences chanceing you'll wind up getting most of wat you need or a potentially infinite number of smaller trips.

III. CHOOSING THE MARKET

This is a trade of off economics vs. safety: Capitol Market gives double-coupons values and the cab ride home is shorter and cheaper, but there are only 2 major intersections to cross to get to Purity Supreme wher selections are more limitied but you are more familiar with the store's layout. (You mya also remember the embarassment of breaking an egg carton, a peanut-butter jar, and knocing over a cereal display the last time you were at P.S. and want not to go there again until you're shure they forget who you are.) (Also, which store is it where the cabbie works who tried to rip-off all your groceries last time when you had a small seizure on the way home?)

IV. GETTING TO THE MARKET

The trip over is relatively uneventful. You walk straght down Victory Rd. (3/4 mile exactly) when you come to Neponset Ave. and you remember you're tendency to space out when you start watching streams of traffic, so you decide to wait fro the lights to be on the safe side. The ligt turns red, traffic stops, and you start to cross the street. The next thing you hear is the squeal of brakes, and you ar in the middle of the street, drivers in both directions coming towards you with horns honking raucously. Briefly immobilizized by situation, suddenly you realize you haev almost been mowed down (again !!!), you were looking at the wrong light, stupid. You run for the opposite curb and do not stop until the corner of the next block. You're heart still pounding you realize you have to cross another street. After several minutes of trying to reason out how to be safe this time you finally read the words "Dead End" on the sign you have been staring at for a minute. This means cars will only come from one direction and you don't have to worry about blanking out between looking to the left and lookig to the right before you cross. Neverthless, it takes a few deep breaths to get up the nerve to step off the sidewalk. From there it's smootth sailing ! No more intersections.

FIGURE 6.1. Excerpts from a narrative proffered by a patient with temporolimbic epilepsy to her neurologist to help him understand events in her life. Spelling, grammar, and punctuation have been preserved as they were provided by the patient.

form. Third, the patient often experiences a significant alteration in sexual behavior. Although this most frequently takes the form of a loss of sexual interest, a reduction in sexual activity, and difficulty becoming aroused or achieving orgasm, it can also include hypersexuality or the development of homosexual, bisexual, or fetishistic interests. One of our female patients found herself more attracted to men when controlled by anticonvulsants and more attracted to women when having frequent seizures.

A fourth aspect is the presence of deepened interpersonal emotions, and particularly increased irritability, aggressiveness, and temper control problems. This is often manifested as an inability to forgive others for what may, in fact, be minor transgressions. From the patient's exaggerated moral perspective, the behavior of others may often be judged shocking or morally reprehensible. This sometimes leads the patient to engage in socially inappropriate or violent behaviors. One male patient was so overcome by his rage concerning litter outside a Boston law school that he marched into the Dean's office, demanded an audience, and began to lecture the Dean while pounding on his desk. The police were called, and the patient was arrested. Such acts are typically impulsive. The patient, however, is not amnestic for them and often expresses equally exaggerated remorse after the event. Similar difficulty can be observed in certain patients' ability to modulate the intensity of a wide range of emotional responses. Most common in our experience have been problems in dealing with sadness, rejection, and suspiciousness, though this obviously varies considerably from patient to patient.

Finally, the fifth and perhaps most striking among the behavioral alterations seen in the interictal behavior syndrome is the development in some patients of "stickiness," "viscosity," or what might best be labeled "social adhesiveness." This takes the form of a persistent drive to sustain or prolong interpersonal contacts and an ability to effectively terminate social interactions. Frequently this is compounded by circumstantiality, as the patient is unable to follow a logical stream of thought in conversation without becoming preoccupied by trivial or irrelevant details or by an exaggerated sense of personal significance, which may become attached to minor events or to the clinician's response. In our experience, this disruption of normal social interchange frequently includes other aspects of social–interpersonal behavior. For example, some patients appear to have deficits in appreciating the significance of nonverbal or paralinguistic communications such as gesture and facial expression unless these are emphatic and convey unmistakable intentions. Many patients also seem unable to perceive or properly observe the boundaries required by certain social roles, and this may be particularly evident in the patient–professional relationship. These patients may be overly familiar or repeatedly challenge their caregivers' intentions or motives. Although they may expect caregivers to react with urgent or extraordinary measures in response to relatively trivial events or symptoms, they often cannot establish a successful therapeutic alliance or relationship, even after years of treatment. On certain occasions, patients with this interictal behavior alteration may be deeply offended or may even become enraged and terminate treatment in response to what they unrealistically perceive as an insufficient mobilization of resources on their behalf.

Mechanism of Interictal Alterations

Various hypotheses have been advanced to account for the occurrence of interictal behavior changes. Surprisingly, the nature of the patient's psychological response to an unpredictable illness has been cited as the causative factor in the development of the interictal behavior syndrome. Although there can be no doubt that this contributes significantly to the patient's behavior patterns, the adoption of this hypothesis would lead to the prediction that all epileptic patients and patients with other diseases having unpredictable courses, such as multiple sclerosis or migraines, should manifest circumstantiality, hypergraphia, and hyposexuality. Although some patient populations have been difficult to distinguish from patients with temporolimbic epilepsy using the Behavior Inventory, notably no cases have been reported in which a particular patient actually manifested a collection of changes that included all of the constituent features of the interictal behavior syndrome without also having temporolimbic epilepsy. Chronic pharmacotherapy with anticonvulsant medications has also been suggested as responsible for these behavior alterations. This explanation can obviously be ruled out by considering the many patients in whom features of the interictal behavior syndrome can easily be discerned who have not yet acquired a diagnosis of temporolimbic epilepsy, much less been exposed to anticonvulsants.

The possibility that seizures mediate the behavioral alterations described in the interictal behavior syndrome cannot be based on the premise that a unitary correlation exists between ictal events and particular instances when these traits are displayed. Patients need not be having sustained paroxysmal discharges whenever they are writing a poem or pondering some philosophical question. At the same time, however, these behavioral alterations may be intensified in some patients during periods of increased seizure frequency (Hermann & Melyn, 1984). More importantly, in certain individuals these traits disappear or become much less pronounced after surgical removal of the site of maximum epileptogenesis. Consider a 23-year-old right-handed single woman who had partial and complex partial seizures from the age of 6 months following an apparent encephalitis. Depth electrode telemetry finally lateralized her seizure focus to the right anterior temporal region, and angiography prior to sodium amobarbital testing demonstrated a partial occlusion of the middle cerebral artery. The patient became seizure-free immediately postoperatively and was rapidly noted to have a significant improvement in her previously irritable, circumstantial personality. Within 6 months, she had her first boyfriend and had become socially outgoing and independent. Some of these changes could be attributed to seizure control facilitating her lifestyle. However, pre- and postoperative measurement with the Behavior Inventory demonstrated a remarkable change not only in her self-rating but most dramatically in her family's rating of her interictal behavior traits.

Although such cases imply that the interictal behavior syndrome may be a function of some underlying structural pathology in temporolimbic structures, this would be contradicted by those patients who have congenitally acquired lesions in temporal lobe structures, such as dyslexics, but who do not evidence these behavioral alterations. It also does not account for fluctuations in the intensity of interictal traits in relation to seizure frequency or for the finding that many patients who display these traits have normal neuropathology when the concerned regions are excised for seizure control. The presence of an underlying structural lesion, however, may contribute to the probability of acquiring features of the interictal behavior syndrome and may act exponentially to facilitate or promote the physiological mechanisms underlying the development of these alterations.

It has been suggested (Bear, 1979) that the presence of a temporal lobe focus acts to produce the interictal behavior syndrome by kindling limbic structures. The state of the temporolimbic network as a result of this kindling has been characterized as "functional hyperconnectivity." The impact of this state on behavior is believed to be an enhancement of affective responses, a loss of the ability to inhibit or reject fortuitous sensory–limbic associations, and an increase in the emotional significance of neutral objects, actions, and events: "As a result of the increasing investment of the environment with limbic significance, external stimuli begin to take on great importance: this leads in turn to increased concern with philosophical, religious, and cosmic matters. Since all events become charged with importance, the patients frequently resort to recording them in written form at great length and in highly charged language" (Geschwind, 1983).

Although this is an attractive hypothesis, it stands in marked contradiction to certain of the physiological mechanisms present in conjunction with a seizure focus that suggest that hyperexcitability is not the only state present in these structures in association with temporolimbic epilepsy. For example, one of the most commonly observed effects of a discharging focus on distal sites with which it is connected has been functional inhibition rather than excitation. At a behavioral level, this process may account for some patients' inability to attach sufficient or appropriate affect to certain relationships or to imprint particular events with the correct affective tone. This may also contribute to the common finding of learning and memory deficits in this population, presumably because the cell assemblies triggered by relevant incoming stimuli cannot be selectively or effectively labeled with the appropriate emotional significance for encoding and storage to occur. If hyperconnection were the only operational mechanism for behavioral alteration, it might actually be more consistent to predict that these patients should have improved memory functioning, at least for those events they consider important. Even for this category of events, however, their memory is often incomplete or inaccurate. Similarly, sexual concerns and interests are generally diminished in the context of the interictal behavior syndrome. This change may be a result of the inhibitory influence of the seizure focus on structures in the hypothalamic–pituitary axis, a hypothesis that is partially corroborated by reports of hormonal abnormalities in this population (Herzog, 1989).

The variety of interictal physiological and behavioral changes that may occur in conjunction with temporolimbic epilepsy lead us to return to the more general concept, introduced earlier in this chapter, that such patients may have a deficit in their ability to assign the appropriate affective tone to environmental experiences. In some patients or under certain circumstances, this deficit may take the form of an enhancement of affective associations. This in turn may prove to be either adaptive or dysfunctional in the context of a variety of other factors. In some instances, the patient's ability to assign affect to experience may be insufficient, inappropriate, or completely lacking. Finally, these problems may not be present all the time or in all patients, and many individuals with temporolimbic epilepsy will function without such behavioral alterations. It should be evident, however, that certain patients will show alterations in their emotions and behavior that are a direct consequence of their neurological condition.

Although it has been repeatedly emphasized that the changes discussed here need not imply psychopathology, there appears to be some persistent concern that accepting the existence of the interictal behavior syndrome may lead to an unfavorable characterization of patients with temporolimbic epilepsy. Such protestations may be well-intentioned, but they may not be in the best interest of this population. In our experience, patients with temporolimbic epilepsy and their families are frequently perplexed—at the very least curious—and often severely distressed by the interpersonal and emotional alterations that may occur in conjunction with a seizure disorder. To attribute these changes solely to reactive psychological causes or to the side effects of medications fails to address the patient's dilemma and concerns in a sensitive or realistic manner. In our opinion, this may not only jeopardize the clinician's credibility but, more importantly, undermine the patient's ability to cope effectively with the illness and achieve an optimal level of functioning.

FUTURE DIRECTIONS

The study of the ictal and interictal behavioral alterations associated with temporolimbic epilepsy is currently an exciting and provocative area of research. The study of these phenomena may not only help to elucidate the etiology of abnormal behavior but may also lead to a better understanding of the neurological basis for the mediation of emotion. Before such goals can be attained, however, fundamental research will be required that relies on a multidisciplinary strategy combining neurological, psychiatric, and neuropsychological perspectives.

Major breakthroughs in relating behavioral alterations to paroxysmal discharges will occur in conjunction with the advancement of neurological technology. This technology must have as its goal the ability to identify reliably the occurrence of discrete, localizable neuronal alterations, which can then be correlated with behavioral observations. Examples of advances in neurophysiology that are leading in this direction are portable, ambulatory telemetry monitoring systems and the broader use of specialized, noninvasive electrodes (Bridgers & Ebersole, 1985; Ives *et al.*, 1990).

The advent of systems capable of recording from up to 128 channels simultaneously will not only refine the detection and localization of significant electrical events, but also allow clinicians to plot the onset and spread of discrete episodes at a structural level, which, in turn, may be correlated with the evolution of particular behavioral manifestations. For example, Figs. 6.2 through 6.5 illustrate the use of the 128-channel computer-based recording device. This patient had 10 depth electrodes stereotactically placed, each of which had eight contact points for recording at different levels. Sixty-three channels are shown in Fig. 6.2, in which the recording has been temporally compressed to obtain an overview of the seizure. In Figs. 6.3 and 6.4, the time base has been expanded for a more detailed review of specific portions of the record.

The probable onset of the seizure is seen in channels LA1–2 and LA2–3, corresponding to the left amygdala nucleus, at 08:36:19.5. At 08:36:35 the first epileptic discharge is noted from LA1–2 and LA2–3. This discharge increases in amplitude and spreads to incorporate the left hippocampal contacts by 08:36:46. At 08:37:10, the patient recognized that an event was occurring and reported a premonition that she was going to have a seizure. In Fig. 6.4 at 08:37:28, the seizure spread to the right amygdala and right hippocampal chains without any observable or reported alteration in behavior. The patient then experienced a secondary generalized major motor seizure at approximately 08:37:42. On previous noninvasive scalp recordings, the first changes observed on EEG were seen when the right temporal lobe structures were involved, suggesting a right hemisphere focus despite the now obvious onset in the left temporal lobe. Figure 6.5 expands only the first 14 channels to demonstrate the intrahemispheric relationships that exist as the seizure starts within the left amygdala and hippocampus. This recording reinforces two points made earlier in this chapter. Scalp-surface recordings can easily lead to false localization, and physiological events that constitute a seizure can occur outside of the individual's self-awareness and certainly without observable behavioral correlates. Numerous left hemisphere electrographic events similar to the one illustrated in Fig. 6.5 were recorded in this same patient. Not all of these progressed to a secondary generalized seizure, and some did not even result in the patient complaining of symptomatic changes. It would appear naive, however, to conclude that such electrophysiological events are benign occurrences in the limbic system. In fact, it seems more probable that such events are related to the long-term behavioral changes discussed above.

In addition to discoveries that are revolutionizing traditional neurophysiology, several new technologies should begin to yield important data in the coming decade. Magmoencephalography (MEG), for example, may soon permit the identification of electrical events from tangential brain structures previously inaccessible to noninvasive electrodes (Rose, Sato, Smith, Porter, Theodore, Friauf, Bonner, & Jabbari, 1987; Sutherling, Crandall, Engel, Darcey, Cahan, & Barth, 1987). In neuroradiology, magnetic resonance imaging (MRI) has improved our ability to identify subtle variations in anatomic structure that may be linked to behavioral outcomes (Jabbari, Gunderson, Wippold, Citrin, Sherman, Bartoszek, Daigh, & Mitchell, 1986). Functional techniques, meanwhile, such as positron emission tomography (PET) (Engel,

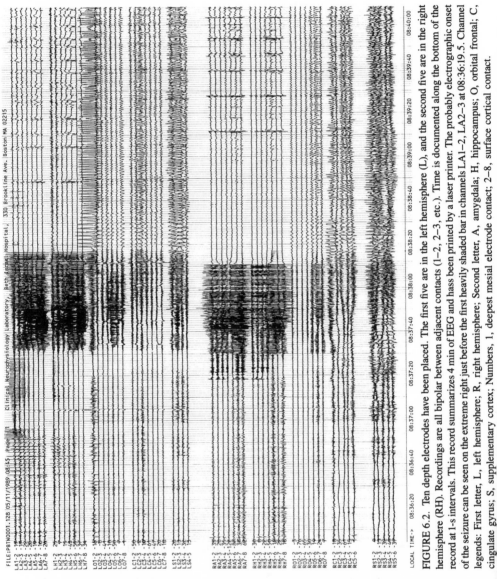

FIGURE 6.2. Ten depth electrodes have been placed. The first five are in the left hemisphere (L), and the second five are in the right hemisphere (RH). Recordings are all bipolar between adjacent contacts (1–2, 2–3, etc.). Time is documented along the bottom of the record at 1-s intervals. This record summarizes 4 min of EEG and hass been printed by a laser printer. The probably electrographic onset of the seizure can be seen on the extreme right just before the first heavily shaded bar in channels LA1–2, LA2–3 at 08:36:19.5. Channel legends: First letter, L, left hemisphere; R, right hemisphere; Second letter, A, amygdala; H, hippocampus; O, orbital frontal; C, cingulate gyrus; S, supplementary cortex; Numbers, 1, deepest mesial electrode contact; 2–8, surface cortical contact.

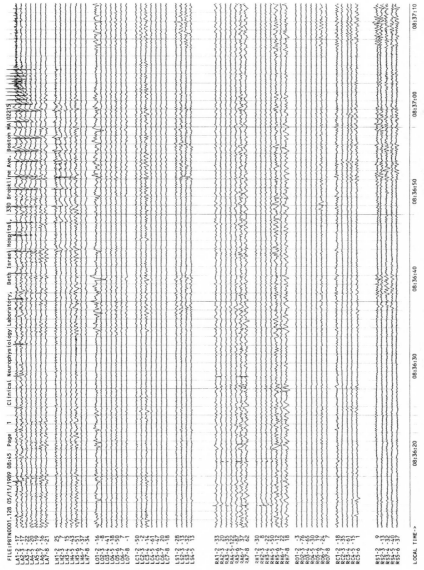

FIGURE 6.3. This is the same patient and event shown in Fig. 6.2. Here the time base has been expanded for ease of analysis, but only the first minute is shown. The electrographic onset can again be seen at 08:36:19.5 in the left amygdala, increasing in amplitude and spreading to the left hippocampus. The patient does not report feeling as if she is going to have a seizure until 08:37:10. Abbreviations as in Fig. 6.2.

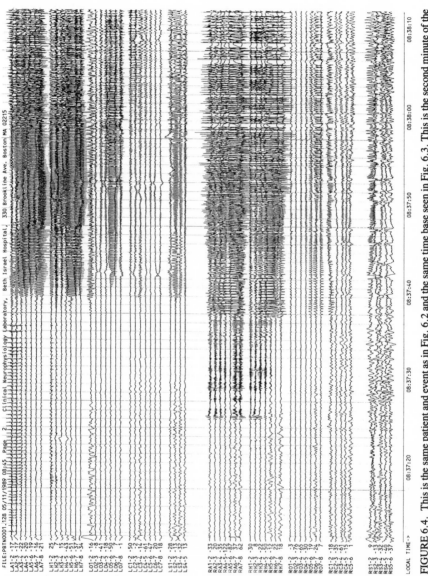

FIGURE 6.4. This is the same patient and event as in Fig. 6.2 and the same time base seen in Fig. 6.3. This is the second minute of the event. The evolution of the seizure can clearly be seen in the left amygdala with the incorporation of the right amygdala and hippocampus at 08:37:28. Previous surface recordings had shown only the right hemisphere activity at the onset on the patient's seizure. Abbreviations as in Fig. 6.2.

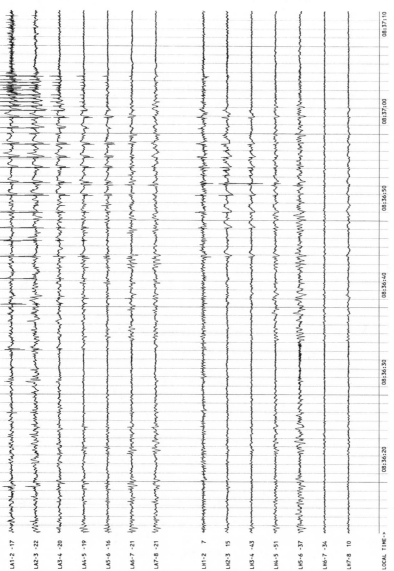

FIGURE 6.5. This is the same patient and event shown in Fig. 6.2. Here the time base is the same as in Fig. 6.3 but the printout has been limited to only the first 14 channels to allow more careful intrahemispheric analysis. The electrographic onset can again be seen at 08:36:19.5, most clearly in LA1–2. The first epileptic discharge is seen in the left amygdala at LA1–2, LA2–3 as 08:36:35 and begins to incorporate the left hippocampus at LH1–2 at 08:36:46. The patient reports nothing at all until 08:37:10. Abbreviations as in Fig. 6.2.

1984; Theodore, Brooks, Sato, Patronas, Margolin, Di Chiro, & Porter, 1984) and single photon emission computerized tomography (SPECT) (Blume, Schomer, Magistretti, Uren, & Spiers, 1982), can presently specify broad zones of ictal and interictal involvement and may ultimately be capable of identifying more discrete behavioral–neurophysiological correlations, particularly if short-acting, rapid-uptake labeling agents are used.

At a cellular and biochemical level, research should focus on specifying the mechanisms underlying the onset and propogation of partial seizures as well as attempting to define the relationship between this evolution and the development of specific behavior problems. The contribution of genetic predisposition and factors such as handedness and learning disabilities should also be more closely controlled and more thoroughly explored. Finally, research is needed to determine those factors related to the misattribution of affect observed in patients with features of the interictal behavior syndrome. The controversy over the existence of this syndrome often seems more political than scientific, and important questions remain to be answered. For example, are these misattributions episodic or continuous in nature, and, if they are episodic, can their occurrence be correlated with reliable EEG changes? In this regard, the lines of investigation already noted here concerning the structural, biochemical, and electrical changes that occur in response to a discharging focus need to be pursued from a broader perspective, one that attempts to relate these changes to the alterations observed at a behavioral level.

The ability of technology to provide detailed neuroanatomical and neurophysiological information can be expected to improve exponentially as we move into the next millennium. For our understanding of the behavior of temporolimbic epilepsy patients to keep pace with these advances, however, a critical reassessment of prevailing dogma will be necessary. If the information supplied by neurophysiologists and neuroradiologists in the next decade is to be applied fruitfully, clinicians in psychiatry and neuropsychology must rediscover their enthusiasm for fundamental scientific observation and explore the possibility of new cause-and-effect relationships. Careful descriptions of patients' actual behaviors and active inquiry regarding their symptoms, experiences, and feelings during episodes or seizures will be central to this process. In addition, the detailed examination of patients' cognitive functioning during, after, and between seizures as well as objective documentation of their emotional functioning will be required in order to map out the interaction between behavior and regions of compromised brain function. In so doing, not only will we arrive at a better understanding of ictal behavioral manifestations in patients with epilepsy, but we may also be able to document the role of paroxysmal discharges or even ictal events in a wide variety of psychiatric conditions and behavior disorders. This, of course, may require that we study patients heretofore excluded from sophisticated, detailed neurophysiological and neuropsychological investigation. It is often the difficult and diagnostically challenging patient, however, whose clinical presentation provides a new insight or significant discovery that, in turn, expands the horizons of our science.

SUMMARY AND CONCLUSION

In this chapter an overview has been provided of the ictal and interictal manifestations of temporolimbic epilepsy. The term "temporolimbic" has been selected to underscore the pivotal role of the temporal lobe in the mediation of emotion and behavior and to remind the reader of the widespread behaviorally relevant reciprocal connections that exist between the limbic system and the rest of the brain. It has been suggested that these connections form the basis for the diverse and often peculiar observations classified as partial seizures, which may run the gamut from simple automatisms to complex hallucinations. It has also been argued that certain predictable, more long-term changes in behavior may occur as a result of the presence of a temporolimbic seizure focus. These are not simply psychological responses to the disease process but, in fact, appear to be a direct outcome of neurochemical and neuroanatomical alterations related to the presence and frequency of abnormal electrical discharges in the limbic system. Although this area of research is surrounded by controversy, there can be no question that such patients exist. Furthermore, it has been our experience to reliably observe five component features that, in various degrees and combinations depending on the individual, constitute an interictal behavior syndrome. These include, but neither require nor are restricted to, increased philosophical interest or hyperreligiosity, irritability and difficulty with the mediation of anger, hypergraphia, social adhesiveness, and altered sexual functioning. The future of research in this area, meanwhile, demands on a return to a truly open-minded, observational, scientific approach that can provide incisive, relevant data for correlation with the information generated by the rapidly evolving technologies in neurophysiology and neuroradiology.

It is a maxim that scientific advancement depends on controversy and the collapse and disintegration of an established paradigm so that a new order and structure for differentiating and classifying phenomena may emerge (Kuhn, 1962; Werner, 1948). The study of temporolimbic epilepsy and behavior is approaching such a crossroads. It is a point where heretical observations replace what has hitherto been accepted as fact and where speculation, of necessity, must take the place of established theory. There are those who will resist such change out of uncertainty and who will continue to rely on traditional methodologies to reinforce time-honored shibboleths concerning this population. To the betterment of our science and our patients, change is, fortunately, inevitable.

ACKNOWLEDGMENTS.   The authors dedicate this chapter to the memory of the late Dr. Norman Geschwind, scholar, teacher, and friend. His breadth of knowledge, geniality, collegiality, and good fellowship are sorely missed. Dr. Geschwind was the James Jackson Putnam Professor of Neurology at Harvard Medical School, Chairman of the Department of Neurology at the Beth Israel Hospital, and founder of the Behavioral Neurology Unit. It was Dr. Geschwind's insight, genius, and enthusiasm for the study of the relationship between the brain and behavior that sustained us, and this work would not have been undertaken except for his influence on all of our careers. The first author would also like to thank Dr. Richard Wurtman of the Massachusetts Institute of Technology for his support and encouragement and for providing an academic environment in which diversity and scholarship can flourish. The preparation of this manuscript was made possible by a grant from the NutraSweet Company to the first two authors.

REFERENCES

Abrams, R., & Taylor, M. A. (1979). Differential EEG patterns in affective disorder and schizophrenia. *Archives of General Psychiatry, 36,* 1355.

Adebimpe, V. R. (1977). Complex-partial seizures simulating schizophrenia. *Journal of the American Medical Association, 237,* 1339.

Allan, T. M., & Stewart, R. S. (1971). Photosensitive epilepsy and driving. *Lancet, 1,* 1125.

Backstrom, T., Zetterlund, B., Blom, S., & Romano, M. (1984). Effects of intravenous progesterone infusions on the epileptic discharge frequency in women with partial epilepsy. *Acta Neurologica Sandinavica, 69,* 240–248.

Ballenger, C. S., King, D. W., & Gallagher, B. (1983). Partial-complex status epilepticus. *Neurology, 33,* 1545.

Baratz, R., & Mesulam, M.-M. (1981). Adult onset stuttering treated with anticonvulsants. *Archives of Neurology, 38,* 132.

Barraclough, B. M. (1987). The suicide rate of epilepsy. *Acta Psychiatrica Scandinavica, 76,* 339–345.

Bear, D. M. (1979). Temporal lobe epilepsy: A syndrome of sensory–limbic hyperconnection. *Cortex, 15,* 357.

Bear, D. M., & Fedio, P. (1977). Quantitative analysis of interictal behavior in temporal lobe epilepsy. *Archives of Neurology, 34,* 454.

Bear, D. M., Levin, K., Blumer, D., Chatman, D., & Reider, J. (1982). Interictal behavior in hospitalized temporal lobe epileptics: Relationship to other psychiatric syndromes. *Journal of Neurology, Neurosurgery & Psychiatry, 45,* 481.

Ben-Ari, Y., & Krnjevic, K. (1981). Actions of GABA on hippocampal neurons with special reference to the etiology of epilepsy. In P. Morselli, K. Lloyd, W. Loscher, B. Meldrum, & E. Reynolds (Eds.), *Neurotransmitters, seizures and epilepsy* (pp. 330–337). New York: Raven Press.

Ben-Ari, Y., Krnjevic, K., & Reinhardt, W. (1979). Hippocampal seizures and failure of inhibition. *Canadian Journal of Physiology & Pharmacology, 57,* 1462.

Bennett, T. L., & Curiel, M. P. (1988). Complex partial seizures presenting as a psychiatric illness: A case study. *International Journal of Clinical Neuropsychology, 10*(1), 41–44.

Berthier, M., Starkstein, S., & Leiguarda, R. (1987). Seizures induced by orgasm. *Annals of Neurology, 22*(3), 394–395.

Bhaskar, P. A. (1987). Scrotal pain with testicular jerking: An unusual manifestation of partial epilepsy. *Journal of Neurology, Neurosurgery, & Psychiatry, 50,* 1233–1243.

Binnie, C. D., Darby, C. E., & Hindley, A. T. (1973). Electroencephalographic changes in epileptics while viewing television. *British Medical Journal, 4,* 378.

Blume, H. W., Schomer, D. L., Magistretti, P., Uren, R., & Spiers, P. A. (1982). Single photon emission computerized tomography in epileptic patients. *Proceedings of the New England Neurosurgical Society* (pp. 25–37). Burlington, MA: New England Neurosurgical Society.

Brandt, J., Seidman, L. J., & Kohl, D. (1984). Personality characteristics of epileptic patients: A controlled study of generalized and temporal lobe cases. *Journal of Clinical and Experimental Neuropsychology, 7,* 25–38.

Bridgers, S. L., & Ebersole, J. S. (1985). The clinical utility of ambulatory cassette EEG. *Neurology, 35,* 166–173.

Commission on Classification and Terminology of the International League Against Epilepsy. (1981).

Proposal for revised clinical and electroencephalographic classification of epileptic seizures. *Epilepsia*, 22, 489–501.

Crowell, R. M. (1970). Distant effects of a focal epileptogenic process. *Brain Research*, 18, 137.

Currier, R. D., Little, S. C., & Suess, J. F. (1971). Sexual seizures. *Archives of Neurology*, 25, 260–264.

Darn, W. M. (1980). Epilepsy and neuron loss in the hippocampus. *Epilepsia*, 21, 617–629.

Delgado-Escueta, A. V. (Ed.). (1988). *Basic mechanisms of the epilepsies*. New York: Raven Press.

Delgado-Escueta, A. V., Mattson, R. H., King, L., Goldensohn, E. S., Spiegel, H., Madsen, J., Crandall, P., Dreyfuss, F., & Porter, R. J. (1981). The nature of aggression during epileptic seizures. *New England Journal of Medicine*, 305, 711.

Delgado-Escueta, A. V., Treiman, D. M., & Walsh, G. O. (1983a). The treatable epilepsies. *New England Journal of Medicine*, 308, 1508.

Delgado-Escueta, A. V., Treiman, D. M., & Walsh, G. O. (1983b). The treatable epilepsies. *New England Journal of Medicine*, 308, 1576.

Devinsky, O., Hafler, D. A., & Victor, J. (1982). Embarassment as the aura of a complex-partial seizure. *Neurology*, 32, 1284.

Devinsky, O., Price, B. H., & Cohen, S. (1986). Cardiac manifestations of complex-partial seizures. *American Journal of Medicine*, 80(2), 195–202.

Drake, M. E. (1983). Isolated ictal autonomic symptoms in complex-partial seizures. *Annals of Neurology*, 14, 100.

Drake, M. E., & Coffey, E. (1983). Complex-partial status epilepticus simulating psychogenic unresponsiveness. *American Journal of Psychiatry*, 140, 800.

Edeh, J., & Toone, B. (1987). Relationship between interictal psychopathology and the type of epilepsy: Results of a survey in general practice. *British Journal of Psychiatry*, 151, 95–101.

Edlund, M. J., Swann, A. C., & Clothier, J. (1987). Patients with panic attacks and abnormal EEG results. *American Journal of Psychiatry*, 144, 508–509.

Efron, R. (1956). The effect of olfactory stimuli in arresting uncinate fits. *Brain*, 79, 267–282.

Efron, R. (1957). The conditioned inhibition of uncinate fits. *Brain*, 80, 251–262.

Engel, J. (1984). The use of positron emission tomographic scanning in epilepsy. *Annals of Neurology*, 15(Supplement), S180–S191.

Escueta, A. V., Buxley, J., & Stubbs, N. (1974). Prolonged twilight state and automatisms: a case report. *Neurology*, 24, 331.

Falconer, M. A. (1971). Genetic and related aetiological factors in temporal lobe epilepsy: A review. *Epilepsia*, 12, 13–31.

Falconer, M. A. (1973). Reversibility by temporal lobe resection of the behavioral abnormalities of temporal lobe epilepsy. *New England Journal of Medicine*, 289, 451–456.

Flor-Henry, P. (1969). Schizophrenic-like reactions and affective psychosis associated with temporal lobe epilepsy. Etiological factors. *American Journal of Psychiatry*, 126, 400.

Flor-Henry, P. (1976). Lateralized temporal–limbic dysfunction and psychopathology. *Annals of the New York Academy of Science*, 280, 777.

Forster, F. M. (1977). Reflex epilepsy. In B. K. Toone (Ed.), *Behavioral therapy and conditioned reflexes* (pp. 115–129). Springfield, Ill.: Charles C. Thomas.

Galaburda, A. M., & Kemper, T. L. (1979). Cytoarchitectonic abnormalities in developmental dyslexia: A case study. *Annals of Neurology*, 6, 94–100.

Galaburda, A. M., Sherman, G. F., Rosen, G. D., Aboitiz, F., & Geschwind, N. (1985). Developmental dyslexia: Four consecutive patients with cortical anomalies. *Annals of Neurology*, 18, 222–233.

Geschwind, N. (1983). Pathogenesis of behavior change in temporal lobe epilepsy. In A. A. Ward, J. R. Penry, & D. Purpura (Eds.), *Epilepsy*. New York: Raven Press.

Geschwind, N. (1984). Dostoevsky's epilepsy. In D. Blumer (Ed.), *Psychiatric aspects of epilepsy* (pp. 75–87). Washington, D.C.: American Psychiatric Press.

Geschwind, N., & Sherwin, I. (1967). Language-induced epilepsy. *Archives of Neurology*, 16, 25.

Gibbs, F. A. (1951). Ictal and non-ictal psychiatric disorders in temporal lobe epilepsy. *Journal of Nervous and Mental Disease*, 113, 522.

Gilchrist, J. M. (1985). Arrhythmogenic seizures: diagnosis by simultaneous EEG/ECG recording. *Neurology, 35,* 1503–1506.

Gilmore, R. L., & Heilman, R. (1981). Speech arrest in partial seizures: Evidence of an associated language disorder. *Neurology, 31,* 1016.

Glista, G. G., Frank, H. G., & Tracy, F. W. (1983). Video games and seizures. *Archives of Neurology, 40,* 588.

Gloor, P., & Feindel, W. (1963). The temporal lobe and affective behavior. In M. Monnier (Ed.), *Physiologie des Vegetativen Nerven Systems,* Volume 2 (pp. 723–741). Stuttgart: Hippokrates-Verlag.

Gloor, P., Olivier, A., Quesney, L. F., Andermann, F., & Horowitz, S. (1982). The role of the limbic system in experiential phenomena of temporal lobe epilepsy. *Annals of Neurology, 12,* 129.

Goddard, G. V. (1983). The kindling model of epilepsy. *Trends in Neurosciences, 7,* 11–23.

Goon, Y., Robinson, S., & Levy, S. (1973). Electroencephalographic changes in schizophrenic patients. *Israeli Annals of Psychiatry and Related Disciplines, 1*(1), 99.

Green, J. B. (1984). Pilomotor seizures. *Neurology, 34,* 837–839.

Hamilton, N. G., & Matthews, T. (1979). Aphasia: The sole manifestation of focal status epilepticus. *Neurology, 29,* 745.

Hebb, D. O. (1966). *A textbook of psychology.* Philadelphia: W. B. Saunders.

Hermann, B. P., & Riel, P. (1981). Interictal personality and behavioral traits in temporal lobe and generalized epilepsy. *Cortex, 17,* 125.

Hermann, B. P., & Melyn, M. (1984). Effects of carbamazepine on interictal psychopathology in TLE with ictal fear. *Journal of Clinical Psychiatry, 45,* 169–171.

Hermann, B. P., Whitman, S., & Arntson, P. (1983). Hypergraphia in epilepsy: Is there a specificity to temporal lobe epilepsy? *Journal of Neurology, Neurosurgery and Psychiatry, 46,* 848.

Hermann, B. P., Whitman, S., Wyler, A. R., Richey, E. T., & Dell, J. (1988). The neurological, psychosocial, and demographic correlates of hypergraphia in patients with epilepsy. *J. Neurology Neurosurgery, and Psychiatry, 51,* 203–208.

Herzog, A. G. (1988). Clomiphene therapy in epileptic women with menstrual disorders. *Neurology, 38,* 432–434.

Herzog, A. G. (1989). A hypothesis to integrate partial seizures of temporal lobe origin and reproductive endocrine disorders. *Epilepsy Research, 3,* 151–159.

Herzog, A. G., Seibel, M. M., Schomer, D. L., Vaitukaitis, J. L., & Geschwind, N. (1986a). Reproductive endocrine disorders in women with partial seizures of temporal lobe origin. *Archives in Neurology, 43,* 341–346.

Herzog, A. G., Seibel, M. M., Schomer, D. L., Vaitukaitis, J. L., & Geschwind, N. (1986b). Reproductive endocrine disorders in men with partial seizures of temporal lobe origin. *Archives of Neurology, 43,* 347–350.

Hirsch, C., & Martin, D. (1971). Unexpected death in young epileptics. *Neurology, 21,* 682–690.

Iivanainen, M., Bergstrom, L., Nuitila, A., & Viukari, M. (1984). Psychosis-like absence status of elderly patients: Successful treatment with sodium valproate. *Journal of Neurology, Neurosurgery, & Psychiatry, 47,* 965–969.

Ives, J., Schachter, S., Drislane, F., Miles, D., & Schomer, D. L. (1990). Comparison of sphenoidal electrode and surface EEGs during focal temporal lobe seizures. In *Proceedings of the American Epilepsy Society.* San Diego: American Epilepsy Society.

Jabbari, B., Gunderson, C. H., Wippold, F., Citrin, C., Sherman, J., Bartoszek, D., Daigh, J. D., & Mitchell, M. H. (1986). Magnetic resonance imaging in partial complex epilepsy. *Archives of Neurology, 43,* 869–872.

Jacome, D. E., & Risko, M. S. (1983). Absence status manifested by compulsive masturbation. *Archives of Neurology, 40,* 523–524.

Jasper, H. H., & Van Gelder, N. (Eds.). (1983). *Basic mechanisms of neuronal hyperexcitability.* New York: Alan R. Liss.

Jay, G., & Leetsma, J. (1981). Sudden death in epilepsy. *Acta Neurologica Scandinavica, 63*(Supplement 82), 1–66.

Jenike, M. A., & Brotman, A. W. (1984). The EEG in obsessive–compulsive disorder. *Journal of Clinical Psychiatry*, *45*, 122–124.

Keilson, M. J., Hauser, W. A., Magrill, J. P., & Goldman, M. (1987). ECG abnormalities in patients with epilepsy. *Neurology*, *37*, 1624–1626.

Kogeorgos, J., Fonagy, P., & Scott, D. F. (1982). Psychiatric symptom patterns of chronic epileptics attending a neurological clinic: A controlled investigation. *British Journal of Psychiatry*, *140*, 236.

Kristensen, O., & Sindrup, E. H. (1979). Psychomotor epilepsy and psychoses: III. Social and psychological correlates. *Acta Neurologica Scandinavica*, *59*, 1.

Krnjevic, K. (1983). GABA-mediated inhibitory mechanisms in relation to epileptic discharges. In H. H. Jasper & N. Van Gelder (Eds.), *Basic mechanisms of neuronal hyperexcitability* (pp. 270–299). New York: Alan R. Liss.

Kuhn, T. S. (1962). *The structure of scientific revolutions*. Chicago: University of Chicago Press.

Laidlaw, J. (1956). Catamenial epilepsy. *Lancet*, *271*, 1235–1237.

Landsborough, D. (1987). St. Paul and temporal lobe epilepsy. *Journal of Neurology, Neurosurgery and Psychiatry*, *50*, 659–664.

Laplante, P., Sainte-Hilaire, J. M., & Bouvier, G. (1983). Headache as an epileptic manifestation. *Neurology*, *33*, 1493.

Lesser, R. P., Lueders, H., Conomy, J P., Furlan, A. J., & Dinner, D. S. (1983). Sensory seizure mimicking a psychogenic seizure. *Neurology*, *33*, 800.

Lewis, D. O., Feldman, M., Greene, M., & Martinze-Mustardo, Y. (1984). Psychomotor epileptic symptoms in six patients with bipolar mood disorders. *American Journal of Psychiatry*, *141*, 1583–1586.

Lifshitz, R., & Gradijan, J. (1974). Spectral evaluation of the electroencephalogram: Power and variability in chronic schizophrenics and control subjects. *Psychophysiology*, *11*, 479.

Lim, J., Yagnik, P., Schraeder, P., & Wheeler, S. (1986). Ictal catatonia as a manifestation of nonconvulsive status epilepticus. *Journal of Neurology, Neurosurgery, & Psychiatry*, *49*, 833–836.

Logsdail, S. J., & Toone, B. K. (1988). Post-ictal psychoses: A clilnical and phenomenological description. *British Journal of Psychiatry*, *152*, 246–252.

Maletzky, B. (1973). The episodic dyscontrol syndrome. *Diseases of the Nervous System*, *34*, 178–185.

Marshall, D. W., Westmoreland, B. R., & Sharbrough, F. W. (1983). Ictal tachycardia during temporal lobe seizures. *Proceedings of the Mayo Clinic*, *58*, 443.

Mallanby, J., Strawbridge, P., Collingridge, G. I., George, G., Rands, G., Stroud, C., & Thompson, P. (1981). Behavioral correlates of an experimental hippocampal epileptiform syndrome in rats. *Journal of Neurology, Neurosurgery, & Psychiatry*, *44*, 1084.

Mark, V. H., & Swelt, W. H. (1974). The role of limbic brain dysfunction in aggression. In S. H. Frazier (Ed.), *Aggression*. Baltimore: Williams & Wilkins.

Mark, V. H. (1982). Epilepsy and episodic aggression. Letters to the editor. *Archives of Neurology*, *39*, 384.

Master, D. R., Toone, B. K., & Scott, D. F. (1984). Interictal behavior in temporal lobe epilepsy. In R. J. Porter (Ed.), *Advances in Epileptology: XVth International Symposium* (pp. 557–565). New York: Raven Press.

Mendez, M. F., Cummings, J. L., & Benson, D. F. (1986). Depression in epilepsy. *Archives of Neurology*, *43*, 766–770.

Mesulam, M.-M. (1981). Dissociative states with abnormal temporal lobe EEG: Multiple personality and the illusion of possession. *Archives of Neurology*, *38*, 176.

Mesulam, M.-M. (1985). Patterns in behavioral neuroanatomy: Association areas, the limbic system, and hemispheric specialization. In M.-M. Mesulam (Ed.), *Principles of behavioral neurology* (pp. 1–58). New York: F. A. Davis.

Mitchell, W. G., Grenwood, R. S., & Mersenheimer, J. A. (1983). Abdominal epilepsy: Cyclic vomiting as the major symptom of simple partial seizures. *Archives of Neurology*, *40*, 251.

Monroe, R. R. (1982). Limbic ictus and atypical psychoses. *Journal of Nervous and Mental Disorders*, *170*, 711.

136   PAUL A. SPIERS *et al.*

Morrell, F. (1988). Secondary epileptogenic lesions in man: Extent of the evidences. In A. V. Delgado-Escueta (Ed.), *Basic mechanism of the epilepsies* (pp. 115–165). New York: Raven Press.

Morselli, P., Lloyd, K., Loscher, W., Meldrum, B., & Reynolds, E. (Eds.). (1981). *Neurotransmitters, seizures and epilepsy.* New York: Raven Press.

Mostofsky, D. A., & Balaschak, B. (1977). Psychobiological control of seizures. *Psychological Bulletin, 84*(4), 723–750.

Mungas, D. (1982). Interictal behavior abnormality in temporal lobe epilepsy: A specific syndrome or nonspecific pathology. *Archives of General Psychiatry, 39,* 108.

Nakada, T., Lee, H., Kwee, I. L., & Lerner, A. M. (1984). Epileptic Kluver–Bucy syndrome: Case report. *Journal of Clinical Psychiatry, 45,* 87–88.

Newman, P. K., & Longley, B. P. (1984). Reading epilepsy. *Archives of Neurology, 41,* 13.

Ounsted, C., & Lindsay, M. (1966). Biological factors in temporal lobe epilepsy. *Clinics in Developmental Medicine, 22,* 17–39.

Peled, R., Harnes, B., Borovich, B., & Sharf, B. (1984). Speech arrest and supplementary motor area seizures. *Neurology, 34,* 110.

Pellegrini, A., Lippmann, S. B., Crump, G., & Manshadi, M. (1984). Psychiatric aspects of complex partial seizures: Case report. *Journal of Clinical Psychiatry, 45,* 269–271.

Penfield, W., & Jasper, H. (1954). *Epilepsy and the functional anatomy of the human brain.* Boston: Little, Brown.

Peppercorn, M. A., Herzog, A. G., & Dichter, M. A. (1978). Abdominal epilepsy: A cause of abdominal pain in adults. *Journal of the American Medical Association, 240,* 2450.

Perez, M., & Trimble, M. R. (1980). Epileptic psychosis: diagnostic comparison with process schizophrenia. *British Journal of Psychiatry, 137,* 245.

Plesner, A. M., Munk-Andersen, E., & Luhdorf, K. (1987). Epileptic aphasia and dysphoria interpreted as endogenous depression. *Acta Neurologica Scandinavica, 76,* 215–218.

Purpura, D., Penry, J., & Walter, R. (Eds.). (1975). *Neurosurgical management of the epilepsies. Advances in Neurology,* Volume 8 (p. 155). New York: Raven Press.

Ramani, V. (1983). Primary reading epilepsy. *Archives of Neurology, 40,* 39.

Ramani, V., & Gumnit, R. J. (1982). Intensive of monitoring of the interictal psychosis of epilepsy. *Annals of Neurology, 11,* 613.

Rasmussen, T. (1979). Cortical resection for medically refractory focal epilepsy: Results, lessons and questions. In T. Rasmussen & R. Marino (Eds.), *Functional neurosurgery* (pp. 68–87). New York: Raven Press.

Reder, A. T., & Wright, F. S. (1982). Epilepsy evoked by eating: The role of peripheral input. *Neurology, 32,* 1065–1069.

Remillard, G. M., Andermann, F., & Gloor, P. (1981). Water-drinking as ictal behavior in complex-partial seizures. *Neurology, 31,* 117.

Remillard, G. M., Andermann, F., Tosta, G. F., Gloor, P., Aube, M., Martin, J. B., Feindel, W., Guberman, A., & Simpson, C. (1983). Sexual ictal manifestations predominant in women with temporal lobe epilepsy: A finding suggesting sexual dimorphism in the human brain. *Neurology, 33,* 323.

Riley, T. L., & Massey, E. W. (1980). The syndrome of aphasia, headaches, and left temporal lobe spikes. *Headache, 20,* 90.

Robb, P. (1975). Focal epilepsy: The problem, prevalence, and contributing factors. In D. Purpura, J. K. Penry, & R. D. Walter (Eds.), *Neurosurgical Management of the Epilepsies* (pp. 11–31). New York: Raven Press.

Robertson, M. M., & Trimble, M. R. (1983). Depressive illness in patients with epilepsy: A review. *Epilepsia, 24* (Supplement 2), S109.

Rodin, E., & Schmaltz, S. (1984). The Bear-Fedio Inventory and temporal lobe epilepsy. *Neurology, 34,* 591–596.

Rodin, E., Schmaltz, S., & Twitty, G. (1984). What does the Bear-Fedio inventory measure? In R. J. Porter (Ed.), *Advances in Epileptology: XVth International Symposium* (pp. 551–555). New York: Raven Press.

Roemer, R. A., Shagass, C., Straumanis, J. J., & Amaded, M. (1978). Pattern evoked potential measurements suggesting laterialized hemispheric dysfunction in chronic schizophrenics. *Biological Psychiatry, 13*, 185.

Rose, D. F., Sato, S., Smith, P. D., Porter, R. J., Theodore, W. H., Friauf, W., Bonner, R., & Jabbari, B. (1987). Localization of magnetic interictal discharges in temporal lobe epilepsy. *Annals of Neurology, 22*, 348–354.

Rosenbaum, A. H., & Barry, M. J. (1975). Positive therapeutic response to lithium in hypomania secondary to organic brain syndrome. *American Journal of Psychiatry, 132*, 1072–1073.

Rosenbaum, D. H., Siegel, M., Barr, W. D., & Rowan, J. A. (1986). Epileptic aphasia. *Neurology, 36*, 822–825.

Sachdev, H. S., & Waxman, S. G. (1981). Frequency of hypergraphia in temporal lobe epilepsy: An index of interictal behaviors syndrome. *Journal of Neurology, Neurosurgery, & Psychiatry, 44*, 358.

Sagar, H. J., & Oxbury, J. M. (1987). Hippocampal neuron loss in temporal lobe epilepsy: correlation with early childhood convulsions. *Annals of Neurology, 22*, 334–340.

Schwartzkroin, P. (1983). Local circuit considerations and intrinsic neuronal properties involved in hyperexcitability and cell synchronization. In H. Jasper & N. Van Gelder (Eds.), *Basic mechanisms of neuronal hyperexcitability* (pp. 236–249). New York: Alan R. Liss.

Schwartzkroin, P., Mutani, R., & Prince, D. A. (1975). Orthodromic and antidromic effects of a cortical epileptiform focus on ventrolateral nucleus of the cat. *Neurophysiology, 38*, 795.

Shalev, R. S., & Amir, N. (1983). Complex partial status epilepticus. *Archives of Neurology, 40*, 90.

Shallice, T. (1979). Case study approach in neuropsychological research. *Journal of Clinical Neuropsychology, 1*, 183–211.

Sherwin, I. (1981). Psychosis associated with epilepsy: Significance of the laterality of the epileptogenic lesion. *Journal of Neurology, Neurosurgery and Psychiatry, 44*, 83.

Silberman, E. K., Post, R. M., Nurnberger, J., Theodore, W., & Boulenger, J.-P. (1985). Transient sensory, cognitive, and affective phenomena in affective illness: A comparison with complex partial epilepsy. *British Journal of Psychiatry, 146*, 81–89.

Slater, E., & Beard, A. W. (1963). The schizophrenic-like psychoses of epilepsy. *British Journal of Psychiatry, 109*, 95.

Somerville, E. R., & Bruni, J. (1983). Tonic status epilepticus presenting as confusional state. *Annals of Neurology, 13*, 549–551.

Sorensen, A. S., Hansen, H., Andersen, R., Hogenhaven, H., Aleerup, P. & Bolwig, T. G. (1989). Personality characteristics and epilepsy. *Acta Psychiatrica Scandinavica, 80*, 620–631.

Spiers, P. A. (1981). Have they come to praise Luria or to bury him? The Luria–Nebraska Battery controversy. *Journal of Consulting and Clinical Psychology, 49*, 331–341.

Spiers, P. A. (1982). The Luria–Nebraska Battery revisited: A theory in practice or just practicing? *Journal of Consulting and Clinical Psychology, 50*, 301–306.

Spiers, P. A., Schomer, D. L., Blume, H. W., & Mesulam, M.-M. (1985). Temporolimbic epilepsy and behavior. In M.-M. Mesulam (Ed.), *Principles of Behavioral Neurology* (pp. 170–195). New York: F. A. Davis.

Stein, T. A., & Murray, G. B. (1984). Complex partial seizures presenting as a psychiatric illness. *Journal of Nervous and Mental Disease, 172*(10), 625–627.

Stevens, J. R., & Hermann, B. P. (1981). Temporal lobe epilepsy, psychopathology, and violence: The state of the evidence. *Neurology, 31*, 1127.

Stevens, J. R., & Livermore, A. (1982). Telemetred in schizophrenia: Spectral analysis during abnormal behaviour episodes. *Journal of Neurology, Neurosurgery and Psychiatry, 45*, 385.

Strauss, E., Risser, A., & Jones, M. W. (1982). Fear responses in patients with epilepsy. *Archives of Neurology, 39*, 626.

Strauss, E., Wada, J., & Kosaka, B. (1983). Spontaneous facial expressions occuring at onset of focal seizure activity. *Archives of Neurology, 40*, 545.

Sutherling, W. W., Crandall, P. H., Engel, J., Darcey, T. M., Cahan, L. D., & Barth, D. S. (1987). The magnetic field of complex-partial seizures agress with intracranial localizations. *Annals of Neurology, 1*, 548–558.

Tarrier, N., Cooke, E. C., & Lader, M .H. (1978). The EEGs of chronic schizophrenic patients in hospitals and in the community. *Electroencephalography and Clinical Neurophysiology*, *44*, 669.

Taylor, D. C. (1975). Factors influencing the occurrence of schizophrenia-like psychosis in patients with temporal lobe epilepsy. *Psychological Medicine*, *5*, 249.

Taylor, D. C., & Lochery, M. (1987). Temporal lobe epilepsy: Origin and significance of simple and complex auras. *Journal of Neurology, Neurosurgery, and Psychiatry*, *50*, 673–681.

Terrence, C., Wisotzkey, H., & Perper, J. (1975). Unexpected, unexplained death in epileptic patients. *Neurology*, *25*, 594–598.

Terzano, M. G., Parrino, L., Manzoni, G. C., & Mancia, D. (1983). Seizures triggered by blinking when beginning to speak. *Archives of Neurology*, *40*, 103–106.

Theodore, W. H., Brooks, R., Sato, S., Patronas, N., Margolin, R., Di Chiro, G., & Porter, R. J. (1984). The role of positron emission tomography in the evaluation of seizure disorders. *Annals of Neurology*, *15* (Supplement), S176-S179.

Toone, B. K., Garralda, M. E., & Ron, M. A. (1982). The psychoses of epilepsy and the functional psychoses: A clinical and phenomenological comparison. *British Journal of Psychiatry*, *141*, 256.

Trevathian, E., & Cascino, G. D. (1988). Partial epilepsy presenting as focal paroxysmal pain. *Neurology*, *38*, 329–330.

Valmier, J., Touchon, J., Daures, P., Zanca, M., & Baldy-Moulinier, M. (1987). Correlations between cerebral blood flow variations and clinical parameters in temporal lobe epilepsy: An interictal study. *Journal of Neurology, Neurosurgery, and Psychiatry*, *50*, 1306–1311.

Van Buren, J. M. (1961). Sensory, motor, and autonomic effects of mesial temporal stimulation in man. *Journal of Neurosurgery*, *18*, 273.

Van Buren, J. M., & Ajmone-Marasan, C. (1960). A correlation of autonomic and EEG components in temporal lobe epilepsy. *Archives of Neurology*, *3*, 683.

Vidaihet, M., Serdaru, M., & Agid, Y. U. (1989). Singing in the brain: A new form of complex-partial seizure? *Journal of Neurology, Neurosurgery, and Psychiatry*, *52*, 1306–1311.

Wall, M., Tuchman, M., & Mielke, D. (1985). Panic attacks and temporal lobe seizures associated with a right temporal lobe arteriovenous malformation: A case report. *Journal of Clinical Psychiatry*, *46*, 143–145.

Wang, R. K., & Traub, R. D. (1988). Cellular mechanisms for neuronal synchronization in epilepsy. In A. V. Delgado-Escueta (Ed.), *Basic mechanisms of the epilepsies* (pp. 97–111). New York: Raven Press.

Waterman, K., Purves, S. J., Kosaka, B., Strauss, E., & Wada, J. A. (1987). An epileptic syndrome caused by mesial frontal lobe seizure foci. *Neurology*, *37*, 577–582.

Waxman, S. G., & Geschwind, N. (1975). The interictal behavior syndrome of temporal lobe epilepsy. *Archives of General Psychiatry*, *32*, 1580.

Weilburg, J. B., Bear, D. M., & Sachs, G. (1987). Three patients with concomitant panic attacks and seizure disorder: Possible clues to the neurology of anxiety. *American Journal of Psychiatry*, *144*(8), 1053–1056.

Weiser, H. G. (1983). Depth recorded limbic seizures and psychopathology. *Neuroscience and Biobehavior Review*, *7*, 427.

Werner, H. (1948). *Comparative psychology of mental development* (rev. ed.). Chicago: Follett.

Wilkins, A. J., Zifkin, B., Andermann, F., & McGovern, E. (1982). Seizures induced by thinking. *Annals of Neurology*, *11*, 608–612.

Wilson, A., Petty, R., Perry, A., & Rose, F. C. (1983). Paroxysmal language disturbance in an epileptic treated with clobazam. *Neurology*, *33*, 652–654.

Woodbury, D. M., Penry, J. K., & Peppenger, C. E. (Eds.). (1982). *Antiepileptic drugs* (2nd ed.). New York: Raven Press.

Young, G. B., & Blume, W. T. (1983). Painful epileptic seizures. *Brain*, *106*, 537.

7

Behavioral Syndromes in Epilepsy
A Multivariate, Empirical Approach

DAN M. MUNGAS

There has been considerable controversy about the association of a specific syndrome of behavior and temporal lobe elilepsy, and this chapter addresses that issue from both a conceptual and an empirical perspective. Previous literature relating to this controversy is reviewed, with particular attention to conceptual and methodological implications for studies to more definitively answer unresolved questions. A study in which an attempt was made to empirically identify behaviorally homogeneous subgroups of patients with epilepsy is presented. Subgroups of a general epilepsy population were derived using cluster analysis procedures and a theoretically derived approach to group definition, and resulting subgroups are compared on seizure, neurological, demographic, behavioral/psychiatric/personality, and past history variables.

HISTORICAL BACKGROUND

Epilepsy is a relatively common disorder that has been recognized throughout recorded history. By virtue of their dramatic, even mystifying presentation, epileptic seizures have historically been poorly understood, and individuals with epilepsy have been widely regarded as deviant (Temkin, 1971), a view often based on ignorance about the disorder in the absence of a scientific body of fact. Over the last half century

DAN M. MUNGAS • Alzheimer's Disease Diagnostic and Treatment Center, University of California, Davis Medical Center, Sacramento, California 95817.

The Neuropsychology of Epilepsy, edited by Thomas L. Bennett. Plenum Press, New York, 1992.

our scientific understanding of epilepsy has dramatically increased, with two major advances making primary contributions. First, the development of the electro-encephalogram (EEG) made possible the objective identification of events within the brain that were associated with seizures and thus provided a crucial diagnostic tool. Second, the development of anticonvulsant medication led to an increasing under-standing of and ability to control seizures, allowing epilepsy to be viewed more as a physical disorder and less as a religious or moral affliction.

The term "epileptic personality" arose near the beginning of the 20th century to describe a pattern of behavior that was felt to be common in epilepsy. This term encompassed characteristics including slowed and perseverative thinking and ego-centric, aggressive, and intrusive interpersonal behavior. This concept was derived almost exclusively from the study of institutionalized populations, where severe forms of epilepsy with marked associated structural brain damage were prominent. The term "epileptic personality" fell out of favor when it was recognized that its purported manifestations were largely a reflection of the relatively severe brain pathology represented in institutional settings and were rarely observed outside of an institutional setting (Lennox & Lennox, 1960).

The "epileptic personality" lost favor, but before fading from awareness it resurfaced in the form of the "temporal lobe epileptic personality." The work of Gibbs and Gibbs (Gibbs, Gibbs, & Fuster, 1948; Gibbs & Gibbs, 1964) provided a major impetus for this conversion. Their extensive *Atlas of Electroencephalography* showed a marked increase of psychopathology associated with psychomotor epilepsy. Several lines of emerging research provided a potentially exciting theoretical explana-tion for this finding. First, with the developing body of neurobiological research on epilepsy came the delineation of temporal lobe, limbic system structures that are frequently the foci of temporal lobe seizures. Second, a large body of research established the importance of the limbic system for mediating emotion. The occur-rence of ictal psychomotor seizure phenomena resembling frank psychiatric symp-toms and research showing dramatic alterations of emotionality and behavior associ-ated with interventions involving the limbic system converged in furthering a model for how temporal lobe seizures could be related to psychopathological manifestations. Viewed in this emerging perspective, temporal lobe epilepsy (TLE) was regarded as a very promising model for facilitating our understanding of the neurobiological basis of abnormal behavior (Stevens, 1966). Within this background came a proliferation of literature, often case reports or uncontrolled studies, showing a broad range of psychopathology in individuals with TLE. Indeed, as described by Stevens (1975), nearly every negative characteristic known to man has been attributed to individuals with TLE.

The convergence of clinical findings and laboratory research provided an exciting and compelling model for understanding the relationship between TLE and behavior, but unfortunately, another body of research was emerging that failed to support the association between temporal lobe seizure disorders and increased psychopathology. A number of controlled studies comparing groups of individuals with temporal lobe or psychomotor epilepsy with appropriately matched groups of individuals with other forms of epilepsy failed to find significant differences (e.g.,

Mathews & Klove, 1968; Mignone, Donnelly, & Sadowsky, 1970; Rodin, Katz, & Lennox, 1976; Small, Millstein, & Stevens, 1962; Standage & Fenton, 1975). Confounding factors that could contribute to the previously reported positive results were identified, such as socioeconomic status, age, and type of medical setting from which samples were obtained (Stevens, 1982), but the net result of the conflicting bodies of research was a heated controversy that has continued to date.

Two highly influential publications in the mid-1970s presented a refinement of the concept of a TLE personality along with arguments to account for the lack of positive evidence from controlled studies. Waxman and Geschwind (1975) described a syndrome of specific behaviors that they felt were directly related to TLE and provided insight into the neuropsychological mechanisms underlying the disorder. Instead of attributing widespread psychopathology to TLE, they focused on three specific traits (hypergraphia, religiosity, and altered sexual behavior) and, in so doing, provided a theoretical model more amenable to being empirically tested.

A second study by Bear and Fedio (1977) continued the attempt to define the TLE personality in a more specific manner. They hypothesized that the lack of positive results from controlled studies resulted from insensitivity of the instruments used to the specific changes in behavior that occur as a consequence of TLE. In particular, they noted that most of the available controlled studies had used traditional measures of psychopathology, such as the Minnesota Multiphasic Personality Inventory (MMPI), and they felt that many of the specific behavior characteristics associated with TLE may not be psychopathological in nature (for example, hypergraphia). They reviewed previous literature examining behavioral characteristics of individuals with TLE and identified 18 separate traits that had had previous support. They then developed an inventory to assess these traits that consisted of five items for each of the 18 traits and an additional 10 items from the MMPI L scale, which were included to control for nonspecific response bias. A version of this instrument was developed to be filled out by patients themselves, and an equivalent version was developed to be completed by an external observer, typically a family member or friend familiar with the patient. This instrument was then used in a study involving four groups: (1) a group of individuals with TLE with a unilateral right temporal lobe focus, (2) a TLE group with a unilateral right temporal lobe focus, (3) a control group consisting of individuals with chronic neurological disease but without epilepsy, and (4) a group of normal controls. They found that the TLE groups were clearly differentiated from the non-TLE groups and, further, that a few variables significantly discriminated the left and right TLE groups.

Bear and Fedio (1977) concluded that these results provided strong evidence of a specific TLE personality syndrome and that their hypothesis about the insensitivity of previously used measures had been verified. Results were interpreted in the context of a theory of "sensory–limbic hyperconnection," which proposed that interictal EEG spikes within temporal lobe, limbic system structures were reflective of a neural process in which incoming stimuli were accorded undue emotional significance, resulting in characteristic changes of emotions and behavior (Bear & Fedio, 1977; Bear, 1979). This study has been widely cited and has been extremely influential in the field. Geschwind (1977), in an editorial in the journal issue in which the study was published, described this study as one of the most important pieces of research that had appeared in recent years.

The Bear and Fedio study had a number of positive features, most notably the systematic attempt to define the TLE personality syndrome in a more specific and testable manner and the intriguing theoretical model to account for the observed findings. Another clear contribution was the instrument, which allowed measurement of theoretically relevant behavioral traits. This subsequently facilitated a number of studies using their instrument or a similar approach, which allowed for a broader understanding of the relationship between TLE and behavior. These subsequent studies also pointed out major weaknesses in the methodology and conclusions of the Bear and Fedio study but, in so doing, may point the way for further research that will more definitively describe the relationship among temporal lobe epilepsy, its underlying neurological substrate, and behavior.

The clearest conclusion that can be drawn from research using the Bear and Fedio instrument or a similar approach is that there has been a very striking lack of positive verification of their findings or, indeed, of any consistent positive findings across studies. Studies have focused on several different questions, including (1) do individuals with TLE differ from normals, (2) do TLE patients differ from individuals with other forms of epilepsy, (3) do TLE patients differ from psychiatric and neurological groups without TLE but with manifest psychopathology, and (4) is there a difference between TLE patients with left and right seizure foci? These questions provide critical information regarding the causal relationship between TLE and behavior and also answer important questions about the Bear and Fedio Inventory and what it measures.

Patients with TLE clearly scored higher than normals across most traits in the Bear and Fedio (1977) study and in a study using the Bear and Fedio Inventory by Rodin and Schmaltz (1984). In contrast, the Bear and Fedio inventory was used in studies by Brandt, Seidman, and Kohl (1985) and Seidman (1980) with much weaker results. In the Brandt *et al.* study, only 5 of 18 variables discriminated a left TLE group from normals, while none of the variables discriminated a right TLE group from normals. Seidman found eight self-report and six rater variables that discriminated a TLE group from normal controls. When comparing patients with TLE with psychiatric controls, two studies have shown no significant differences (Mungas, 1982; Rodin & Schmaltz, 1984), and one, using a structured interview format for assessing most of the traits from the Bear and Fedio Inventory, showed significant differences on 7 of 14 variables (Bear, Levin, Blumer, Chetham, & Ryder, 1982).

Four studies have compared temporal lobe and generalized epilepsy groups. One showed significant differences on 4 of 18 variables (Hermann & Riel, 1981), whereas one showed differences on only 1 of 18 variables (Rodin & Schmaltz, 1984). Brandt *et al.* (1985) found differences on 2 of 18 variables, but the generalized epilepsy group was significantly more elevated on both. Bear *et al.* (1982) found differences on 4 of 14 variables using their structured interview. What is particularly striking is that only one variable, philosophical interest, significantly differentiated TLE and generalized epilepsy groups in two studies, and no variable showed overlap across more than two studies.

The picture for comparisons between left and right TLE groups is even more unfavorable. In five studies (Bear & Fedio, 1977; Brandt *et al.*, 1985; Nielsen & Kristensen, 1981; Rodin & Schmaltz, 1984; Seidman, 1980) in which such comparisons have been made using both self-report (all five studies) and rater (three of the five) data (143 comparisons overall), only 12 individual comparisons (8%) have been statistically significant. Obsessionalism was greater for the left group for both self-report and rater data in the Seidman study but was found to be greater for the right group using rater data from the Bear and Fedio study. No other comparisons were replicated across studies or within studies across self-report and rater data. Further, Bear and Fedio's finding that patients with right TLE underreported symptoms in comparison with raters was not replicated by Rodin and Schmaltz.

There has also been a lack of consistent positive findings using different methods to assess specific traits purported to be associated with TLE. Sachdev and Waxman (1981) studied the relationship between TLE and hypergraphia in a more naturalistic manner by writing to patients with epilepsy and asking them to reply to a question about their health and effects and understanding of their seizure disorder. More of the TLE patients than non-TLE epilepsy patients were responders, wrote significantly longer letters, and manifested more of the interictal syndrome in the content of their responses. This finding was not replicated in a similar study by Hermann, Whitman, and Arnston (1983). The relationship between religiosity and TLE was studied by Tucker, Novelly, and Walker (1987), with results failing to differentiate left and right TLE groups from each other or from non-TLE comparison groups. A recent study by Hermann, Whitman, Wyler, Richey, and Dell (1988) examined the relationship between TLE and two measures of hypergraphia. Hypergraphia was not related to a temporal lobe seizure focus, although it did show multidimensional correlates with other variables, particularly measures of psychopathology.

The research reviewed above has provided little empirical support for a specific syndrome of behavior associated with TLE, and to a large extent, our substantive knowledge of the relationship between TLE and behavior has not substantially increased since the publication of the Bear and Fedio (1977) paper. On the other hand, this body of research has served as an important catalyst for identifying and stimulating discourse on theoretical and methodological issues that have important significance for our ultimate understanding of the relationship between the brain and behavior. A number of these important issues are reviewed.

CONCEPTUAL AND METHODOLOGICAL ISSUES AND IMPLICATIONS FOR FURTHER RESEARCH

Specification of the Temporal Lobe Epilepsy Personality Syndrome

Bear and Fedio (1977) and Waxman and Geschwind (1975) made an important theoretical contribution to the study of a specific behavior syndrome in TLE by narrowing the range of behavior of interest and focusing attention on particular characteristics that had been observed in clinical practice. The Waxman and Geschwind paper described a very specific theoretical model of the TLE personality syndrome, but unfortunately, their description was at a qualitative level without specific guidelines for assessing and quantifying the proposed characteristics. Bear and Fedio did provide instrumentation for assessing the traits within their formulation, but their study also had limitations. These included psychometric limitations of their instrument, which are discussed later, but also a more basic conceptual problem in that the 18 traits they identified encompassed a very broad range of behavior including a large number of categories of traditionally defined psychopathology. Inclusion of such a broad range of behavior tends to water down the significance of any "syndrome" that might be found.

In order for the concept of an interictal personality syndrome to be adequately studied, it must first be defined in such a manner that it can be objectively identified and thus empirically tested. This goes beyond just defining relevant personality characteristics. The interrelationships among specific personality characteristics and their potential relationship to etiological factors also need to be stated explicitly before the proposed syndrome can be empirically tested. The meaning of the term "syndrome," in particular, needs to be clearly specified. It has been suggested that it is a constellation of commonly elevated personality characteristics that defines a syndrome (Bear, 1983), as opposed to abnormalities in terms of individual characteristics. However, this has generally not been directly tested, with the typical research design involving between-group comparisons on a number of separate, individual variables.* This requires an underlying assumption that common group elevations are also likely to reflect common individual elevations, which may or may not be viable. Alternate research designs may be more appropriate for directly testing the presence of a proposed syndrome and are discussed below.

Measures of Personality

Controlled studies using traditional measures such as the MMPI and Rorschach Inkblot Test have typically failed to identify characteristics specific to TLE, which Bear and Fedio (1977) attributed to lack of sensitivity of these instruments to characteristics relevant to TLE, particularly those that are not necessarily psychopathological in nature. Indeed, this was a very important consideration in the development of their inventory, as they tried to construct an instrument designed specifically to assess TLE-relevant behavior. Although their criticism of traditional measures has potential value, it has to date not been adequately validated. In this regard, it is noteworthy that a number of the personality traits measured by the Bear and Fedio Inventory reflect classically psychopathological characteristics that are also measured by the MMPI, for example, depression, paranoia, and obsessionalism. Why the Bear and Fedio Inventory would present any advantage over the MMPI, or how the criticism of insensitivity of the MMPI for these characteristics would apply,

*When the number of commonly elevated traits has been directly assessed, there has been no evidence of an increased incidence of a "syndrome" in temporal lobe epilepsy (Mungas, 1983; Stark-Adamec & Adamec, 1986).

is not at all clear. More importantly, however, the Bear and Fedio Inventory has never been directly compared with other tests such as the MMPI in terms of relative sensitivity. Until it can be empirically demonstrated that the Bear and Fedio Inventory, or for that matter any other instrument, has discriminative power lacking in previously used tests, it seems premature to discount negative findings from controlled studies using those tests.

Regardless of the psychological test used, psychometric characteristics are important. The Bear and Fedio Inventory has been used in a number of studies and lends itself to use because it can be easily obtained. However, basic psychometric characteristics such as reliability and validity have not been adequately demonstrated. Reliability data are lacking, and, based on a large body of psychometric literature, it appears that having five items per scale is questionable in terms of establishing adequate levels of reliability.

With respect to validity, data regarding construct validity of the instrument are either notably lacking or negative. This test was developed using a relatively unsophisticated rational–intuitive construction strategy in which there was no attempt to demonstrate that the test was actually measuring 18 independent dimensions or to establish convergent and discriminant validity (Campbell & Fiske, 1959) of these dimensions. Indeed, data that are available, including a factor analysis reported in the initial study (Bear & Fedio, 1977), suggest that the instrument is strongly influenced by a compelling dimension of nonspecific psychopathology (Mungas, 1982; Rodin & Schmaltz, 1984) and has limited discriminative power beyond this general factor. Nonspecific influences in personality inventories have long been recognized in psychometric literature, and very sophisticated procedures have been developed to deal with this problem (Wiggins, 1973), but such procedures were not used in the development of the Bear and Fedio Inventory. When one goes beyond the issue of construct validity to other forms of validity, the body of literature comparing TLE groups with a variety of controls is predominantly either negative or strikingly inconsistent, as has been previously discussed.

In addition to the need for more clearly specifying relevant dimensions of the temporal lobe epilepsy personality syndrome, there is also a need for psychometrically sound measures of those dimensions. The influence of nonspecific factors needs to be considered in a particularly careful manner, not only in test construction but also in research design. It should be noted that use of items from the L Scale of the MMPI (Bear & Fedio, 1977; Brandt et al., 1985) is not an adequate correction for nonspecific response bias. This scale appears to be sensitive only to a relatively naive and unsophisticated response distortion in a positive direction and not to more subtle and prevalent response bias. Indeed, the MMPI K scale was developed as a result of inadequacies of the L scale for this purpose (Meehl & Hathaway, 1946).

Research Design

Subject Selection

It has been well documented in research on behavioral correlates of TLE that different findings emerge when sampling is from different populations. Lennox and

Lennox (1960) noted that the degree of behavioral and brain pathology seen in institutionalized epilepsy patients was not representative of the epilepsy population as a whole. Stevens (1966) has addressed the implications of selecting epileptic patients from psychiatric hospitals, and other studies have shown differences in psychopathology when comparing subjects from teaching hospitals associated with medical schools with those being followed in private practice settings (Stevens, 1975), presumably because the more difficult patients gravitate toward medical school settings. Significant differences have also been found in comparing patients with epilepsy who are receiving treatment with those not receiving treatment (Zielinski, 1974). More subtle factors might also be present. For example, when it is known that a particular investigator is conducting a study on behavioral characteristics of TLE, it is quite possible that patients with behavioral characteristics similar to those frequently posited are more likely to be referred by colleagues. Given the obvious potential for subject selection factors to influence results, it is crucial that careful consideration go into subject selection procedures and equally important that such procedures be carefully described in research reports so that the nature of the sample is well defined (cf. Hermann & Whitman, 1984).

Control Groups

Selection of control groups with which to compare TLE groups has profound implications for interpretation of results both at a clinical level and at a more theoretical, etiological level. Normal control groups are frequently employed, but they are of limited value for answering questions about behavioral characteristics associated with TLE that go beyond the presence or absence of abnormal behavior, in a normative sense.* In order to establish that certain characteristics are specific to TLE, other controls must also be used. The precise meaning of the term "specific" in this context has also been the subject of some discussion as to whether it refers to characteristics that are specific to or occur only in TLE or to a specific constellation or group of characteristics that occurs in TLE but may also be present in other disorders (Bear, 1983; Silberman, 1983). The latter usage is clearly less restrictive, but if it can be established that such a constellation occurs in TLE, that would be an important clinical and theoretical finding. However, even if such a "specific" constellation can be identified, a causal relationship between that constellation or syndrome and TLE cannot be established without some degree of specificity in the other sense of the term.

To the degree that such features are present in other disorders, other etiological hypotheses that may have no relationship to the neuroanatomical substrate of TLE are possible and need to be ruled out. It is possible that different disorders with shared behavioral features may point to a final common pathway in a neuroanatomical sense (Bear, 1983), but it becomes more complex and difficult to make such an argument

---

*When normal controls are used, careful attention must be paid to utilizing selection factors similar to those used in selecting patient groups (Hermann & Whitman, 1984) in order for valid inferences to be made.

when the behavioral features are found in increasingly diverse disorders. For example, if a symptom constellation could be found in common between TLE and unipolar depression but not between TLE and other psychopathological conditions, that might have important theoretical significance. On the other hand, if the constellation also applies to schizophrenia, anxiety disorders, and the borderline personality syndrome, then it becomes much more difficult to identify and support the notion of a final common pathway.

For these reasons, the selection of non-TLE control groups becomes critical with regard to any neurobiological inferences. Epileptics who do not have a temporal lobe seizure focus are particularly important for comparison purposes, as they allow for some determination of the significance of the seizure focus lying in the temporal lobes. There is a strong rationale for considering patients with temporal lobe plus generalized seizures separately from those with only temporal lobe seizures, since there appears to be greater behavioral pathology in the former (Rodin *et al.*, 1976). The technology for determining the presence of temporal lobe electrical abnormality is far from perfect in the sense that individuals who show no temporal lobe abnormality on one or several EEGs may indeed have temporal lobe abnormalities demonstrable at other times or by other methods, such as special leads or activation techniques. However, this methodological limitation does not negate the need to employ epilepsy groups without demonstrable temporal lobe EEG abnormalities. Even when the inadequacies of EEG criteria are considered, it is eminently reasonable to expect that there are valid differences between patients with and without temporal lobe EEG abnormalities, even though the validity is less than perfect.

Other control groups also have important theoretical significance. Psychiatric control groups consisting of patients with heterogeneous disorders can be valuable for ruling out influences of nonspecific psychopathology. Such groups are particularly important when instruments are used that, like the Bear and Fedio Inventory, are strongly influenced by nonspecific psychopathology. As previously discussed, there is also potential theoretical significance in determining if specific psychiatric syndromes share characteristics with TLE patients. Ultimately, utilizing both heterogeneous psychiatric groups to control for nonspecific effects and well-defined homogeneous groups of patients with specific psychiatric disorders might lead to the most meaningful results in this regard. Other kinds of control groups and extraneous variables that need to be controlled for are discussed by Hermann and Whitman (1984).

Research Design

The traditional design used to perform separate between-groups comparisons on a number of individual variables has limitations when one is concerned with a constellation of behavioral characteristics that purportedly occur together. It is possible for two groups to differ on all relevant variables being considered but for no common profile to exist across individuals from either group. This problem becomes more salient in dealing with groups that are heterogeneous by nature, and it seems clear that patients with TLE are a heterogeneous group whether or not a subgroup exists that manifests a specific behavioral syndrome. A more promising way of approaching this problem might be to first identify individuals who show a particular behavioral constellation and then compare these individuals with others without this constellation. In this manner, the hypothesis of a specific behavioral syndrome occurring in TLE could be tested by defining the relevant behavioral characteristics and how they relate to each other in defining the overall syndrome, identifying a homogeneous subgroup of epileptic patients (without regard to seizure focus) who manifest this syndrome, and then comparing this group with other groups, including seizure and nonseizure patients, to identify potential etiological variables. Cluster analysis procedures could be used to identify homogeneous subgroups in the absence of a clearly articulated theory, or alternatively, the syndrome could be defined on an *a priori* basis, and patients could be assigned to groups according to specific criteria derived from the history.

Statistical Considerations

The sample size of most previous research in the area has generally been characterized by 10–20 subjects per group. A relatively small sample size not only limits degrees of freedom for statistical tests and increases the probability of capitalizing on chance variation when using multivariate statistical procedures but also limits sensitivity or statistical power. For example, if 20% of patients with TLE manifest a specific behavioral syndrome (a figure most would probably agree is generous), only four subjects out of a group of 20 would be expected to show that syndrome. When the score is averaged in with the other subjects in the group, any specific behavioral features might well be obscured. Thus, in order to adequately represent the syndrome, one would need a much larger sample size so that a suitably sized group of patients with the specific syndrome could be identified. One of the advantages of studying epilepsy is that it is a relatively common disorder, so that it is clearly within the realm of reality to obtain larger samples than have typically been studied. The need to consider subjects manifesting a specific constellation of characteristics separately from others is still crucial even given a large sample size, since specific behavioral characteristics would be diluted by the larger number of subjects without the syndrome of interest regardless of sample size.

A second area where statistical considerations are important has to do with the judicious use of multivariate statistics. Personality research in general, and research on personality characteristics of patients with epilepsy in particular, tends to be multivariate in nature and lends itself to multivariate statistical procedures. When the ratio of sample size to number of variables is not adequately considered, the potential for capitalization on chance variation becomes quite problematic. The Bear and Fedio (1977) study has been used as an example of inappropriate usage of discriminant analysis in neuropsychological research (Fletcher, Rice, & Ray, 1978) for failure to take this ratio into account. This issue is far more than an academic debate about statistical assumptions, as the reproducibility of statistical findings is intimately dependent on the appropriate use of these very powerful multivariate procedures. As with all multivariate research, there is no substitute for an adequate sample size for the number of variables being tested or, preferably, for cross-validation of results.

EMPIRICAL SEARCH FOR SPECIFIC BEHAVIOR PATTERNS IN EPILEPSY

In the remainder of this chapter I describe some of the findings from a study conducted in collaboration with George Palma and Dale Blunden in which we have tried to address some of the as yet not satisfactorily answered questions about TLE and specific patterns of behavior. Our primary interest was to determine if it is possible to identify subgroups of patients with epilepsy that are homogeneous with respect to specific patterns of behavior or personality characteristics. In doing so, we attempted to take the conceptual and methodological issues previously discussed into account in designing the study and analyzing data.

Briefly, we obtained a sample of 75 outpatients of an epilepsy clinic who were selected only for a diagnosis of epilepsy and willingness to participate in the study and, in particular, were not selected with respect to variables such as seizure type or location. We then attempted to empirically derive homogeneous subgroups of this overall sample with respect to behavioral characteristics, with the goal of then comparing these subgroups in order to identify variables that show a specific relationship with these specific patterns of behavior. We used multiple measures assessed via multiple methods to assess behavioral characteristics, including the Bear and Fedio Inventory (BF), the MMPI, the Eysenck Personality Questionnaire (EPQ) (Eysenck & Eysenck, 1973), and a structural interview developed to assess behavioral characteristics that have been the focus of recent formulations of specific patterns of behavior in TLE. Using these multiple methods, we were able to compare directly different measures with respect to their relevance to epilepsy in general and TLE in particular. Use of multiple methods assessing a broad range of behavior allowed us to identify psychopathological as well as nonpsychopathological aspects of epilepsy and relatively specific kinds of behavior in addition to more nonspecific response tendencies. Instead of the more traditional research design in which groups are defined on an *a priori* basis, for example, by seizure type or location, we used cluster analysis to empirically identify behaviorally homogeneous subgroups. In this manner, an empirical approach to syndrome definition was followed. In this process, we made a concerted effort to maintain adequate subject-to-variable ratios and to ensure reproducibility of findings.

Methodology

Subjects

Subjects were outpatients who were being followed through the Neurology Clinic of the UC Davis Medical Center in Sacramento, California with an unequivocal diagnosis of epilepsy. This hospital is the teaching hospital for the UC Davis School of Medicine and serves a population that is similar in many ways to teaching hospitals in other urban areas. Inclusion criteria for subjects consisted of a diagnosis of epilepsy supported by a clinical history of seizures and an abnormal EEG consistent with a seizure disorder. Three subjects were included who had unequivocal clinical seizures but had normal EEG findings. Exclusion criteria were age less than 18, a history of mental retardation, or a documented IQ from an individually administered intelligence test of less than 80. In the initial phase of recruitment, patients were referred to the study by Neurology Department faculty and residents who were following them. Patients interested in participating were then contacted by study personnel and scheduled for subsequent procedures. A second phase of recruitment was also carried out to ensure that we reached as broad a range of this patient population as possible. A computerized data base of all patients being followed in this clinic with a diagnosis of epilepsy was used to generate a mailing list, and a request for volunteers was then mailed to all individuals on the list. Those interested in participating were asked to call and, on doing so, were scheduled for the rest of the study. Subjects were paid $20 for participation in the study.

A total of 80 subjects initially became involved in the study, compared with a total of about 210 subjects on the mailing list. Of the 80, five did not complete the self-report paper-and-pencil data collection procedures. This left a sample of 75 individuals with complete data. Demographic characteristics of the subject sample are shown in Table 7.1. Seizure variables and neurological variables are shown in Table 7.2.

Variables

Measures of Behavior and Personality. Multiple measures obtained from multiple methods of measurement were used to assess behavior and personality characteris-

TABLE 7.1.   Demographic Characteristics of Subject Sample

Age	Race
Mean: 38.8	White: 88%
S.D.: 12.5	Nonwhite: 12%
Range: 19–69	Marital status
Education	Single: 42%
Mean: 12.8	Married: 31%
S.D.: 2.6	Separated/divorced: 21%
Range: 2–20	Widow/widower: 6%
Monthly household income	Employment
Mean: 1,118.6	Full-time: 28%
S.D.: 1,449.1	Homemaker/full-time student: 4%
Range: 0–9,600	Part-time: 7%
Sex	Part-time student: 1%
Male: 50%	Unemployed: 60%
Female: 50%	

TABLE 7.2. Seizure Characteristics of Subject Sample

Seizure type[a]	Seizure diagnosis
Elementary partial: 12%	Temporal lobe: 36%
Elementary partial 2° generalized: 8%	Generalized: 11%
Complex partial: 62%	Other: 53%
Complex partial 2° generalized: 34%	Seizure etiology
Generalized convulsive: 34%	Idiopathic: 43%
Generalized nonconvulsive: 11%	Symptomatic: 57%
Epileptiform discharges	Number of anticonvulsant medications
Left temporal: 34%	0: 7%
Right temporal: 29%	1: 37%
Focal nontemporal: 19%	2: 32%
Generalized: 14%	3: 18%
Nonepileptiform discharges	4: 6%
Left temporal: 39%	Age of seizure onset
Right temporal: 33%	Mean: 21.1
Focal nontemporal: 11%	S.D.; 15.2
Generalized: 12%	Range: < 1–59
Seizure control	Duration of seizure disorder
Good: 42%	Mean; 17.8
Fair: 37%	S.D.: 13.1
Poor: 21%	Range: <1–54

[a]Percentages do not add to 100 becaues more than one category was possible for each subject.

tics. An attempt was made to include a broad range of measures of characteristics that have been attributed to patients with TLE as well as measures of psychopathology and normal personality. These data were obtained from self-report, from the report of a friend or relative of the subject, and from objective ratings made by research personnel. The specific instruments used were as follows.

1. MMPI. Variables used included the 10 clinical scales, the three validity scales, and two supplemental scales, the Ego Strength Scale (Barron, 1953) and the Goldberg Index (Goldberg, 1965). The 13 Wiggins Content Scales (Wiggins, 1966) were also scored and used in data analysis.
2. Bear and Fedio Inventory. A modified version of the Bear and Fedio Inventory, developed by Stark-Adamec and Adamec (1986a) to provide more favorable psychometric characteristics, was used to assess the 18 personality traits included in the inventory. This version used the same items but differed from the original mainly in that instead of a yes-or-no response to each item, a seven-point rating scale was used to indicate the degree to which that particular item was applicable. A self-report version of this inventory was filled out by patients, and in addition, a version for external raters was used to be completed by a friend or relative. At the time of initial contact with subjects, they were asked if they had a friend or relative who would be willing to come in and complete this survey and a brief interview about the subject's behavior. If so, this individual was then scheduled to come in for completion

of these procedures and was subsequently paid $5 for his or her participation. External rater data were obtained for 55 of the overall sample of 75 subjects.

3. EPQ. This is an instrument that has been developed to assess three dimensions of personality (neuroticism, psychoticism, and introversion–extraversion) that have been shown to have strong relevance to both normal and abnormal behavior (Eysenck & Eysenck, 1973). There is considerable clinical support for the reliability and validity of this instrument, and of particular interest, it has also been used in research exploring biological factors underlying personality.

4. Washington Psychosocial Seizure Inventory (WPSI) (Dodrill, Batzel, Queisser, & Temkin, 1980). This is a self-report instrument developed to assess the following dimensions of behavior relevant to individuals with epilepsy: family background, emotional adjustment, interpersonal adjustment, vocational adjustment, financial status, adjustment to seizures, medicine and medical management, overall psychosocial functioning, impairment, and intelligence.

5. Semistructured interview ratings of behavior. Ratings of the following eight behavior parameters were obtained within a structured interview format: (1) hypergraphia, (2) sexual interest/activity, (3) religious belief, (4) philosophical interest, (5) physical aggression, (6) verbal aggression, (7) viscosity/stickiness, and (8) circumstantiality. A semistructured interview was used in which a standardized group of questions was presented to assess each of these characteristics, with the interviewer being allowed to ask further probing questions to clarify answers. Each behavior was rated according to a five-point rating scale with specific guidelines for each rating. The structured interview format and the rating alternatives were patterned after the Schedule for Affective Disorders and Schizophrenia (SADS) (Endicott & Spitzer, 1978). This procedure was administered to all subjects, and a version for external observers was administered to the friend or relative who accompanied the subject. Independent ratings were made by the rater who administered the instrument and by three other independent raters who rated from an audiotape of the interview. With only one exception, the scores of all four raters were averaged in order to derive the score used in subsequent analyses. The one exception was the circumstantiality measure, where inadequate interrater reliabilities were obtained for one of the raters. For that variable, the ratings of the other three raters were used, and the final score was the average of the three raters. Interrater reliability was determined by comparing each pair of raters using Pearson correlation coefficients and then averaging the correlation coefficients across all of the combinations of raters. These average correlation coefficients were corrected for number of raters using the Spearman–Brown formula (Lord & Novick, 1968). The final, corrected interrater reliability estimate for the circumstantiality measure fell at a marginal level ($r = .62$), whereas all others were quite respectable: hypergraphia, .97; sexual interest/activity, .97; religious interest, .98; philosophical interest, .89; verbal aggression, .93; physical aggression, .94; and stickiness/viscosity, .81.

6. Schedule for Affective Disorders and Schizophrenia—Change Version (SADS-C) (Spitzer & Endicott, 1978). This instrument represents a subset of items from the SADS that assess symptoms of affective disorders and schizophrenia that have occurred in the past week. From these items, the following composite scales are derived: depressive syndrome, endogenous features, manic symptoms, anxiety, psychotic features, miscellaneous symptoms, Hamilton Rating Scale for Depression (HRSD), and sum of HRSD items. The latter two variables are based on the same items but use different procedures for assigning scores to each item. The SADS-C is administered in a semistructured interview format with specific, objective guidelines for rating each item.

Seizure and Neurological Variables. Data pertaining to the following seizure and neurological parameters were obtained from a review of each subject's medical records: (1) age of onset of seizures, (2) duration of seizures, (3) etiology (idiopathic versus symptomatic), (4) seizure control, (5) seizure type, (6) type and location of EEG abnormality, (7) rate of focal epileptiform discharges (EFD), (8) rate of generalized EFD, (9) amount of background slow-wave activity, (10) neurological exam (normal versus abnormal), (11) CT scan and other neuroradiological findings, (12) neurological diagnosis other than epilepsy, (13) blood levels of anticonvulsant medications, and (13) current psychiatric medications.

Seizure control was rated according to a three-point rating scale developed by Karnes and described by Hermann, Schwartz, Karnes, and Vahdat (1980) in which an overall rating is made according to both the frequency of seizures and their severity. All EEG data were abstracted from the report of clinical EEGs. Rate of focal and generalized EFD referred to the respective frequencies of spike and sharp-wave abnormalities considered epileptiform in nature, and background slow-wave activity referred to the amount and frequency range of background slow-wave activity.

Demographic and Past History Variables. The following variables were obtained via a semistructured interview with the subject following explicit, objective guidelines for rating each variable: (1) age, (2) sex, (3) race, (4) marital status, (5) education, (6) current employment, (7) monthly income of immediate family, (8) number of children at home, (9) number of children total, (10) handedness, (11) history of birth abnormalities, (12) history of delay of developmental milestones, (13) history of febrile seizures, (14) history of repeated grades, (15) history of learning disabilities, (16) psychosocial adjustment as a child, (17) history of psychiatric treatment, (18) history of legal problems, (19) history of alcohol abuse, (20) history of drug abuse, (21) history of head trauma, and (22) family history.

Procedure

Subjects who expressed interest in the study were contacted by research personnel, the study was described further, any questions were answered, and those who elected to participate were scheduled for an appointment to complete data collection procedures. The external rater was also scheduled for an appointment at this time. At the time of the appointment the subject and rater each signed informed consent. The paper-and-pencil tests were completed under supervision of research personnel at the time of the appointment. A second appointment was scheduled when necessary to complete data collection procedures. The interview to collect behavior-rating data and demographic and past history data was conducted during the same appointment.

Empirical Identification of Behaviorally Homogeneous Subgroups

A cluster analysis approach was used to empirically identify subgroups of the overall sample that were homogeneous according to behavior/personality variables. Separate cluster solutions were obtained using measures from four different instruments—the MMPI, the Bear and Fedio Inventory, the EPQ, and the ratings from the semistructured interview with the patients (PR)—in order to allow for assessing the cross-measure reproducibility of obtained cluster solutions. The first step in the cluster analysis process was to reduce the large number of variables from the three instruments excluding the EPQ into a smaller number of variables on which to base cluster analysis but, at the same time, to include as broad a range of variance on which to categorize groups as possible. To do so, independent principal-components analyses with varimax rotation of components with eigenvalues greater than 1.0 were performed for the 18 variables of the BF, the eight PR variables, and nine MMPI clinical scales (the Mf scale was not included since high scores have different meaning for males and females), plus the three validity scales. These analyses and subsequent cluster analyses were based on 66 subjects for whom complete data on all instruments were available. Then, for each of the three methods of measurement, one variable that strongly defined each derived component but showed minimal loadings on other components was selected to serve as the basis for subsequent cluster analysis. The N, P, and IE scales of the EPQ were used as the basis for subsequent cluster analysis without modification.

For the MMPI, four principal components were retained and rotated, accounting for 76% of the total variance. Component 1 (accounting for 27% of the total variance) was defined by Sc (loading = .83), F (.82), Pa (.77), Ma (.69), and Pt (.63). Component 2 (23% of variance) was defined by Hy (.95), Hs (.88), and D (.66). Component 3 (16% of variance) was defined by Si (−.93), K (.63), and D (−.59). Component 4 (10% of variance) was defined by L (.91). The F, Hy, Si, and L scales were selected as the variables on which cluster analysis was performed.

Four BF components were retained and rotated, accounting for 62% of the total variance. Component 1 (accounting for 35% of total variance) was most strongly defined by depression/sadness (.86), guilt (.70), anger (.65), paranoia (.62), and dependency (.60). Component 2 (13% of variance) was defined by religiosity (.84), philosophical interest (.79), and personal destiny (.66). Component 3 (9% of variance) was primarily defined by hypergraphia (.84). Component 4 (6% of variance) was defined by obsessionalism (.75), circumstantiality (.73), and elation (.71).

Depression, religiosity, hypergraphia, and circumstantiality were selected as the variables on which to base cluster analysis.

Three PR components, accounting for 56% of the total variance, had eigenvalues greater than 1.0 and were retained and rotated. Component 1 (25% of total variance) was defined by verbal aggression (.79), physical aggression, (.76), and stickiness (.71). Component 2 (16% of variance) was defined by religion ($-.77$) and philosophical interest ($-.77$). Component 3 (16% of variance) was defined by hypergraphia (.78) and circumstantiality (.70). Verbal aggression, religion, and hypergraphia were selected as the three variables to represent these factors and serve as the basis for cluster analysis. Sexual interest/activity was not well accounted for by the three-component solution, with a communality of .23. Since this has been a very significant variable in previous research and was not well accounted for by the other variables selected, it was also included in the group for cluster analysis, making a total of PR four variables on which cluster analysis was performed.

Cluster Analysis Procedure

An independent cluster analysis process was performed for the sets of variables from the MMPI, the BF, the EPQ, and the PR. Multiple procedures were carried out in order to test the reliability of derived cluster solutions. First, a K-means clustering algorithm (Hartigan, 1975; Morris, Blashfield, & Satz, 1981) was used to obtain solutions for three clusters, four clusters, etc., up to 12 clusters. The overlap between each consecutive pair of solutions was examined by looking at the degree to which group membership was shared across the two solutions. Through this process, it was possible to identify an optimal number of clusters, after which adding further clusters did not substantially alter cluster membership. The solution with this number of clusters was then selected as the cluster solution that subsequent comparisons were based on.

The reliability of the cluster solutions derived as described was then tested in two ways. First, a hierarchical partitioning clustering algorithm (Hartigan, 1975) was used to establish independent cluster solutions, and results of these solutions were compared with results from the K-means procedure according to shared group membership. Four hierarchical cluster analyses were performed on each set of variables, representing the possible combinations of a euclidean distance measure versus a Pearson correlation measure and a complete linkage versus average linkage method (Wilkinson, 1987). The overlap of solutions from each of these four analyses with the K-means solution was then assessed. This was done by determining the percentage of subjects from each cluster in the K-means solution who were classified in the same group in the hierarchical cluster solution. The average percentage overlap was then calculated for each cluster across the four methods of hierarchical clustering. A second measure of stability was derived by applying a K-means clustering approach to randomly selected subsamples of the overall sample. Five different subsamples were identified by dropping a unique, randomly selected one-fifth of the total sample of subjects so that each group consisted of four-fifths of the total sample.

Separate K-means procedures were performed using each of the five subsamples, with number of clusters established in the manner previously described. The overlap of solutions from each of the five subsamples with the solution from the total sample was then assessed by determining the percentage of subjects from each cluster in the subgroup analyses who were classified in the same group in the solution from the overall sample. The average percentage overlap was also calculated for each cluster across the five subsamples.

Cluster Analysis of the MMPI

The K-means cluster analysis solution based on the MMPI scales F, Hy, Si, and L was found to stabilize after an eight-group solution, with only two subjects changing cluster membership from the eight- to the nine-cluster solution. Two of the clusters from the eight-cluster solution contained only one subject each, and a third contained two. These subjects were considered unclassified in subsequent analyses, resulting in 62 of the 66 subjects (94%) entered into the analysis being classified. The number of subjects in each of the derived clusters and the indices of average overlap across the solutions from the whole sample and the five subsamples and across the K-means and hierarchical solutions are presented in Table 7.3. Reliability indices show relatively good reproducibility of all five clusters.

Definition of these five clusters was attempted by comparing the groups on all 12 MMPI variables (three validity scales and 10 clinical scales excepting My). A multivariate analysis of variance (MANOVA) was performed comparing the five groups across the 12 variables. The overall Wilk's lambda was significant (approximate $F = 8.09$; $df = 48, 179$; $p < .001$). Cluster means and results of univariate analyses of variance (ANOVAs) across variables are shown in Table 7.4. Results show that the derived cluster solution was very successful in accounting for variance in the MMPI. Cluster 1 appears to be interpretable as reflecting generalized psychopathology. Cluster 2 is defined by mild depression as well as introversion and seems interpretable in these terms. Cluster 3 reflects a relative absence of psychopathology, though there is an indication of increased energy or need for achievement. Cluster 4 is defined more by the "psychotic" scales and represents more severe psychopathology, while cluster 5 is defined by the "neurotic" scales and likely reflects more internalized psychopathology.

Cluster Analysis of the Bear and Fedio Inventory

A stable K-means cluster analysis solution based on the BF variables hypergraphia, religiosity, depression, and circumstantiality was found using seven clusters. One cluster contained only one subject, and that subject was considered unclassified, resulting in classification of 65 of 66 subjects (98%). Table 7.3 shows numbers of subjects within clusters and reliability indices for the BF cluster solution. The derived clusters were quite stable across the different clustering procedures. A MANOVA involving these variables yielded a highly significant Wilk's lambda (approximate

TABLE 7.3. Cluster Size and Reliability

Method	Cluster	n	K-means index of reliability	Hierarchical index of reliability
MMPI	1	14	.80	.66
	2	13	.86	.63
	3	11	.73	.82
	4	12	.71	.92
	5	12	.81	.83
BF	1	9	1.00	.72
	2	20	.89	.73
	3	14	.85	.89
	4	9	.81	.97
	5	7	.93	.96
	6	6	.92	1.00
EPQ	1	10	.88	.75
	2	8	.75	.88
	3	11	.80	.64
	4	5	.81	.75
	5	5	1.00	.90
	6	8	.91	1.00
	7	11	.84	1.00
PR	1	14	.84	.91
	2	11	.93	.95
	3	23	.66	.73
	4	7	.89	.68
	5	9	.72	1.00
	6	11	.95	.93

$F = 4.74$; $df = 90, 208$; $p < .001$). Cluster means and results of univariate ANOVAs for each variable are shown in Table 7.5. As with the MMPI results, the obtained cluster solution was very successful in accounting for variance in the BF variables.

Cluster 1 appears to be defined by a relative absence of elevations on any of the 18 traits. Cluster 2 is defined by high elevations overall, with particular elevations on circumstantiality, obsessionalism, stickiness, depression, and emotionality, and appears to represent a group with generalized psychopathology. Cluster 6 is similar to cluster 2 in that it has elevations on circumstantiality, obsessionalism, elation, and stickiness but shows much less prominent elevations on other variables, so that it seems interpretable as representing more specific ideational changes that have been attributed to TLE in past literature. Cluster 3 is defined by religiosity and personal destiny and seems interpretable in those terms. Cluster 4 is defined by hypergraphia and circumstantiality with elevations also on hypermoralism and stickiness and appears to represent a perception of one's ideas as important combined with a need to present those ideas at length and in detail. Cluster 5 is defined by aggression,

TABLE 7.4.   MMPI and EPQ Cluster Means

MMPI scale	Cluster[a] 1	2	3	4	5	F[b]
L	*47.9*	*52.6*	*48.0*	*50.3*	*52.7*	2.09[†]
F	*73.1*	*58.0*	*57.9*	*85.3*	*61.3*	36.97***
K	42.9	45.7	55.0	46.8	56.8	6.63***
Hs	78.8	56.1	57.0	58.2	79.7	18.48***
D	86.2	67.9	62.0	65.0	76.3	9.04***
Hy	*71.6*	*55.5*	*59.7*	*56.6*	*78.2*	21.70***
Pd	71.6	58.7	62.9	69.2	72.5	4.52**
Pa	69.1	59.9	62.5	69.3	63.8	2.76*
Pt	73.7	62.4	59.7	72.7	63.8	5.06***
Sc	84.8	61.3	67.8	85.0	74.0	11.68***
Ma	65.7	56.8	69.5	74.2	68.6	4.79**
Si	*70.7*	*66.7*	*45.0*	*55.9*	*53.4*	40.49***

EPQ scale	Cluster[a] 1	2	3	4	5	6	7	F
P	43.9	50.8	56.6	41.2	52.2	47.9	57.9	21.27***
IE	45.9	48.3	56.2	61.6	59.4	32.3	46.6	36.65***
N	59.7	44.5	57.5	53.0	36.6	63.1	62.7	27.90***

[a]The means for variables used as a basis for cluster derivation are shown in italics.
[b]Significance: [†]$p < .10$; *$p < .05$; **$p < .01$; ***$p < .001$.

depression, stickiness, and emotionality and appears to represent intense and varied emotionality.

Cluster Analysis of EPQ Variables

A stable K-means solution for the EPQ was found using 10 clusters. Four subjects were considered unclassifiable, two comprising their own clusters and two being included in one other cluster, resulting in 62 of 66 (94%) of subjects being classified. Table 7.4 shows number of subjects and reliability indices for the EPQ cluster solution. Again, clusters are reliably found across clustering methods. The Wilk's lambda for the MANOVA comparing the derived groups across clusters was significant ($F = 33.15$; $df = 18, 133$; $p < .001$), and all individual variables significantly discriminated groups at beyond the .001 level.

Cluster 1 is defined by a relative elevation of the N scale with average scores on the other two scales and so appears to represent relatively specific neuroticism. Cluster 6 is also defined by high N but, in contrast, shows low IE and appears to represent high neuroticism combined with introversion. Cluster 7 combines neuroticism and psychoticism as its defining characteristics. Cluster 2 is defined by moderate elevations on all variables and as such represents a relatively normal group. Cluster 3 is defined by moderately high elevations on all variables and thus combines

TABLE 7.5.   BF and PR Cluster Means

Scale	Cluster[a]						F^b
	1	2	3	4	5	6	
BF							
Hypergraphia	*2.47*	*4.01*	*3.48*	*5.56*	*2.54*	*2.90*	11.69***
Altered sex	2.82	3.76	3.05	3.60	2.91	2.47	2.98*
Hypermoralism	2.91	4.55	4.16	4.80	3.69	3.73	2.60*
Religiosity	*1.80*	*4.65*	*5.71*	*2.56*	*1.71*	*3.17*	29.88***
Aggression	2.49	4.11	2.66	4.11	5.06	3.07	4.30*
Obessional	2.81	5.35	4.13	4.33	4.29	5.03	5.56***
Paranoia	2.40	4.68	4.11	4.33	3.77	3.13	6.81***
Guilt	2.31	4.66	3.51	3.02	4.14	2.50	5.74***
Humorless	2.82	4.33	4.25	4.09	3.57	3.53	2.89*
Depression	*1.76*	*5.12*	*2.96*	*3.07*	*4.97*	*2.20*	28.80***
Emotion	3.02	5.06	3.51	4.67	4.66	3.80	4.88***
Circumstantial	*2.96*	*6.02*	*4.01*	*5.02*	*3.38*	*6.07*	20.21***
Philosophical	2.22	3.91	3.96	3.31	2.49	3.27	4.63***
Personal destiny	2.16	3.79	4.78	4.24	3.23	2.73	6.34***
Stickiness	2.40	5.28	4.06	4.56	4.83	4.70	8.52***
Dependency	2.76	4.88	3.83	3.73	4.26	3.37	4.30**
Elation	3.31	4.46	3.70	4.47	3.54	4.97	2.01†
Anger	1.80	4.74	2.87	4.42	4.06	3.18	8.49***
PR							
Hypergraphia	*1.98*	*3.63*	*1.59*	*3.95*	*1.00*	*1.52*	48.96***
Sexual	*2.68*	*2.49*	*2.61*	*3.07*	*2.86*	*1.71*	7.00***
Religion	*1.63*	*1.84*	*2.79*	*4.00*	*2.81*	*4.33*	39.16***
Philosophical	2.30	2.71	2.14	2.31	2.56	2.82	1.90†
Physical aggression	2.16	1.64	1.41	1.95	2.61	1.74	14.09***
Verbal aggression	*3.20*	*2.49*	*1.78*	*2.54*	*3.53*	*3.10*	2.84*
Stickiness	3.21	3.21	2.93	3.18	3.25	3.19	1.61
Circumstantial	3.00	3.11	2.95	3.14	3.00	2.87	0.57

[a]The means for variables used as a basis for cluster derivation are shown in italics.
[b]Significance: †$p < .10$; *$p < .05$; **$p < .01$; ***$p < .001$.

neuroticism, psychoticism, and extraversion at moderate degrees. Cluster 4 is defined by high N and relatively low P and appears to represent relatively low psychoticism, while cluster 5 shows extraversion coupled with low neuroticism.

Cluster Analysis of PR Variables

A stable solution was found using seven clusters for the PR variables hypergraphia, sexual activity/interest, religion, and verbal aggression. One subject was the sole member of one group and was considered unclassifiable. This left 65 of 66 subjects (98%) classified within the obtained solution. Table 7.3 shows number of subjects and reliability indices for these clusters, and elevations on the means of variables used to define these clusters are presented in Table 7.5. Clusters could again be derived with consistency across methods of cluster extraction. The MANOVA comparing clusters across PR measures showed a significant overall Wilk's lambda (approximate $F = 11.06$; $df = 40, 238$; $p < .001$). Three of the measures, stickiness/viscosity, circumstantiality, and philosophical interest, did not significantly discriminate groups.

Cluster 1 was defined by verbal and to a lessor extent physical aggression, with a relative absence of other traits at an unusual level. Cluster 5 also showed elevated amounts of verbal and physical aggression but in contrast showed greater interest in religion. Cluster 6 showed clear verbal aggression, pronounced preoccupation with religion, and decreased sexual interest/activity. These three clusters appear to represent increased aggressiveness/irritability with varying levels of religious preoccupation and sexual hypoactivity. Cluster 2 was defined by relatively pure hypergraphia. Cluster 3 showed a general lack of the traits at an unusual level. Cluster 4 was defined by the combination of hypergraphia and strong religious interest.

Derivation of a Cluster with the Purported TLE Syndrome

A different approach to cluster derivation was also used in an attempt to maximize the likelihood of finding a specific syndrome of behavior, should it exist. This approach used preexisting theory as the basis for cluster identification. Based on the Waxman and Geschwind (1975) formulation, the hypergraphia, religion, and sexual interest/activity scales from the PR were selected as a basis for syndrome identification. The philosophical interest scale was added to this group, as it has also frequently been associated with TLE. Subjects were then classified as to whether they were above or below the means on each of these four variables. For each subject, a composite index ranging from 0 to 4 was established, with one point added each time the subject's score exceeded the overall mean for the first three variables or was below the mean for the sexuality variable. Thus, this index represented the total number of these four variables on which the subject scored in the direction that would be predicted by previous formulations of the TLE behavior syndrome. From the total sample of 80 subjects, eight received a score on this index of 0, 24 of 1, 31 of 2, 16 of 3, and one of 4. A cutoff of 3 was used to define a group of subjects with the proposed behavioral syndrome ($n = 17$) versus a group without the behavioral syndrome ($n = 63$).

Psychological and Neurological Characteristics of Clusters

The clusters from the MMPI, BF, EPQ, and PR were derived with careful attention to issues of internal validity (Morris *et al.*, 1981), and as a result, most of the derived clusters showed strong evidence of reliability or reproducibility across different methods of cluster extraction. In order to have any scientific value, however, the derived clusters must also be related to external variables or must have external validity. In this regard, the relationship of the cluster solutions to each other is important, as is their relationship to other, external variables.

Relationships among Derived Clusters

Two-way contingency tables were used to assess the association of each possible pair of cluster solutions. The Pearson chi-square statistic was computed to assess whether there was a significant association between each pair, and Cramer's V was used to compare the degree of association across the different pairs. The obtained Cramer's V values for each possible pair of cluster solutions are presented in Table 7.6 along with the associated levels of significance of the chi-square tests. The MMPI and EPQ solutions were significantly related, as were the BF and EPQ solutions and the BF and PR solutions. The behavioral syndrome categorization was related to those for the EPQ and PR but not the MMPI or BF. The magnitude of relationships was generally modest at best, indicating there was not strong reproducibility of the same subject clusters across different methods of measurement.

A second approach was used to test the comparability of clusters from different methods of measurement. A variable corresponding to each derived cluster was formed by giving a subject a score of 1 if he or she was classified in that cluster and a score of 0 if not classified in that cluster. Then, correlation coefficients were computed to assess the association of each of these variables with each of the others. The variable pairs for which the obtained correlation coefficients exceeded .30 were as follows: MMPI CL 1 with BF CL 5 ($r = .32$), MMPI CL 2 with BF CL 4 (.38) and EPQ CL 1 (.35), MMPI CL 3 with EPQ CL 5 (.50), MMPI CL 5 with EPQ CL 4 (.33), BF CL 1 with EPQ CL 5 (.56), BF CL 4 with PR CL 2 (.32) and EPQ CL 1 (.34), and BF CL 5 with PR CL 1 (.32) and EPQ CL 6 (.34).

Relationship of Derived Clusters to External Variables

The next step in data analysis involved assessing the relationship of the derived cluster solutions to external variables, including measures of psychological/behavioral/psychiatric variables, seizure disorder and EEG parameters, other neurological variables, and demographic and past history variables. In this process a large number of external variables were of potential interest, and the number of subjects within some of the derived clusters was relatively small, so special attention needed to be paid to avoiding capitalization on chance variation. This was done in several

TABLE 7.6. Cramer's V Values Comparing Clustering Solutions[a]

	MMPI	EPQ	BF	PR
EPQ	.49***			
BF	.34†	.49***		
PR	.27	.37	.38**	
BEHSYN	.18	.48*	.32	.59***

[a]Probability values refer to significance levels of chi-square tests: $†p < .10$; $*p < .05$; $**p < .01$; $***p < .001$.

ways. First, the external variables to be tested were organized into groups of related variables. When these groups of variables were relatively large, principal components analysis was performed to reduce the large number of variables to a more manageable number of underlying dimensions. Second, the error rate for comparisons was set at the level of groups of variables as opposed to individual variables. For groups of continuous or ordered variables this was done by using a MANOVA and requiring a significant overall Wilk's lambda before assessing effects pertaining to individual variables using univariate ANOVAs. For categorical or dichotomous variables, a Bonferroni procedure was used in which the criterion p value for determining significance was calculated by dividing .05 by the number of variables within the group; for example, if there were five variables in a given group, a criterion p value of .01 would be required. The relationship of cluster membership and categorical variables was assessed using the chi-square statistic. In a further attempt to avoid capitalization on chance, whenever possible categorical variables were made into dichotomous variables to maximize sample size within each cell of the contingency table. This was particularly important since the cluster solutions defined a relatively large number of groups.

Measures of Psychological/Behavioral/Psychiatric Parameters

The relationship of each cluster solution with measures from the MMPI, BF, EPQ, PR, Wiggins Content Scales of the MMPI, SADS-C, and WPSI was assessed. Each of these groups of measures was first reduced to a smaller number of variables by principal components analysis, and then cluster differences in component scores were tested using MANOVAs. The principal components analyses previously described for the MMPI, BF, and PR were used as the basis for derivation of component scores for these analyses. The EPQ variables P, IE, and N were used without modification.

Four principal components of the Wiggins Content Scales of the MMPI (WIGG) were retained and rotated using the varimax method. These four components accounted for 71.7% of the total variance. The first component (accounting for 26.0% of total variance) was defined by hostility (.84), authority (.78), hypomania (.74), psychosis (.73), depression (.58), poor morale (.52), and family conflict (.48). This component seems to represent interpersonal conflict/psychiatric symptoms. Component 2 (12.5% of variance) was defined by religion (.75), feminine interest (.72), and secondarily by family conflict (.52) and appears to represent religious/aesthetic interest. Component 3 (16.9% of variance) was defined by social maladjustment (.88), poor morale (.67), and depression (.62) and appears to represent general psychosocial maladjustment. Component 4 (16.2% of variance) was defined by organic symptoms (.89), phobias (.72), and poor health (.66) and appears interpretable as somatic/health concern.

The composite scales of the SADS-C were entered into a principal components analysis, with two components accounting for 70.7% of the overall variance retained for varimax rotation. Component 1 (50.8% of total variance) had high loadings on

HRSD items (.93), depressive syndrome (.91), endogenous features (.87), the HRSD (.86), and miscellaneous symptoms (.76). This components seems clearly definable as a dimension representing depression. Component 2 (19.9% of total variance) was defined by psychotic features (.77), manic symptoms ($-.75$), and anxiety (.62) and seems interpretable as a measure of nondepressed psychopathology.

The scales of the WPSI excepting the validity scales were subjected to principal components analysis with two components accounting for 65.6% of the total variance retained for rotation. Component 1 (33.5% of variance) was defined by psychosocial (.89), emotion (.85), background (.84), intelligence ($-.73$), and adjustment to seizures (.68). This component appears to represent general level of adjustment. Component 2 (32.1% of variance) was defined by medication (.82), interpersonal (.80), financial (.76), vocational (.73), and impairment (.58) and appears to represent interpersonal/role adjustment.

Table 7.7 summarizes results comparing derived clusters across components from the MMPI, BF, PR, WIGG, SADS-C, and WPSI and the P, IE, and N scales of the EPQ. This table shows the p values associated with the approximate F test of the significance of the Wilk's lambda from the overall multivariate test and, when that test was significant, shows significance levels of subsequent univariate ANOVAs. A more detailed description of these results follows.

MMPI Components. The four MMPI components as a whole significantly discriminated the BF and EPQ clusters at a .001 level but were not significantly different across PR and behavioral syndrome clusters. Component 3 (measuring social ease/lack of depression) was significantly related to both the BF and EPQ, while the other components were not. Table 7.8 shows means of this component for BF and EPQ clusters. Tukey's HSD test was used for pairwise comparisons of cluster means from the BF and EPQ, and significant differences are also indicated in Table 7.11.

BF Components. The four principal components derived from the BF were significantly related to the clusters from all of the four other methods of measurement. Component 1 (measuring depression/dysphoria) was significantly related to MMPI and EPQ clusters. PR and behavioral syndrome groups were significantly different on component 2, and PR groups also significantly differed on component 3 (hypergraphia). Cluster means of BF components and significance levels of pairwise comparisons using Tukey's HSD test are shown in Table 7.9.

EPQ Components. EPQ variables significantly discriminated MMPI clusters and BF clusters. IE was significantly related to MMPI clusters, and N was related to BF clusters. Cluster means on these variables and significance levels of pairwise comparisons are presented in Table 7.8.

PR Components. Principal components from PR were significantly related to MMPI and BF clusters and to the behavioral syndrome groups but not to the EPQ. Component 2 (lack of religious/philosophical interest) significantly differed across

TABLE 7.7. Summary of MANOVAs Comparing
Behavioral/Personality Variables across Clusters

Variables	MMPI clusters	BF clusters	EPQ clusters	PR clusters	Behavioral syndrome
MMPI Fac.[a]	.001	.001	.001	.080	ns
Fac 1[b]		ns	.056		
Fac 2[b]		ns	ns		
Fac 3[b]		.001	.001		
Fac 4[b]		ns	ns		
BF Fac.[a]	.01		.001	.001	.010
Fac 1[b]	.001		.001	ns	ns
Fac 2[b]	ns		.07	.001	.001
Fac 3[b]	ns		.08	.009	ns
Fac 4[b]	ns		ns	ns	ns
EPQ[a]	.001	.001		.08	ns
P[b]	ns	ns			
IE[b]	.001	ns			
N[b]	.001	.001			
PR Fac.[a]	.05	.001	ns		.001
Fac 1[b]	ns	.021			ns
Fac 2[b]	.015	.006			.001
Fac 3[b]	ns	ns			ns
WIGGS Fac.[a]	.001	.001	.001	.001	.04
Fac 1[b]	.001	.001	.005	ns	ns
Fac 2[b]	.001	.022	.001	.082	ns
Fac 3[b]	.001	ns	ns	.045	ns
Fac 4[b]	ns	.001	ns	.001	.002
SADS Fac.[a]	ns	.030	.030	ns	ns
Fac 1[b]		.012	.012		
Fac 2[b]		ns	ns		
WPSI Fac.[a]	.001	.001	.001	ns	ns
Fac 1[b]	.005	.069	.019		
Fac 2[b]	.003	.002	.035		

[a]Table values represent p values for approximate F test of significance of Wilk's lambda from MANOVA.
[b]Table values represent p values from univariate ANOVAs.

MMPI clusters, BF clusters, and the behavioral syndrome groups. Component 1 (aggression/stickiness) differed across BF clusters. Means of these components across relevant clusters and associated significance levels of pairwise comparisons are shown in Table 7.9.

WIGG Components. Principal components from WIGG significantly differentiated clusters from the MMPI, BF, EPQ, and PR in addition to the behavioral syndrome groups. MMPI, BF, and EPQ clusters significantly differed on component 1 (interpersonal conflict/psychiatric symptoms) and on component 2 (religious/esthetic interest). Component 3 (psychosocial maladjustment) significantly differed across

TABLE 7.8.   Cluster Means for MMPI Components and EPQ Scales[a]

		MMPI				EPQ		
		Comp.1	Comp.2	Comp.3	Comp.4	P	IE	N
MMPI	CL 1						43.8[45]	62.9[35]
	CL 2						42.1[45]	58.2[3]
	CL 3						42.6[45]	47.9[12]
	CL 4						52.5[123]	54.9
	CL 5						53.3[123]	49.3[1]
BF	CL 1			0.65[25]				40.3[2456]
	Cl 2			−0.54[16]				61.4[13]
	CL 3			0.20				48.6[245]
	CL 4			−0.02				59.3[13]
	CL 5			−0.82[16]				63.4[136]
	CL 6			0.96[25]				52.3[15]
EPQ	CL 1			−0.38[45]				
	CL 2			0.71[6]				
	CL 3			0.15[56]				
	CL 4			0.95[167]				
	CL 5			1.46[1367]				
	CL 6			−1.19[2345]				
	CL 7			−0.37[45]				

[a]Superscript numbers denote clusters whose means significantly differ from the indicated cluster mean using Tukey's HSD test.

MMPI and PR clusters. Component 4 (somatic/health concern) significantly differed across BF and PR clusters and behavioral syndrome groups. Means of these components across relevant clusters and associated levels of significance of pairwise comparisons are shown in Table 7.10.

SADS-C Components. Component 1 of the SADS-C significantly differed across BF and EPQ clusters, but SADS-C components were not related to groups derived from the other measures. Means of component 1 across BF and PR clusters and significance levels of pairwise comparisons are presented in Table 7.10.

WPSI Components. Both principal components of the WPSI were significantly related to the MMPI and EPQ clusters, and component 2 significantly differed across BF clusters. These components did not discriminate PR clusters or behavioral syndrome groups. Component means for MMPI, BF, and EPQ clusters and significance levels of pairwise comparisons are shown in Table 7.10.

Demographic, Neurological, and History Variables

Table 7.11 summarizes MANOVA and ANOVA results for the other external continuous/ordered variables. A more specific description of results follows:

TABLE 7.9.   Cluster Means for BF and PR Components[a]

		BF				PR		
		Comp.1	Comp.2	Comp.3	Comp.4	Comp.1	Comp.2	Comp.3
MMPI	CL 1	0.89^{35}					-0.01	
	CL 2	0.15^{3}					0.22	
	CL 3	-0.86^{12}					-0.62^{4}	
	CL 4	0.00^{5}					0.76^{3}	
	CL 5	-0.38^{1}					-0.26	
BF	CL 1					-0.74^{56}	0.75^{3}	
	CL 2					0.07	-0.05	
	CL 3					-0.46	-0.87^{15}	
	CL 4					0.26	0.22	
	CL 5					0.62^{1}	0.56^{3}	
	CL 6					0.43^{1}	0.15	
EPQ	CL 1	0.31^{5}						
	CL 2	-0.47						
	CL 3	0.21^{5}						
	CL 4	-0.94^{6}						
	CL 5	-1.20^{1367}						
	CL 6	0.90^{45}						
	CL 7	0.36^{5}						
PR	CL 1		-0.91^{346}	-0.16				
	CL 2		-0.47^{46}	0.67				
	CL 3		0.17^{1}	-0.47				
	CL 4		0.63^{12}	0.39				
	CL 5		-0.17^{6}	0.62				
	CL 6		0.98^{125}	-0.41				
Behav.	GRP 1		0.87				-1.24	
synd.	GRP 2		-0.87				1.24	

[a]Superscript numbers denote clusters whose means significantly differ from the indicated cluser mean using Tukey's HSD test.

Seizure and EEG Severity Variables. These variables jointly significantly discriminated the behavioral syndrome groups but were not related to any of the other derived clusters. There was less background slow-wave activity in the subjects manifesting the behavioral syndrome (mean = 1.000) than in the group without the syndrome (mean = 1.704).

Demographic Variables. MMPI clusters and behavioral syndrome groups significantly differed across these measures in multivariate tests. MMPI clusters significantly differed in education, and cluster means and associated significance levels of pairwise comparisons are shown in Table 7.12. Behavioral syndrome was related to age, with the group with the behavioral syndrome (mean = 46.81) being significantly older than the group without the syndrome (mean = 27.38).

TABLE 7.10. Cluster Means for WIGG, SADS-C, and WPSI Components[a]

		WIGG				SADS-C		WPSI	
		Comp.1	Comp.2	Comp.3	Comp.4	Comp.1	Comp.2	Comp.1	Comp.2
MMPI	CL 1	0.20	0.89[345]	0.87[73]		0.68[3]		0.66[3]	0.10[3]
	CL 2	0.07	0.44[35]	-0.44[1]		-0.07		-0.26	-0.21
	CL 3	-0.21[4]	-0.97[12]	-0.68[15]		-0.49[1]		-0.75[1]	-0.87[14]
	CL 4	0.88[35]	-0.40[1]	-0.02		-0.27		0.18	0.41[3]
	CL 5	-0.73[4]	-0.50[12]	0.38[3]		-0.02		-0.29	0.09
BF	CL 1	-1.10[2456]	-0.33		-0.73[3]	-0.76[5]			-0.83[2]
	CL 2	0.61[1]	0.38[2]		0.09	0.33			0.42[1]
	CL 3	-0.46	0.02		0.74[15]	-0.11			-0.39
	CL 4	0.37[1]	-0.12		-0.39	-0.14			0.12
	CL 5	0.26[1]	0.60[2]		-0.67[3]	0.78[1]			0.14
	CL 6	0.26[1]	-0.99[25]	-0.21	-0.24			-0.43	
EPQ	CL 1	0.34	0.26[45]			-0.01		-0.07	0.15
	CL 2	-0.55	-0.48[6]			-0.07		-0.72	-0.57
	CL 3	0.72[5]	-0.34[6]			-0.51		-0.15	0.27[5]
	CL 4	-0.58	-1.34[167]			-0.23		-0.56	-0.26
	CL 5	-0.75[3]	-1.38[167]			-0.73[7]		-0.95	-1.21[3]
	CL 6	0.32	1.24[2345]			0.30		0.56	0.00
	CL 7	0.32	0.30[45]			0.84[5]		0.51	0.10
PR	CL 1			-0.23	-0.60[6]				
	CL 2			-0.52[5]	-0.75[46]				
	CL 3			0.13	0.02				
	CL 4			0.35	0.29[2]				
	CL 5			0.89[2]	0.21				
	CL 6			0.21	1.16[12]				
Behav. synd.	GRP 1		-1.24						
	GRP 2		1.24						

[a]Superscript numbers denote clusters whose means significantly differ from the indicated cluster mean using Tukey's HSD test.

168   DAN M. MUNGAS

TABLE 7.11. Summary of MANOVAs Comparing Continuous/Ordered
External Variables across Clusters

Variables	MMPI clusters	BP clusters	EPQ clusters	PR clusters	Behavioral syndrome
Seizure and EEG severity[a]	ns	ns	ns	ns	.01
Sz control[b]					ns
Rate foc. EFD[b]					ns
Rate gen. EFD[b]					ns
Amt. background slowing[b]					.011
Duration of epilepsy[b]					.092
Num. meds.[b]					ns
Demographic[a]	.02	ns	ns	ns	.01
Age[b]	ns				.006
Age onset[b]	ns				ns
Education[b]	.003				ns
Income[b]	ns	.075			
Develop. Hx[a]	ns	ns	ns	ns	ns
Birth trauma[b]					
Dev. milestones[b]					
Febrile sz[b]					
Rept. grades[b]					
Social Hx[a]	.09	ns	ns	ns	ns
Social adj.[b]					
Sch. achvmnt[b]					
Beh. prob.[b]					
Psych. Rx[b]					
Current Hx[a]	ns	ns	ns	ns	.04
Psych. Hx[b]					ns
Legal Hx[b]					ns
EtOH Hx[b]					ns
Drug Hx[b]					.006

[a]Table values represent p values for approximate F test of significance of Wilk's lambda from MANOVA.
[b]Table values represent p values for univariate ANOVAs.

TABLE 7.12. MMPI Cluster and Behavioral Syndrome Group Means
on Continuous/Ordered Variables that Discriminated Groups[a]

		EEG background slowing	Age	Education	Drug Hx
MMPI	CL 1			12.1[43]	
	CL 2			14.2[4]	
	CL 3			14.8[14]	
	Cl 4			11.5[23]	
	CL 5			13.0	
Behav.	GRP 1	1.00	46.8		1.47
synd.	GRP 2	1.70	27.3		0.69

[a]Superscript numbers denote clusters whose means significantly differ from the indicated
cluster mean using Tukey's HSD test.

Social and Developmental History Variables. None of these variables were significantly different across clusters associated with any of the four measures or across behavioral syndrome groups.

Current History Variables. These variables jointly discriminated only the two behavioral syndrome groups, and of the four variables, only the drug history variable differed across groups. The group with the behavioral syndrome (mean = 1.471) scored significantly higher than the group without (mean = 0.693).

Categorical/Dichotomous Variables

Table 7.13 shows results of chi-square tests performed on seizure and EEG parameters, seizure disorder diagnosis, demographic variables, and neurological variables. Only two variables showed a significant relationship to any of the derived clusters or groups, and only one of these was significant after application of the Bonferroni correction. Sex was significantly different in the behavioral syndrome groups, with 82% of the group with the behavioral syndrome being females in comparison with 41% of the group without the syndrome being females. Sex also showed a trend toward differing across PR clusters, with percentage male by cluster as follows: 1, 57; 2, 60; 3, 52; 4, 14; 5, 89; 6, 27. There was a trend for a significant relationship between complex partial seizures and behavioral syndrome groups.

TABLE 7.13. Summary of Chi-Square Tests Comparing Categorical/Dichotomous External Variables across Clusters[a]

Variables	MMPI clusters	BF clusters	EPQ clusters	PR clusters	Behavioral syndrome
Seizure and EEG					
Compl. Part. Sz.	ns	ns	ns	ns	.04
Gen. Sz.	ns	ns	ns	ns	ns
RTEFD	ns	ns	ns	ns	ns
LTEFD	ns	ns	ns	ns	ns
Seizure Dx					
Temporal lobe	ns	ns	ns	ns	ns
Generalized	ns	ns	ns	ns	ns
Demographic					
Sex	ns	ns	ns	.035	.003
Employment	ns	ns	ns	ns	ns
Neurological					
Hx head trauma	ns	ns	ns	ns	ns
Seizure etiology	ns	ns	ns	ns	ns
Neuro Dx	ns	ns	ns	ns	ns
Neuro exam	ns	ns	ns	ns	ns
CT temp.	ns	ns	ns	ns	ns
CT lat.	ns	ns	ns	ns	ns

[a]Table values represent p values associated with respective chi-square tests.

Eighty-eight percent of the group with the syndrome had complex partial seizures, while 62% of the group without the syndrome had complex partial seizures.

IMPLICATIONS AND FUTURE DIRECTIONS

Methodology for Assessing Behavior in Epilepsy

Measures of Behavior/Personality

Measures for assessing behavior have played a major role in the controversy regarding a specific behavior syndrome in TLE, with some interpreting the lack of positive findings with instruments such as the MMPI as indicating lack of sensitivity to behavior that occurs in epilepsy. Several instruments assessing a variety of variables with different methods of measurement were used in this study, allowing for cross-method comparisons.

Clusters derived from the MMPI were related to variables from all of the other psychometric measures of behavior/personality. Clusters defined by high Si scores were associated with high EPQ IE scores, and the cluster showing generalized psychopathology of relatively mild degree (cluster 1) had a very high mean EPQ N score. MMPI clusters were related to only one BF component, the depression/ dysphoria component. This component is defined by BF variables that are clearly psychopathological in nature, so it is not surprising that the two extremes in group means on this component were found for the generalized psychopathology cluster (cluster 1) and the cluster with a relative absence of MMPI abnormalities (cluster 3). It is noteworthy that cluster 4, defined by more severe psychopathology in the psychotic spectrum, did not show extreme scores on this BF component, suggesting that the variables defining it assess less severe forms of behavior. The MMPI was also related to only one PR component, the lack of religious/philosophical interest component, with cluster 4 showing a lack of religious/philosophical interest and cluster 3 showing relatively strong religious/philosophical interest.

The MMPI was strongly related to all WIGG components but component 4, assessing somatic/health concern. Cluster 1 showed high scores on the social mal-adjustment component, with cluster 3 showing low scores, as would be predicted. The cluster defined by psychopathology more in the psychotic spectrum (cluster 4) showed the highest scores on the interpersonal conflict/psychiatric symptoms compo-nent (component 1), whereas the cluster characterized by denial, inhibition, and somatic expression of conflict (cluster 5) showed the lowest scores on this component, again consistent with expectations. The MMPI cluster solution was related to the SADS-C depression component (component 1) and to both WPSI maladjustment components, with cluster 3, characterized by a relative lack of MMPI abnormalities, showing low scores on both components. Taken as a whole, external correlates of MMPI clusters show a relationship with other measures of psychopathology and, with the exception of the PR cluster, no significant relationship with measures of parame-ters that are less inherently psychopathological in nature.

The EPQ cluster solution related significantly only to MMPI component 3 (social extraversion). As expected, the clusters with high scores on this component were defined by high EPQ IE, and the cluster with a low score by low IE. The EPQ also was related to only one BF component (depression/dysphoria). Cluster means on this component were highly correlated with the cluster means of the EPQ N variable ($r = .87$), further substantiating the interpretation of this component as assessing neurotic spectrum behavior. EPQ clusters did not relate to PR components. The EPQ was related to WIGG, SADS-C, and WPSI components. WIGG component 2 (religious/aesthetic interest) was related to EPQ N ($r = .78$), and component 1 (interpersonal conflict/psychiatric symptoms) appeared to have a more complex relationship to EPQ scales. The SADS-C depression component had the highest mean score on the EPQ cluster defined by high P and high N, with the lowest score on the group defined by low N and moderate P. Both WPSI maladjustment components had cluster means that were highly correlated with mean N ($r = .92$ and $.95$, respectively). Overall, the EPQ clusters were generally sensitive to measures of psychopathology (N) and to measures associated with introversion/extraversion (IE).

The BF clusters related only to the MMPI social extraversion component, with cluster means on this component highly correlated with means on the BF depression scale ($r = -.94$). BF clusters also related to the EPQ N scale, again with a high correlation between cluster means on the N scale and mean BF depression scores ($r = .85$). There was a clear relationship between the BF clusters and the PR aggression and religious/philosophical interest components but not the PR hypergraphia component. As would be expected, there was a clear relationship between mean PR aggression and mean BF aggression and anger scores ($r = .79$ and $.71$, respectively) and between PR lack of religious/philosophical interest and BF religiosity ($r = -.95$).

The BF clusters were related to two WIGG components. The interpersonal conflict/psychiatric symptoms component had high scores on the BF cluster characterized by generally high scores on all BF scales, and it had an extremely low mean for the BF cluster defined by low scores overall. Somewhat unexpectedly, the means of the religious/esthetic interest component showed a strong correlation with the BF depression scale ($r = .85$) and not with BF religiosity ($r = .07$). The WIGG somatic/health concern component means showed a very strong relationship to BF religiosity ($r = .98$). As would be expected, cluster means on the SADS-C depression component correlated highly with mean BF depression ($r = .93$), and means of the WPSI interpersonal/role maladjustment component correlated highly with BF aggression ($r = .85$). Overall, these results show that the BF, particularly the depression scale and most likely other scales that it correlates with, shares a considerable amount of variance with measures of psychopathology, although there is evidence of a relationship between religiosity and behavioral measures of religious interest that is relatively independent of psychopathology.

PR clusters were not related to either the MMPI, EPQ, SADS-C, or WPSI, suggesting that the PR shares relatively little variance with measures of psychopathology. These clusters did differ on two WIGG components. As would be expected, the cluster with high verbal and physical aggression (cluster 5) had high scores on the WIGG psychosocial maladjustment component. Mean WIGG somatic/health concern scores were highly correlated with mean PR religion ($r = .93$). This replicates the relationship between this component and the BF measure of religiosity.

PR clusters were related to two BF components assessing religious/philosophical interest and hypergraphia. As expected, means of the religious/philosophical interest component correlated highly with PR religion ($r = .97$), but the BF hypergraphia component showed a less clear relationship to PR variables, including hypergraphia ($r = .46$).

Results of this study show relative advantages and disadvantages of each method of measurement for assessing behavior in individuals with epilepsy. Results show that the patients in this sample clearly can be differentiated according to a number of measures of psychopathology and general dimensions of personality, so that such measures are relevant to the assessment of behavior in epilepsy. On the other hand, patients could also be differentiated according to dimensions that are less inherently psychopathological in nature, in particular, hypergraphia, religious interest, and philosophical interest. Results suggest that the most appropriate measure for assessing behavior in epilepsy would depend on the kind of behavior one would want to assess. If one is interested in general dimensions of normal and abnormal personality, the EPQ would have clear advantages, but the MMPI might also be applicable. The MMPI would probably be most appropriate to measure psychopathology because of the range of manifestations it covers, but the EPQ might also be appropriate. The BF has a considerable amount of variance related to psychopathology but seems to be a poorer choice for assessment in this realm because it most likely is not as reliable as the MMPI or EPQ and undoubtedly does not have the extensive validation of these two instruments. For assessing nonpsychopathological manifestations of interest in epilepsy, there is evidence from this study that both the BF and PR would be applicable. The PR appears to be preferable since it shows relatively little contamination by nonspecific psychopathology, unlike the BF, and since there are empirical estimates of the reliability of its scales. It is noteworthy that the WIGG showed a strong relationship to all four methods used for cluster derivation and thus may have considerable utility for assessment of behavior of individuals with epilepsy. Since the WIGG scales and MMPI scales are derived from the MMPI, one can assess a broad range of behavior relevant to epilepsy using the MMPI.

Empirical Definition of Behavioral Clusters

The cluster analysis procedure used in this study resulted in derivation of clusters within each method of measurement that could be reproduced using other methods of cluster extraction or using different subsamples of subjects. A few of the clusters were moderately reproduced according to one reliability estimate, but these were generally more reliable using the other reliability measure, and most of the derived clusters were strongly reproducible using both reliability estimates. Overall, the results indicate that clusters can be derived that have internal validity.

Results were also favorable in terms of external validity. Each cluster solution showed relationships to external variables not involved in cluster extraction, and these relationships generally fit well with theoretical expectations. It was quite apparent that derived clusters were associated with measures of parameters similar to those used to derive clusters but showed relatively little association with parameters that are less directly related to variables used for cluster extraction. More specifically, derived clusters show strong relations to other psychometric measures of behavior/personality/psychopathology but showed minimal relationships with measures of demographic variables, past history, or neurological, seizure, or EEG variables.

One striking aspect of the results of this study was that there was very little correspondence between clusters derived from different methods of measurement. The way subjects were categorized into groups appeared to be highly dependent on the measures used. One interpretation of this finding is that behavior in epilepsy is complex and multidimensional, and the more variables one considers, the less likely one is to find clearly separable groups. An alternative interpretation could be that the cluster analysis approach used in this study was inadequate in terms of identifying clusters that are robust across methods of measurement. One clear methodological limitation of this study was the relatively small sample size, particularly of derived clusters. Using a cluster analysis approach with a much larger sample size, preferably 400–500 subjects, would much more clearly answer the question of whether robust clusters can be found. These considerations aside, results of this study did not show evidence of robust clusters across measures.

Implications for a TLE Behavior Syndrome

Clusters resembling the personality syndrome proposed for TLE were identified, particularly using measures from the BF and PR, despite the lack of robust cross-method clusters. Identification of such clusters with the BF and PR is not surprising given that these instruments were developed to assess behavior that has been purported to occur with some specificity in TLE. Further, the behavioral syndrome variable specifically defined a group based on theoretical considerations regarding a TLE behavior syndrome. Even though groups consistent with previous formulations of the TLE personality syndrome were identified, results were unequivocal in that, with only two exceptions, groups derived from any set of variables did not differ on any variables related to seizure type, seizure severity, or seizure location. Both exceptions involved the behavioral syndrome group, where the group with the syndrome was found to have less background slowing and a relatively higher frequency of complex partial seizures. Epileptiform discharges arising within the temporal lobes did not discriminate groups from any method of measurement, nor did a diagnosis of temporal lobe epilepsy. In addition to the multiple appropriately controlled studies that have failed to find differences between groups of TLE patients and controls on a wide variety of measures including the BF and MMPI, this study failed to find a relationship when groups were derived on the basis of behavior and compared with respect to frequency of TLE or temporal lobe EFD.

The dearth of positive findings relating temporal lobe seizures to derived clusters is even more striking given the large number of comparisons that were performed for the sample size available for this study. A very deliberate attempt was made to avoid capitalizing on chance variation, so one possible explanation for the lack of positive results is that the sample size did not allow for adequate power to detect meaningful differences. This does not seem to be a viable explanation for several reasons. First, differences were found on other variables, and these differences generally followed theoretical expectations. Second, the power for some of the relevant comparisons was quite satisfactory. Third, the differences that were obtained generally did not come close to being statistically significant. Indeed, if a p level of .10 based on individual comparisons had been used instead of a p level of .05 based on groups of comparisons, results would not have differed.

Results of this study also fail to support the hypothesis that previous negative results have been caused by insensitive instruments, as no one instrument was clearly superior to others even though two of the instruments used, employing different methods of measurement, had been developed specifically to be sensitive to theoretically relevant behavior. This conclusion is consistent with the predominantly negative results, discussed in an earlier section, that have been obtained with the BF. These considerations make it much more likely that the lack of significant TLE–behavior relationships found in this study reflects a true absence of such a relationship as opposed to methodological inadequacies of this study and of the number of previous studies with negative findings.

This study did not use controls without epilepsy, so it cannot address questions about how behavior in epilepsy differs or doesn't differ from behavior in a normal population or behavior associated with other chronic illnesses, neurological disorders, or psychiatric disorders. The behavioral clusters identified in this study may well prove to have meaning with respect to understanding behavior in epilepsy, even though results do not favor the hypothesis that specific patterns of behavior are associated with specific parameters of the seizure disorder. Further study using nonepilepsy control groups may be very valuable for a better understanding of the determinants of both normal and abnormal behavior in epilepsy.

Future Directions

Epilepsy, and more recently TLE, have long been regarded as important models for understanding the way that abnormalities of brain function relate to behavior. For this reason, there has been considerable effort devoted to identifying behavioral variables that have a specific relationship to TLE, and much of the intellectual energy in the field has been focused on the debate about whether there are or are not behaviors or constellations of behaviors that are unique to TLE. This has had an unfortunate effect in that questions about causes of behavior that are not directly related to the neurological substrate have been relatively neglected. There clearly seems to be a need for further research, as recommended by Hermann and Whitman (1986), that systematically tries to identify risk factors for specific kinds of behavior that occur in epilepsy. Research of this kind that compares a broad range of potential epilepsy and nonepilepsy variables with specific behavior variables of interest will be very important for a better understanding of how behavior in patients with epilepsy has both common and different determinants than behavior in individuals without epilepsy. Hermann and Whitman (1984) have made an important conceptual step in this direction with their model identifying kinds of behavior that occur in epilepsy that are relatively independent or epilepsy parameters (e.g., aggression) and behaviors that do appear to have a specific relationship to parameters of epilepsy (e.g., hyposexuality).

The approach followed in this study in which groups were defined on the basis of behavior may also have utility for further study of determinants of behavior in epilepsy. Several recommendations appear to be appropriate in terms of maximizing the significance of such research. First, variables should be selected to span as broad a range of normal and abnormal behavior as possible. Careful consideration should be given to the psychometric properties of measures of these variables. The MMPI would appear to be a good candidate for such research, as it spans a very broad range of behavior, particularly with the use of the Wiggins Content Scales, has established psychometric properties, and has been widely used with both normal and abnormal populations. Whatever instrument is used, it is important to identify a parsimonious number of variables that adequately represent the entire range of behavior of interest. This can be done empirically through factor analytic or cluster-analytic procedures or using *a priori* theoretical considerations in the context of the body or research on behavior/personality assessment.

Second, this kind of research, by its very nature, requires a large sample in order to assure that meaningful numbers of subjects will be found in some of the less frequent but reliable and valid categories. A third, related issue deals with the subject sample from which groups are derived. Selecting epilepsy patients from different populations (e.g., teaching hospital and private practice) would provide for much greater heterogeneity of both behavior and parameters of epilepsy. In addition to patients with epilepsy, it would also be very useful to include groups of normal subjects, groups of patients with other chronic illnesses, groups with other neurological illnesses, and groups with psychiatric illness. Deriving behaviorally homogeneous clusters from a large, heterogeneous sample would allow for much broader characterization of factors that relate to different homogeneous clusters.

Both this approach and the risk factor approach advocated by Hermann and Whitman (1986) would inherently require at least several hundred subjects to maximize the impact of the study. Either approach followed in a comprehensive manner would require considerable effort and time to complete. On the other hand, epilepsy is a relatively prevalent disorder, and large numbers of patients with epilepsy can be found. Further, personality inventories can assess a broad range of behavior in a relatively short period of time, and behavioral rating scales such as that used in this study can also be used in a time-effective manner. Comprehensive study of the relationship between epilepsy and behavior is feasible and is likely to be far more revealing than the multitude of studies that have occurred in the last 30 years involving small sample sizes and addressing only the question of existence of behaviors unique to TLE.

One final caveat about future research in this area is appropriate. Although research on behavioral correlates of TLE may have considerable significance for understanding the neuropsychological organization of higher-level adaptive behavior, there is a need for appropriate caution in interpreting research findings, particularly when attempting to make brain–behavior links. The field of neuropsychology has been very successful in identifying brain–behavior relationships, but these generally involve relatively discrete perceptual–motor and cognitive processes. It is widely acknowledged that complex cognitive functions are difficult to localize discretely (Luria, 1966), and it should come as no surprise that higher-level adaptive behavior that involves an integration of simple and complex perceptual and motor abilities, higher cognitive abilities, and emotions should be complexly organized within the brain. In the area of TLE, the neurological substrate of the disorder is quite heterogeneous and complex (Kligman & Goldberg, 1975; Tizard, 1962), and this complexity is further compounded by the complexity of the limbic system. The limbic system is composed of numerous separate nuclei and their interconnections, and widely divergent and unpredictable behavioral effects can result from manipulation of closely spaced structures or from manipulation of the same structure under different circumstances (cf. Valenstein, 1973).

Given the extreme complexity of the problem of the neuropsychological organization of behavior in TLE and the relatively primitive nature of empirical data in the area, inferences about possible neurobiological mechanisms that could account for behavioral characteristics of TLE appear to be premature. With the present state of knowledge, it would appear to be more appropriate to focus efforts on better defining the range and quality of behavior that occurs in epilepsy. Lack of theory has not historically been a problem in this field—future research needs to provide the empirical data base from which meaningful theory can be derived.

CHAPTER SUMMARY

A number of recent studies have addressed the issue of a specific syndrome of behavior associated with temporal lobe epilepsy, but conceptual and methodological limitations have left a number of important questions not adequately answered. One particular problem is that the issue of a syndrome of behavior has not typically been directly addressed in research design. Cluster analysis offers a potentially valuable methodology for empirically and directly identifying subgroups of patients with epilepsy who are homogeneous according to specific patterns of behavior. This chapter describes an attempt to use cluster analysis procedures based on a broad range of behavioral variables to identify subgroups. An attempt was then made to determine if these subgroups differed from each other on relevant seizure, neurological, demographic, and psychosocial variables.

Measures used as a basis for cluster derivation were selected in an attempt to broadly sample normal and abnormal behavior and personality characteristics, psychiatric symptoms, and specific parameters of behavior that have been attributed to patients with temporal lobe epilepsy. These measures included the MMPI, the Eysenck Personality Questionnaire, the Bear and Fedio Personality Inventory, and a behavior rating scale developed to assess behavior characteristics that have played a prominent role in the controversy about specific patterns of behavior in temporal lobe epilepsy. For each of these measurement methods, a cluster analysis procedure was independently performed to derive homogeneous subgroups from a sample of general epilepsy outpatients. In addition, using a theory-guided approach, subjects were divided into groups with and without behavioral characteristics matching previous theoretical formulations about temporal lobe epilepsy.

The cluster analysis solutions for each method of measurement showed good evidence for internal validity or reproducibility of the obtained clusters across different clustering methods. On the other hand, the derived clusters showed modest, at best, correspondence to clusters derived from other methods of measurement. The theory-based groups also showed only modest association with derived clusters. External validity of the identified subgroups was tested by comparing groups on a broad spectrum of variables not used in group derivation. There was strong evidence for external validity in that groups did differ on a number of behavior/personality/psychiatric variables that assessed characteristics similar to those assessed by the variables that served as a basis for subgroup derivation. Several of the derived subgroups were defined by characteristics that have often been attributed to temporal lobe epilepsy. There was limited association between derived subgroups and external variables not directly related to the behavior in question. In particular, there was no relationship between temporal lobe epilepsy or a seizure focus within the temporal lobes and any of the derived groups.

Results fail to support the hypothesis that there is a specific syndrome of behavior that can be identified in temporal lobe epilepsy. Subgroups with prominent characteristics that have been attributed to temporal lobe epilepsy were identified, but these groups were not differentially associated with temporal lobe epilepsy. Results suggest that behavior in patients with epilepsy is complexly determined and cannot easily be categorized according to seizure focus. Future research attempting to relate important behavior in epilepsy to a broad range of potential etiological variables, including but not limited to seizure and neurological variables, is recommended to further our understanding of the behavioral effects of epilepsy and to provide an empirical base for a better theoretical understanding of neuropsychological mechanisms underlying adaptive behavior.

ACKNOWLEDGMENTS.   This research was supported by NIMH Grant No. 1 RO3 MH39700-01A1. This study was conducted in collaboration with George Palma and Dale Blunden. Kent Bentington and Andrea Lasken made major contributions, particularly involving the behavioral ratings. Faculty, residents, and staff of the U.C. Davis Medical Center Neurology Outpatient Clinic assisted with subject recruitment. This study was made possible by the patients who volunteered their time as subjects.

REFERENCES

Barron, F. (1953). An ego-strength scale which predicts response to psychothereapy. *Journal of Consulting Psychiatry, 17*, 327–333.

Bear, D. M. (1979). Temporal lobe epilepsy: A syndrome of sensory–limbic hyperconnection. *Cortex, 15*, 357–384.

Bear, D. (1983). Behavioral symptoms in temporal lobe epilepsy. *Archives of General Psychiatry, 40*, 467–468.

Bear, D. M., & Fedio, P. (1977). Quantitative analysis of interictal behavior in temporal lobe epilepsy. *Archives of Neurology, 34*, 454–467.

Bear, D., Levin, K., Blumer, D., Chetham, D., & Ryder, J. (1982). Interictal behavior in hospitalized temporal lobe epileptics: Relationship to idiopathic psychiatric syndromes. *Journal of Neurology, Neurosurgery, and Psychiatry, 45*, 481–488.

Brandt, J., Seidman, L. J., & Kohl, D. (1985). Personality characteristics of epileptic patients: A controlled study of generalized and temporal lobe cases. *Journal of Clinical and Experimental Neuropsychology, 7*, 25–38.

Campbell, D. T., & Fiske, D. W. (1959). Convergent and discriminant validation by the multitrait–multimethod matrix. *Psychological Bulletin, 56*, 81–105.

Dodrill, C. B., Batzel, L. W., Queisser, H. R., & Temkin, N. R. (1980). An objective method for the assessment of psychological and social problems among epileptics. *Epilepsia, 21*, 123–135.

Endicott, J., & Spitzer, R. L. (1978). A diagnostic interview: The schedule for affective disorders and schizophrenia. *Archives of General Psychiatry, 35*, 837–844.

Eysenck, H. J., & Eysenck, S. B. G. (1973). *Eysenck Personality Inventory, ETIS manual*. San Diego: Educational and Industrial Testing Service.

Fletcher, J. M., Rice, W. J., & Ray, R. M. (1978). Linear discriminant function analysis in neuropsychological research: Some uses and abuses. *Cortex, 14*, 564–577.

Geschwind, N. (1977). Behavioral change in temporal lobe epilepsy. *Archives of Neurology, 34*, 453.

Gibbs, F. A., & Gibbs, E. L. (1964). *Atlas of electroencephalography*, Volume 3. Reading, MA: Addison-Wesley.

Gibbs, F. A., Gibbs, E. L., & Fuster, B. (1948). Psychomotor epilepsy. *Archives of Neurology and Psychiatry, 60*, 331–339.

Goldberg, L. R. (1965). Diagnosticians vs. diagnostic signs: The diagnosis of psychosis vs. neurosis from the *MMPI*. *Psychological Monographs, 79*, (No. 602).

Hartigan, J. A. (1975). *Clustering algorithms*. New York: John Wiley & Sons.

Hermann, B. P., & Riel, P. (1981). Interictal personality and behavioral traits in temporal lobe and generalized epilepsy. *Cortex, 17*, 125–128.

Hermann, B. P., & Whitman, S. (1984). Behavioral and personality correlates of epilepsy: A review, methodological critique, and conceptual model. *Psychological Bulletin, 95*, 451–497.

Hermann, B. P., & Whitman, S. (1986). Psychopathology in epilepsy: A multietiologic model. In S. Whitman & B. P. Hermann (Eds.), *Psychopathology in epilepsy: Social dimensions* (pp. 5–37). New York: Oxford University Press.

Hermann, B. P., Schwartz, M. S., Karnes, W. E., & Vahdat, P. (1980). Psychopathology in epilepsy: Relationship of seizure type to age of onset. *Epilepsia, 21*, 15–23.

Hermann, B. P., Whitman, S., & Arnston, P. (1983). Hypergraphia in epilepsy: Is there a specifity to temporal lobe epilepsy? *Journal of Neurology, Neurosurgery, and Psychiatry, 46*, 848–853.

Hermann, B. P., Whitman, S., Wyler, A. R., Richey, T. T., & Dell, J. (1988). The neurological, psychosocial, and demographic correlates of hypergraphia in patients with epilepsy. *Journal of Neurology, Neurosurgery, and Psychiatry, 51*, 203–208.

Kligman, D., & Goldberg, D. A. (1975). Temporal lobe epilepsy and aggression: Problems in clinical research. *Journal of Nervous and Mental Disease, 160*, 324–341.

Lennox, W. G., & Lennox, M. A. (1960). *Epilepsy and related disorders*. Boston: Little, Brown.

Lord, F. M., & Novick, M. R. (1968). *Statistical theories of mental test scores*. Reading, MA: Addison-Wesley.

Luria, A. R. (1966). *Higher cortical functions in man* (B. Haigh, trans.). New York: Basic Books.

Mathews, C. G., & Klove, H. (1968). MMPI performance in major motor, psychomotor and mixed seizure classifications of known and unknown etiology. *Epilepsia, 9,* 43–53.

Meehl, P. E., & Hathaway, S. R. (1946). The K factor as a supressor variable in the MMPI. *Journal of Applied Psychology, 30,* 525–564.

Mignone, R. J., Donnelly, E. F., & Sadowsky, D. (1970). Psychological and neurological comparisons of psychomotor and nonpsychomotor epileptic patients. *Epilepsia, 11,* 345–359.

Morris, R., Blashfield, R., & Satz, P. (1981). Neuropsychology and cluster analysis: Potentials and problems. *Journal of Clinical Neuropsychology, 3,* 79–99.

Mungas, D. (1982). Interictal behavior abnormality in temporal lobe epilepsy: A specific syndrome or non-specific psychopathology? *Archives of General Psychiatry, 39,* 108–111.

Mungas, D. (1983). Behavioral symptoms in temporal lobe epilepsy. In reply. *Archives of General Psychiatry, 40,* 468–469.

Nielsen, H., & Kristensen, O. (1981). Personality correlates of sphenoidal EEG foci in temporal lobe epilepsy. *Acta Neurologica Scandinavica, 64,* 289–300.

Rodin, E., & Schmaltz, S. (1984). The Bear–Fedio Personality Inventory and temporal lobe epilepsy. *Neurology, 34,* 591–596.

Rodin, E. A., Katz, M., & Lennox, C. (1976). Differences between patients with temporal lobe seizures and those with other forms of epileptic attacks. *Epilepsia, 17,* 313–320.

Sachdev, H. S., & Waxman, S. G. (1981). Frequency of hypergraphia in temporal lobe epilepsy: An index of interictal behavior syndrome. *Journal of Neurology, Neurosurgery, and Psychiatry, 44,* 358–360.

Seidman, L. (1980). *Lateralized cerebral dysfunction, personality, and cognition in temporal lobe epilepsy*. Dissertation, Boston University: University Microfilms International.

Silberman, E. K. (1983). Behavioral symptoms in temporal lobe epilepsy. *Archives of General Psychiatry, 40,* 468.

Small, J. G., Millstein, V., & Stevens, J. R. (1962). Are psychomotor epileptics different? A controlled study. *Archives of Neurology, 7,* 187–194.

Spitzer, R. L., & Endicott, J. (1978). *Schedule for affective disorders and schizophrenia—change version (SADS-C)* (ed. 3). New York: Biometrics Research, New York State Psychiatric Institute.

Standage, K. F., & Fenton, G. W. (1975). Psychiatris symptom profiles of patients with epilepsy: A controlled investigation. *Psychological Medicine, 5,* 152–160.

Stark-Adamec, C., & Adamec, R. E. (1986). Psychological methodology versus clinical impressions: Different perspectives on psychopathology and seizures. In B. K. Doane & K. E. Livingstone (Eds.), *The limbic system: Functional organization and clinical disorders* (pp. 217–227). New York: Raven Press.

Stevens, J. R. (1966). Psychiatric implications of psychomotor epilepsy. *Archives of General Psychiatry, 14,* 461–471.

Stevens, J. R. (1975). Interictal clinical manifestations of complex partial seizures, In J. K. Penry & D. D. Daly (Eds.), *Complex partial seizures and their treatment, Vol. 11, Advances in Neurology* (pp. 85–112). New York: Raven Press.

Stevens, J. R. (1982). Risk factors for psychopathology in individuals with epilepsy. In W. P. Koella & M. R. Trimble (Eds.), *Advances in Biological Psychiatry* (Volume 8, pp. 56–80). Basel: S. Karger.

Temkin, O. (1971). *The falling sickness: A history of epilepsy from the Greeks to the beginnings of modern neurology*, (ed. 2). Baltimore, MD: Johns Hopkins University Press.

Tizard, B. (1962). The personality of epileptics: A discussion of the evidence. *Psychological Bulletin, 59,* 196–210.

Tucker, D. M., Novelly, R. A., & Walker, P. J. (1987). Hyperreligiosity in temporal lobe epilepsy: Redefining the relationship. *Journal of Nervous and Mental Disease, 175,* 181–184.

Valenstein, E. (1973). *Brain control: A critical examination of brain stimulation and psychosurgery*. New York: John Wiley & Sons.

Waxman, S. G., & Geschwind, N. (1975). The interictal behavior syndrome of temporal lobe epilepsy. *Archives of General Psychiatry, 32*, 1580–1586.

Wiggins, J. S. (1966). Substantive dimensions of self-report in the MMPI item pool. *Psychological Monographs, 80*(22, whole No. 630).

Wiggins, J. S. (1973). *Personality and prediction: Principles of personality assessment*. Reading, MA: Addison-Wesley.

Wilkinson, L. (1987). *SYSTAT: The system for statistics*. Evanston, IL: SYSTAT, Inc.

Zielinski, J. J. (1974). Epileptics not in treatment. *Epilepsia, 15*, 203–210.

8

Psychological and Psychosocial Outcome of Anterior Temporal Lobectomy

LINDSEY J. ROBINSON and ANDREW J. SAYKIN

It is now generally recognized that the outcome of epilepsy surgery must be measured not just in terms of relief from seizures but also with respect to psychosocial functioning, including psychiatric, vocational, and interpersonal factors (Taylor, 1987; Fenwick, 1988; Dodrill, 1986). In this chapter, common methods of measuring psychological and psychosocial outcome are reviewed, including representative studies that have employed each method. We also examine methodological issues and present preliminary data from our laboratory that illustrate the importance of adequate experimental control. Finally, we propose several directions for future research.

Domains of interest in assessing psychosocial outcome include affective, vocational, and interpersonal functioning as well as functioning with respect to activities of daily living (see Table 8.1). Several methods for measuring psychological and psychosocial outcome have been employed in previous studies. These include psychiatric diagnoses, experimenter-designed rating scales, structured interviews developed to assess patients' own perceptions of their functioning, and objective, standardized measures of personality and psychopathology developed for use with epileptic patients or general clinical populations. More "external" indices of functioning including vocational status, rates of psychiatric hospitalization, and incidence of suicide have also been examined.

LINDSEY J. ROBINSON and ANDREW J. SAYKIN • Brain Behavior Laboratory, Department of Psychiatry, University of Pennsylvania School of Medicine, Philadelphia, Pennsylvania 19104-4283.

The Neuropsychology of Epilepsy, edited by Thomas L. Bennett. Plenum Press, New York, 1992.

TABLE 8.1.   Psychosocial
Outcome Domains

I. Affective
   A. Diagnosable psychiatric disorder
   B. Other affective symptoms
   C. "Epileptic personality" traits
   D. Psychological well-being
II. Vocational
   A. Type of employment
   B. Hours worked (percentage of full time)
III. Interpersonal
   A. Relationships with family members
   B. Relationships with others
   C. Sexual functioning
IV. Activities of daily living
   A. Self-care
   B. Functioning in the home
   C. Functioning in the community

PSYCHIATRIC DIAGNOSES AND RATING SCALES

In an early study, Green, Steelman, Duisberg, McGrath, and Wick (1958) followed 38 patients for 18 months to 8.5 years after temporal lobectomy. All were economically dependent and exhibited "mild to severe disturbances of behavior" prior to surgery. Following surgery, 17 patients (45%) were independent and self-supporting. Changes in "thinking," "feeling," and "action" were rated by clinicians on a five-point scale; improvements in affect and behavior were reported to be greatest in those patients obtaining the best postoperative seizure control. However, there was no control group, no statistical tests were performed on the ratings, and effects of side of surgery were not considered.

Taylor and Falconer (1968; Taylor, 1972; Falconer, 1973) reported on psycho-social outcome in the second Maudsley Hospital series of 100 patients, who were followed for 2 to 12 years. Outcome data were obtained from record reviews and semistructured interviews with patients and with their relatives when possible. Patients were rated on 64 variables including degree of independence in living arrangements, quality of family and nonfamily relationships, vocational status, use of leisure time, and sexual adjustment. "Reliability" of the rating system, assessed by rerating 10 patients with different raters, was found to be adequate (i.e., no significant differences between raters by ANOVA). The authors also compared the distribution of ratings for the first 50 and second 50 cases and found no significant difference. Only 13 of 100 patients (13%) were considered psychiatrically normal before surgery. The remainder were diagnosed as "neurotic," "psychopathic," "psychotic," or "epileptic personality." The criteria for these diagnoses were not specified. Following surgery, 32 (32%) patients were considered normal. However, whereas 16 patients were diagnosed as "psychotic" before surgery, 19 received this diagnosis after surgery. Examination of ratings of social adjustment indicated that patients improved with respect to family and nonfamily relationships and vocational adjustment but not use of leisure time or sexual adjustment. Quality of social adjustment was significantly related to relief from seizures and findings of mesial temporal sclerosis on neuropathological examination. Poor outcome was associated with the presence of preoperative psychosis, adolescent onset, low IQ, family history of mental illness, and nonspecific neuropathological findings. Patients receiving a preoperative diagnosis of "psychopathic" were more likely to have a left temporal focus, whereas those diagnosed "neurotic" were more likely to have a right focus; however, this trend failed to reach statistical significance. Although Taylor and Falconer's use of a structured rating system and statistical tests of their findings were strengths, it should be noted that most of their patients were referred through a psychiatric hospital. Thus, descriptions of psychiatric and social outcome in this group may not be representative of the general surgical epilepsy population.

Walker and Blumer (1977, 1984) presented observations of 50 patients followed from 12 to 30 years after surgery. Information was obtained from interviews with patients and family members and observations of patients during hospitalizations, with particular emphasis on characteristics believed to be associated with the "epileptic personality" (Bear & Fedio, 1977; Geschwind, 1983). Walker and Blumer reported that temporal lobectomy resulted in improvements in aggressiveness, irritability, and hyposexuality but not in cognitive viscosity or hyperreligiosity. These improvements appeared to be related to degree of seizure control after surgery. In this series, five patients (10%) were characterized as psychotic preoperatively; following surgery, three additional patients developed psychoses. Walker and Blumer present no statistical tests of their findings.

Horowitz and Cohen (1968) made subjective ratings of adaptive functioning of 17 patients who had undergone temporal lobectomy 1 to 12 years earlier: 53% to 59% were rated as improved in overall functioning. Rankings of level of functioning were correlated highly with scores on a memory test. The authors noted that patients whose adaptive functioning did not improve tended to have more cognitive deficits or preexisting psychopathology. Laterality effects were not examined.

Horowitz, Cohen, Skolnikoff, and Saunders (1970) used a similar rating system to evaluate 19 epileptic patients before and 6 months after surgery. Some of these patients had stereotactic temporal lobe lesions, some had standard temporal lobectomies, and some underwent both procedures. They found no changes in level of adaptive functioning after 6 months but noted that some patients were improved when reevaluated at a later date. Again, laterality effects were not examined.

In a study of Danish patients, Jensen and Larsen (1979) followed 74 temporal lobectomy patients for 1 to 11 years after surgery. Outcome data consisted of subjective ratings by the experimenters and retrospective review of medical records. Prior to surgery, 63 patients (85%) were noted to have "behavioral disturbances," including 11 patients (15%) who were psychotic. After surgery, only 50 (68%) were reported as having psychiatric disturbances; however, 20 of these (27%) were psychotic. Sixty patients had marked reduction in seizures or were completely seizure-free following surgery; of these, 18 (30%) had "markedly improved" psychiatrically, and 17 (28%) had deteriorated or were unchanged. The authors drew the conclusion that temporal lobectomy resulted in improved psychiatric functioning, especially with relief from seizures. Flor-Henry (1983), in contrast, has interpreted this study as supporting the hypothesis that "forced normalization" secondary to removal of epileptogenic tissue may result in *increased* psychopathology. Laterality effects, again, were not examined. Jensen and Larsen reported no statistical tests of their findings.

Rausch and Crandall (1982) examined psychosocial functioning in 31 patients before and at 1 and 12 months after temporal lobectomy. Rating scales similar to those used by Taylor and Falconer (1968) and Horowitz and Cohen (1968) were completed by two raters with good interrater reliability (.84 to .97), based on interviews with patients and family members. Patients were grouped according to degree of seizure control following surgery. Only patients who were seizure-free showed significant improvement in psychosocial functioning (degree of dependency, work performance, and nonfamily relationships). However, these patients also had lower seizure frequencies and better psychosocial functioning before surgery. Patients with left- and right-sided resections did not differ significantly.

Finally, Polkey (1983) presented intellectual and psychiatric observations of 40 patients followed for 2 to 6 years after surgery. Prior to surgery, 23 patients (58%) had some form of "mental disorder," including aggressive and obsessional behavior, phobias, and depression. After surgery, 28 patients (70%) were unchanged, 8 (20%) improved (predominantly because of decreases in aggressiveness), and 4 (10%) worsened. Postoperative complications included depression, psychosis, ruminant obsessions, and pseudoseizures. Patients who developed psychosis all had nondominant resections. Polkey did not specify the criteria used for psychiatric diagnosis, nor were statistical analyses employed.

STRUCTURED INTERVIEWS

Patients' perceptions of changes in psychosocial functioning following surgery have been assessed using structured interviews designed for this purpose. Savard and Walker (1965) interviewed 39 patients 2 to 5 years after surgery. Patients were first asked to describe changes they had noticed and then were questioned about change (negative, positive, or no change) in six areas of functioning: self (self-care, attitude toward self), home physical environment, home interpersonal environment, vocational functioning, participation in community activities, and sexual behavior. Most patients (81%) reported that their overall social functioning had improved, and the number of positive changes reported exceeded the number of negative changes. The most frequent changes reported were increased self-esteem and greater involvement in activities outside the home. Positive changes were greatest in patients with the best seizure outcome, although even those with no change in seizure frequency reported some positive changes. The authors note that these were patients whose seizures changed in their qualitative characteristics so as to become less socially incapacitating. Laterality effects were not examined. In half of the cases, a family member was also interviewed. Savard and Walker report that there was "substantial agreement" between patients and relatives, but this was not evaluated statistically.

In our laboratory, a structured neurobehavioral interview was developed to assess patient and family perception of change following cortical resection surgery (Reinecke, Saykin, Sperling, Roberts, Kester, Gur, & O'Connor, 1989). Global perceptions of change in cognitive, affective, and overall functioning were assessed. Patients also rated themselves as improved, unchanged, or worsened in nine areas of cognitive functioning (e.g., memory, expressive and receptive language, attention, and alertness) and 20 affective/psychiatric symptoms (e.g., depression, anxiety, hallucinations, delusional thinking, agitation). Family members made analogous ratings. To date, 47 patients and 31 relatives have completed the interview. Preliminary analyses indicate that most patients reported improved cognitive functioning (64%), improved emotional functioning (64%), and improved overall functioning (74%). Distributions of ratings by patients and relatives did not differ significantly. However, patients undergoing left compared to right temporal lobectomy were more likely to rate themselves as worsened with respect to overall cognitive functioning (15% versus 0%, $p < .02$), expressive language functioning (27% versus 0%, $p < .01$), and attention and alertness (15% versus 0%, $p < .03$). These findings suggest that, although most patients report improved functioning following surgery, patients undergoing left temporal resections are more likely to perceive and report negative changes than are patients undergoing right temporal resections (see Fig. 8.1). It is unclear whether left temporal patients actually experience more deficits or, alternatively, that right temporal patients are more likely to deny or minimize difficulties. A more detailed discussion of this study will be presented in a separate publication.

"EXTERNAL" INDICES

Experimenter biases and distortions in patients' impressions of their own functioning may be circumvented by examining external, more objective indicators of psychosocial functioning. One such indicator is employment status. Taylor and Falconer (1968) noted that only 7 (7%) of their patients were working with no difficulty before surgery, whereas 36 (36%) were employed after surgery. Of 37 patients who were unemployed before surgery, 13 (35%) became employed after surgery.

Augustine, Novelly, Mattson, Glaser, Williamson, Spencer, and Spencer (1984) classified the vocational status of 32 surgical epilepsy patients as employed (75–100% of full time), underemployed (25–74%), or unemployed (0–24%) before surgery and at three postoperative intervals (first year, second year, and most recent year). Across these intervals, the number employed increased from 14 (44%) to 23 (72%), and the number underemployed decreased from 8 (25%) to 0. Rate of unemployment did not

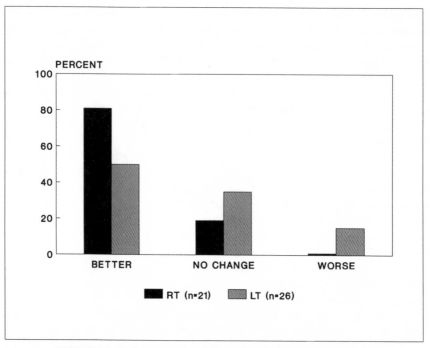

FIGURE 8.1. Patient perception of change in overall cognitive functioning.

change. Most shifts in employment status occurred during the first postoperative year. Degree of seizure control after surgery was significantly better for the employed group than the unemployed, but "vocationally improved" patients and those who continued to be unemployed did not differ in this respect. Continued unemployed patients were more likely to have a nondominant seizure focus, lower PIQ, and preoperative psychiatric disorder.

Occurrences of psychiatric hospitalizations before and after surgery may also serve as an indicator of outcome. For example, Walker and Blumer (1984) reported that 14 of their 50 patients (28%) were hospitalized at some point: six both before and after surgery, four before surgery only, and four after surgery only. They note that other patients were never hospitalized, although they had experienced psychiatric difficulties of equal severity.

Rate of suicide among patients with epilepsy has been examined by several investigators. Among nonsurgical epileptic patients, suicide rates up to 25 times higher than the general population have been observed (Barraclough, 1981; Hawton, Fagg, & Marsack, 1980). Taylor and Marsh (1977) reported nine suicides following surgery in a series of 193 patients, a rate (4.7%) they describe as 45 times greater than expected based on population statistics. Walker and Blumer (1984) reported two probable suicides (4%) in their series of 50 surgical patients. Fenwick (1988), in a survey of 14 surgical epilepsy centers, found rates of suicide ranging from 0 to 2%, approximately consistent with population expectations. He noted that rates may vary considerably from study to study and underscored the need for clear description of patient characteristics, criteria for inclusion and exclusion, and rates of psychiatric morbidity. In fact, a problem with the use of any external index as an outcome criterion is that it may be influenced by a variety of uncontrolled environmental, economic, and historical factors (Walker & Blumer, 1984).

STANDARDIZED INSTRUMENTS

In an attempt to reduce the subjectivity inherent in use of psychiatric diagnoses, rating scales, and clinical observations as outcome criteria, many investigators have employed standardized measures of psychopathology developed for use in general clinical populations. The Minnesota Multiphasic Personality Inventory (MMPI) is one such instrument. Use of the MMPI in epilepsy research has been criticized by some (Flor-Henry, 1972; Trimble, 1983; Bear & Fedio, 1977) as being insensitive to the unique psychological characteristics of epileptic patients. Although it has been suggested that elevations on Scale 8 (Sc) simply reflect accurate reporting of neurological symptoms rather than the presence of psychopathology, the validity of the MMPI as a measure of psychopathology in epilepsy has been empirically demonstrated (Dikmen, Hermann, Wilensky, & Rainwater, 1983).

Meier and French (1965) examined MMPI clinical scales, the MMPI Caudality scale, and a global MMPI-based index of psychopathology (Ip) in 40 temporal lobectomy patients before and after surgery. Mean group scores were compared via multiple t-tests. The length of the follow-up period was unclear. After surgery, the group as a whole obtained significantly higher scores on Scale K and lower scores on Scales 6 (Pa), Caudality, and Ip. Patients with left temporal resections obtained higher postoperative scores on Scale K and lower scores on Scales 6 (Pa), O (Si), and Caudality, whereas right temporal patients obtained higher postoperative scores on Scale L and lower scores on Scales 8 (Sc) and Caudality. This study was unusual in that a control group of 19 nonsurgical epileptic patients was retested after 1 year; mean MMPI t-scores for this group were not significantly different on retesting. The authors concluded that their findings indicated mild declines in personality disturbance following temporal lobectomy.

Lansdell (1968) administered the MMPI before and 2 weeks after temporal lobectomy to 37 patients. Postoperative scores on MMPI Scales F and 8 (Sc), the Taulbee–Sisson score, Welsh's A scale, and the Goldberg index were examined using preoperative scores and extent of tissue removal as covariates. Left temporal cases obtained significantly higher scores than right temporal cases on Scale F and the Goldberg index. There was a nonsignificant trend for left temporal cases to score higher on Scale 8 (Sc) as well. Welsh's A scale was negatively correlated with size of tissue resection ($r = -.42$). It was concluded that left temporal lobectomy was associated with nonspecific psychological abnormality, whereas large right temporal resections were associated with decreased emphasis on some neurotic symptoms. However, no control group was employed.

Rausch, McCreary, and Crandall (1977) studied 10 patients who had undergone temporal lobectomy at least 1 year earlier. This sample was restricted to patients who had no history of psychiatric treatment, no cognitive changes following surgery, and who had experienced at least a 50% decrease in seizure frequency following surgery. An attempt was made to predict postoperative level of psychosocial functioning from subjective clinical evaluations of preoperative MMPI profiles. It was concluded that patients with evidence of "rigid, well-organized" psychopathology on the MMPI had poor psychosocial adjustments after surgery. Patients with left and right lobectomies did not differ in level of postoperative adjustment. Although this study is unique in that individual MMPI profiles were examined rather than group means, other methodological limitations (particularly restriction of the sample to patients with no psychiatric history) may limit the generalizability of their findings.

Other standardized measures of personality and psychopathology have also been employed. Serafetinides (1975) assessed 31 temporal lobectomy patients before and after surgery. The length of the follow-up period was unclear, and the degree of seizure relief obtained by each patient was not specified. Nonsignificant trends toward decreased scores on the Brief Psychiatric Rating Scale and the Zung Depression Inventory were noted. Laterality effects were not examined.

Taylor and Marsh (1979) administered the Eysenck Personality Questionnaire to 31 surgical patients from the Maudsley series who had "alien tissue" lesions (e.g., small tumors, hamartomas, focal dysplasia). Patients were divided into four groups on the basis of gender and side of operation. Although all patients had elevated Lie scores, other scores were compatible with Eysenck's normative data. Males with left temporal resections scored lower than males with right temporal resections on the Extraversion scale, and females with left temporal resections scored higher than females with right temporal resections on the Lie scale. Interpretation of these findings is difficult for several reasons. Patients studied were restricted to those with structural lesions and were tested after surgery only. Group sizes were very small (4 to 11 patients per group), and within-group variability was high. In addition, the authors noted that the female left temporal group was significantly older than the other groups.

Hermann, Wyler, Ackerman, and Rosenthal (1989) tested 41 patients before and 1, 3, and 6 months after surgery with the Mental Health Inventory (MHI), a 38-item questionnaire assessing psychological distress and well-being. Significant decreases in psychological distress and increases in well-being were observed at 1 and 3 months after surgery for seizure-free patients but not for those with continued seizures. Laterality effects were not examined. In addition, the seizure-free patients demonstrated more psychopathology on the MHI preoperatively, a finding that the authors minimize but that may have affected postoperative between-group comparisons.

Hermann and Wyler (1989) examined the relationship between depression and locus of control in 37 patients tested before and 6 months after surgery with the Center for Epidemiological Studies of Depression Scale (CES-D) and Rotter's internal–external control of reinforcement (I–E) scale. Before surgery, level of depression was positively correlated with external locus of control ($r = .38$); the correlation after surgery was nonsignificant ($r = .02$). The CES-D scores decreased significantly for patients who were seizure-free after surgery but not for those with continued seizures; I–E scores did not change.

Bear and Fedio's Temporal Lobe Personality Inventory (TLPI; Bear & Fedio, 1977) was developed to assess 18 personality traits believed to characterize patients with temporal lobe epilepsy. Subsequent studies have suggested, instead, that scores on the TLPI reflect degree of nonspecific psychopathology rather than the presence of a behavioral syndrome specific to temporal lobe epilepsy (Mungas, 1982; Reinecke, Saykin, Sperling, & Gur, 1988). Fedio and Martin (1983) administered the TLPI to patients who had undergone left ($n = 9$) or right ($n = 10$) temporal lobectomy 3 to 19 years earlier and to six normal controls. "Ideative" and "emotive" indices were computed based on the results of factor analysis of Bear and Fedio's (1977) original sample of 27 subjects. Although differences were not statistically significant, left temporal patients tended to rate themselves higher on "ideative" traits (religiosity, philosophical interests, sense of personal destiny), whereas right temporal patients rated themselves higher on "emotive" traits (anger, aggression, sadness). In addition, both groups of lobectomy patients rated themselves lower overall than Bear and Fedio's original sample of nonoperated temporal lobe epileptics. The authors interpret this difference as indicative of a positive effect of lobectomy on psychosocial functioning. Two problems limit the interpretability of the Fedio and Martin (1983) study. First, their "ideative" and "emotive" indices were based on factor analysis of a very small sample and were not cross-validated on their own (even smaller) sample. Second, they compare postoperative data on their own subjects with "preoperative" data on an entirely different group of subjects (who were not actually surgical candidates). The "improvement" they report as an effect of surgery may actually reflect other unknown and uncontrolled differences between the two samples.

METHODOLOGICAL ISSUES

Four classes of methodological issues can be identified in the studies reviewed above: subject selection, methods of measuring outcome, consideration of potential mediating variables, and use of appropriate control groups (see Table 8.2).

The first issue is subject selection. In some studies, patient groups were selected on the basis of psychiatric status or other variables known to influence psychological functioning. This practice confounds dependent and independent variables. Taylor and Falconer (1968; Taylor, 1972; Falconer, 1973) studied patients who were referred for surgery from a psychiatric hospital, most likely resulting in an overrepresentation of psychiatric difficulties in comparison with other, unselected surgical populations. In contrast, Rausch et al. (1977) selected patients for study who had no history of psychiatric treatment before or after surgery. Taylor and Marsh (1979) examined only patients with "alien tissue" lesions, although their previous work suggested differ-

TABLE 8.2.   Methodological Issues in Psychosocial Outcome Research

I. Subject selection
  A. Selection on the basis of psychiatric status
  B. Restriction of sample on the basis of clinical variables known to influence outcome
II. Outcome measures
  A. Vague or unspecified diagnostic criteria
  B. Retrospective review of records to obtain outcome data
  C. Some measures influenced by external factors unrelated to outcome
  D. Lack of generalizability to "real-world" functioning
III. Lack of control for mediating or extraneous variables
  A. Medication
  B. Side of surgery
  C. Seizure outcome
  D. Neuropathology
  E. Length of time since surgery
  F. Age of seizure onset or first risk factor
  G. Preoperative psychopathology
  H. Preoperative and postoperative neuropsychological functioning
IV. Absence of appropriate control groups
  A. Nonoperated epileptic patients
  B. Healthy normal control subjects

ences in social adjustment in patients with different forms of neuropathology (Taylor, 1972). These differences in subject selection limit the generalizability of findings of outcome studies and make comparisons between studies difficult.

Second, problems are inherent in each of the methods of measuring outcome as described above. Several studies employed psychiatric diagnoses as primary outcome criteria (e.g., Taylor & Falconer, 1968; Walker & Blumer, 1984; Polkey, 1983). However, diagnostic criteria were vague or unspecified and may have differed markedly between centers. Often, subjective ratings were based on retrospective review of records, which may be subject to inaccuracy and experimenter biases. As noted above, external indices of functioning (e.g., employment, incidence of psychiatric hospitalization) are influenced by numerous environmental and historical variables. For example, change in employment status after surgery may be affected by the availability of disability compensation and/or vocational rehabilitation services. Standardized measures of psychopathology are objective and generally reliable, allowing for greater comparability across studies. However, the relationship of performance on these measures to "real-world" functioning in patients with epilepsy has yet to be clearly demonstrated.

Third, many studies failed to control for variables that may influence psychological and psychosocial outcome in either systematic or nonsystematic ways. The effects of anticonvulsant medication on psychological functioning has been virtually ignored in surgical outcome studies, although many anticonvulsants have known psychotropic effects (Reynolds, 1981, 1986). For example, Robertson (1986) found that depressed epileptic patients taking carbamazepine obtained lower scores on measures of depression and anxiety than did patients taking other medications. The outcome studies reviewed failed to control for changes in medication regimen after surgery, which may have influenced results. Similarly, many of the studies reviewed did not consider side of surgery as a variable, although laterality effects have been demonstrated by several investigators (e.g., Lansdell, 1968; Taylor, 1972; Augustine *et al.*, 1984; Reinecke *et al.*, 1989). Other potentially important variables include length of time since surgery, age at onset of seizures, and nature of neuropsychological impairments before and after surgery.

Finally, the most important methodological problem in virtually all of the outcome studies reviewed (with the exception of Meier & French, 1965) is the lack of control groups. Without a control group of nonoperated subjects evaluated on two occasions, it is impossible to be certain that postoperative changes observed in patient groups are attributable to the surgery rather than to other factors. Data collected in our laboratory during the past 2 years illustrate this point.

The MMPI and TLPI were administered to 37 patients before and 2 weeks after right (*n* = 18) or left (*n* = 19) temporal lobectomy (Robinson, 1990; Reinecke, Saykin, Kester, Sperling, & Gur, 1990). In addition, these instruments were administered at a similar interval to a group of 20 epileptics with complex partial seizures (primarily temporal in origin) who did not undergo surgery. These control subjects were mixed with respect to side of seizure focus but did not differ from right or left temporal surgical groups in age, education, duration of seizure disorder, or test–retest interval. Mean preoperative MMPI profiles for right and left temporal surgical patients and controls are presented in Fig. 8.2; the three groups did not differ significantly with respect to profile elevation or shape. To evaluate change in test performance after surgery, difference score profiles were computed for each subject

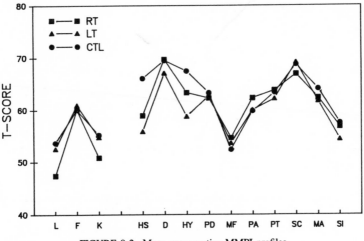

FIGURE 8.2. Mean preoperative MMPI profiles.

by subtracting the preoperative from the postoperative score for each MMPI scale. Mean difference score profiles are presented in Fig. 8.3.

Repeated-measures MANOVA, with patient group as the between-subject factor and pre–post and scale as within-subject factors, yielded a significant pre–post main effect for the validity scales [$F(1,54) = 6.03, p < .02$] and a significant pre–post by scale interaction, with scores for all three groups increasing on Scales L and K and decreasing on Scale F. For clinical scales, there was a trend toward a pre–post main effect [$F(1,54) = 3.27, p < .08$], indicating decreases in reported psychopathology for all three groups. However, there was no significant pre–post by group interaction for validity or clinical scales, indicating that control subjects did not differ significantly from surgical patients in their pattern of change across testings. Similarly, examination of TLPI total scores yielded a significant pre–post main effect [$F(1,48) = 22.98, p < .001$], with a total score decreasing in all three groups. In addition, there was a significant pre–post by group interaction [$F(2,48) = 3.58, p < .04$]; decomposition of this interaction indicated that scores for right temporal patients decreased significantly more than those for left temporal patients or controls. Controls did not differ from left temporal patients in their pattern of change.

To summarize, all groups showed reductions in psychopathology on posttesting, including the nonoperated control group. This finding was unexpected and warrants further consideration. As a group, control subjects did not differ from surgical patients on any demographic variable. At the time of posttesting, controls continued to experience frequent seizures, whereas most surgical patients experienced significant reductions in seizure frequency. It is unlikely that this difference accounts for the observed change in control subjects, however, as continued frequent seizures would be expected to be associated with continued, if not increased, psychological distress.

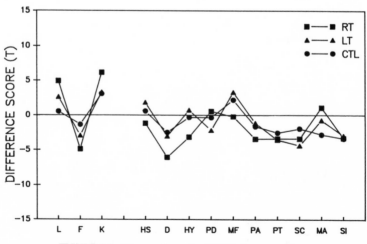

FIGURE 8.3. Mean postoperative MMPI change profiles.

Another possible explanation for this observed improvement is the statistical phenomenon of regression toward the mean. This phenomenon is a result of measurement error: scores that are extreme in value relative to the population tend to become less extreme on retesting (Spector, 1981). In this study, most mean MMPI scale elevations at pretesting are elevated relative to the "population" mean t-score of 50 and approach the population mean more closely on retesting. However, regression toward the mean cannot account for the significant interaction effect indicating greater improvement in TLPI scores for right temporal patients than for left temporal patients or controls, which again suggests lateralized differences in patient perception of change following surgery.

CONCLUSION

Studies of psychological and psychosocial outcome reviewed in this chapter are summarized in Table 8.3. In general, these studies have yielded results that are difficult to interpret. Many demonstrated mild improvements in functioning following surgery. This improvement may be related to the degree of seizure control achieved. However, data presented above suggest that the degree of improvement may not differ significantly from that seen in a control group retested at a similar interval. Other studies suggest that psychiatric difficulties, particularly psychosis, may increase following temporal lobectomy in some patients. Many of the studies reviewed did not address the question of laterality effects. Those that did (e.g., Lansdell, 1968; Reinecke et al., 1989) suggest greater postoperative psychological and psychosocial dysfunction following left temporal lobectomy. Patients undergoing right lobectomy, conversely, may demonstrate greater improvement in functioning or may be more likely to minimize difficulties.

DIRECTIONS FOR FUTURE RESEARCH

Review of the literature and experiences in our laboratory suggest several important considerations for future studies. First, the data presented above (Reinecke et al., 1990) clearly indicate the need for a nonoperated control group in any future study of the effects of surgery. Use of nonsurgical epileptic patients as controls is considered more desirable than healthy normal individuals for two reasons. First, an epileptic control group more closely resembles the experimental groups with respect to important demographic and clinical variables (e.g., education, medication, duration of chronic medical disorder). Second, in order to provide adequate control for regression toward the mean, it is important that the control group resemble the experimental groups with respect to baseline level of functioning. For this reason, healthy normal control subjects are not considered appropriate, because their initial test performance would not be as deviant from the population mean as that of the

TABLE 8.3. Summary of Psychosocial Outcome Studies

Authors	Sample size	Length of follow-up	Methods employed[a]	Findings
Green et al. (1958)	38	1.5–8.5 years	2, 4	Improvements in affect, behavior related to seizure control
Meier & French (1965)	40	Unknown	7	Mild declines in personality disturbance
Savard & Walker (1965)	39	2–5 years	3	Improved overall social functioning related to seizure control
Horowitz & Cohen (1968)	17	1–12 years	2	Majority improved in overall functioning
Lansdell (1968)	37	2 weeks	7	LT[b] results in nonspecific psychological abnormality; RT decreased neurotic symptoms
Taylor & Falconer (1968)	100	2–12 years	1, 2	Improved social adjustment; increase in diagnoses of psychosis
Horowitz et al. (1970)	19	6 months	2	No change in level of functioning
Serafetinides (1975)	31	Unknown	7	Trends toward decreased psychopathology
Rausch et al. (1977)	10	≥ 1 year	2, 7	Poor adjustment related to preoperative psychopathology
Walker & Blumer (1977, 1984)	50	12–30 years	1, 5, 6	Improvements in some personality traits but increased occurrence of psychosis; 2 suicides
Jensen & Larsen (1979)	74	1–11 years	1	Increased diagnoses of psychosis
Taylor & Marsh (1979)	31	Unknown	2, 7	LT males less extraverted than RT; scores consistent with psychosocial adjustment
Rausch & Crandall (1982)	31	1, 12 months	2	Improvement in psychosocial functioning related to seizure control
Fedio & Martin (1983)	19	3–19 years	7	LT report more "ideative" personality traits; RT report more "emotive" traits
Polkey (1983)	40	2–6 years	1	Majority of patients unchanged; only RT developed psychoses after surgery
Augustine et al. (1984)	32	1–10 years	1, 4	Increase in employment, decrease in "underemployment"; unemployment related to RT focus, preoperative psychiatric disorder
Hermann et al. (1989)	41	1–6 months	7	Improved psychological functioning related to seizure control
Hermann & Wyler (1989)	37	6 months	7	Depression correlated with external locus of control before but not after surgery; decreased depression related to seizure control
Reinecke et al. (1989)	47	2 weeks to 2 years	3	Majority report improved functioning; LT more likely than RT to report worsened cognitive functioning
Reinecke et al. (1990)	37	2 weeks	7	Surgical patients did not differ from controls in degree of improvement; RT improve more than LT or controls on TLPI

[a]1, psychiatric diagnosis; 2, clinical ratings; 3, patient/family interview; 4, employment status; 5, suicide rate; 6, psychiatric hospitalization rate; 7, objective personality tests.

[b]RT, right temporal lobectomy; LT, left temporal lobectomy.

experimental groups. Normal controls are also likely to show smaller variances on outcome measures. In a longitudinal research design, each patient could serve as his own control by being tested on at least three occasions: twice, at predetermined intervals, before surgery and at least once after surgery. A second control group, composed of healthy normal individuals, would ideally be included to permit examination of baseline level and changes in psychosocial functioning relative to the healthy population.

Second, the type of outcome measure selected should be considered carefully. Ideally, multiple measures of different types should be employed. When psychiatric diagnosis is used, diagnostic criteria should be clearly specified (e.g., DSM-III-R, ICD-9, RDC). Structured diagnostic interviews such as the SCID, although time-consuming, increase the reliability of diagnosis and should be used more frequently. In addition, it is important to assess the perceptions of family members and others who have close contact with the surgical patient, as their perceptions of postoperative changes in functioning may be quite different from those of the patient. In the future, it will be important to devote increased effort to development of new objective measures of psychosocial outcome that are sensitive and specific to the unique characteristics of the epileptic population and are "ecologically" valid in that they accurately assess the patient's "real-world" functioning. An example of such a measure is the Neurobehavioral Function and Activities of Daily Living scale (NBF-ADL; Saykin, 1988), which was developed in our laboratory to assess a broad range of higher cortical symptoms and their consequences for daily psychosocial functions. An application of the NBF-ADL to surgical epilepsy will be presented in a later report.

Third, systematic consideration of variables that may predict or mediate surgical outcome is needed. Such variables may include, but are not limited to, degree of seizure control achieved after surgery, side of surgery, type of neuropathology, preoperative level of functioning, and nature of neuropsychological impairments sustained after surgery. In addition, it is important to control for, or at least systematically assess, other "confounding" variables such as number and types of anticonvulsant medications used before and after surgery and location and size of tissue resection.

Finally, as our understanding of the postoperative course following temporal lobectomy increases and suggests treatment strategies, there will be need for clinical trials examining the effectiveness of various approaches (e.g., psychopharmacology, psychotherapy, cognitive rehabilitation, vocational training) for remediating the psychosocial impairments that are so prevalent in these patients before and after surgery.

ACKNOWLEDGMENTS. The authors wish to thank Michael R. Sperling, M.D., Michael J. O'Connor, M.D., and Delight Roberts, B.S.W., of the Comprehensive Epilepsy Center, Graduate Hospital, Philadelphia, PA for their helpful comments and collaboration in the original research described in this chapter. Partial support for this work was provided by NIH grant NS-28813 and by an EFA fellowship (LJR).

REFERENCES

Augustine, E., Novelly, R., Mattson, R., Glaser, G., Williamson, P., Spencer, D., & Spencer, S. (1984). Occupational adjustment following neurosurgical treatment of epilepsy. *Annals of Neurology, 15,* 68–72.

Barraclough, B. (1981). Suicide and epilepsy. In E. H. Reynolds & M. Trimble (Eds.), *Epilepsy and psychiatry* (pp. 72–76). New York: Churchill Livingstone.

Bear, D., & Fedio, P. (1977). Quantitative analysis of interictal behavior in temporal lobe epilepsy. *Archives of Neurology, 34,* 454–467.

Dikmen, S., Hermann, B., Wilensky, A., & Rainwater, G. (1983). Validity of the MMPI to psychopathology in patients with epilepsy. *Journal of Nervous and Mental Disease, 171,* 114–122.

Dodrill, C. (1986). Psychosocial consequences of epilepsy. In S. Filskov & T. Boll (Eds.), *Handbook of clinical neuropsychology,* Vol. 2 (pp. 338–363). New York: Wiley-Interscience.

Falconer, M. (1973). Reversibility by temporal lobe resection of the behavioral abnormalities of temporal lobe epilepsy. *New England Journal of Medicine, 289,* 451–455.

Fedio, P., & Martin, A. (1983). Ideative–emotive behavioral characteristics of patients following left or right temporal lobectomy. *Epilepsia, 24*(Supplement 2), S117–S130.

Fenwick, P. (1988). Psychiatric assessment and temporal lobectomy. *Acta Neurologica Scandinavica, 117* (Supplement), 96–102.

Flor-Henry, P. (1972). Ictal and interictal psychiatric manifestations in epilepsy: Specific or non-specific? *Epilepsia, 13,* 773–783.

Flor-Henry, P. (1983). Hemisyndromes of temporal lobe epilepsy: Review of evidence relating psychopathological manifestations in epilepsy to right- and left-sided epilepsy. In M. Myslobodsky (Ed.), *Hemisyndromes: Psychobiology, neurology, psychiatry* (pp. 149–174). New York: Academic Press.

Geschwind, N. (1983). Pathogenesis of behavior change in temporal lobe epilepsy. In A. Ward, J. Penry, & D. Purpura (Eds.), *Epilepsy* (pp. 355–370). New York: Raven Press.

Green, J., Steelman, H., Duisberg, R., McGrath, W., & Wick, S. (1958). Behavior changes following radical temporal lobe excision in the treatment of focal epilepsy. *Research Publication of the American Association of Nervous and Mental Disease, 36,* 295–315.

Hawton, K., Fagg, J., & Marsack, P. (1980). Association between epilepsy and attempted suicide. *Journal of Neurology, Neurosurgery, and Psychiatry, 43,* 168–170.

Hermann, B., & Wyler, A. (1989). Depression, locus of control, and the effects of epilepsy surgery. *Epilepsia, 30,* 332–338.

Hermann, B., Wyler, A., Ackerman, B., & Rosenthal, T. (1989). Short-term psychological outcome of anterior temporal lobectomy. *Journal of Neurosurgery, 71,* 327–334.

Horowitz, M., & Cohen, F. (1968). Temporal lobe epilepsy: Effect of lobectomy on psychosocial functioning. *Epilepsia, 9,* 23–41.

Horowitz, M., Cohen, F., Skolnikoff, A., & Saunders, F. (1970). Psychomotor epilepsy: Rehabilitation after surgical treatment. *Journal of Nervous and Mental Disease, 150,* 273–290.

Jensen, I., & Larsen, J. (1979). Mental aspects of temporal lobe epilepsy: Follow-up of 74 patients after resection of a temporal lobe. *Journal of Neurology, Neurosurgery, and Psychiatry, 42,* 256–265.

Lansdell, H. (1968). Effect of extent of temporal lobe surgery and neuropathology on the MMPI. *Journal of Clinical Psychology, 24,* 406–412.

Meier, M., & French, L. (1965). Changes in MMPI scale scores and an index of psychopathology following unilateral temporal lobectomy for epilepsy. *Epilepsia, 6,* 263–273.

Mungas, D. (1982). Interictal behavior abnormality in temporal lobe epilepsy: A specific syndrome or nonspecific psychopathology? *Archives of General Psychiatry, 39,* 108–111.

Polkey, C. (1983). Effects of anterior temporal lobectomy apart from the relief of seizures: A study of 40 patients. *Journal of the Royal Society of Medicine, 76,* 354–358.

Rausch, R., & Crandall, P. (1982). Psychological status related to surgical control of temporal lobe seizures. *Epilepsia, 23,* 191–202.

Rausch, R., McCreary, C., & Crandall, P. (1977). Psychosocial functioning following successful surgical relief from seizures: Evidence of prediction from preoperative personality characteristics. *Journal of Psychosomatic Research, 21,* 141–146.

Reinecke, L. J., Saykin, A. J., Sperling, M. R., & Gur, R. C. (1988). Bear and Fedio inventory and MMPI in temporal lobe epilepsy. *Journal of Clinical and Experimental Neuropsychology, 10,* 82.

Reinecke, L. J., Saykin, A. J., Sperling, M. R., Roberts, D., Kester, D. B., Gur, R. C., & O'Connor, M. J. (1989). Neurobehavioral changes following anterior temporal lobectomy: Patient and family perception assessed with a structured interview. *Epilepsia, 30,* 727.

Reinecke, L. J., Saykin, A. J., Kester, D. B., Sperling, M. R., & Gur, R. C. (1990). Decrease in psychopathology following temporal lobectomy: Evidence from a prospective study using the Bear and Fedio inventory and MMPI. *Journal of Clinical and Experimental Neuropsychology, 12,* 33.

Reynolds, E. H. (1981). Biological factors in psychological disorders associated with epilepsy. In E. Reynolds & M. Trimble (Eds.), *Epilepsy and psychiatry* (pp. 264–290). New York: Churchill Livingstone.

Reynolds, E. H. (1986). Antiepileptic drugs and personality. In M. Trimble and T. Bolwig (Eds.), *Aspects of epilepsy and psychiatry.* New York: John Wiley & Sons.

Robertson, M. (1986). Ictal and interictal depression in patients with epilepsy. In M. Trimble & T. Bolwig (Eds.), *Aspects of epilepsy and psychiatry.* New York: John Wiley & Sons.

Robinson, L. J. (1990). *Personality and psychosocial functioning before and after temporal lobectomy.* Unpublished doctoral dissertation, Purdue University, West Lafayette, IN.

Savard, R., & Walker, E. (1965). Changes in social functioning after surgical treatment for temporal lobe epilepsy. *Social Work, 10,* 87–95.

Saykin, A. J. (1988). Neurobehavioral Function and Activities of Daily Living Scale. Unpublished data, University of Pennsylvania, Philadelphia.

Serafetinides, E. (1975). Psychosocial aspects of neurosurgical management of epilepsy. In D. Purpura, J. Penry, & R. Walter (Eds.), *Advances in neurology,* Volume 8 (pp. 323–332). New York: Raven Press.

Spector, P. (1981). *Research designs. Sage University Paper series on Quantitative Applications in the Social Sciences, 07-023.* Beverly Hills: Sage Publications.

Taylor, D. (1972). Mental state and temporal lobe epilepsy. *Epilepsia, 13,* 727–765.

Taylor, D. (1987). Psychiatric and social issues in measuring the input and outcome of epilepsy surgery. In J. Engel (Ed.), *Surgical treatment of the epilepsies* (pp. 485–503). New York: Raven Press.

Taylor, D., & Falconer, M. (1968). Clinical, socio-economic, and psychological changes after temporal lobectomy for epilepsy. *British Journal of Psychiatry, 114,* 1247–1261.

Taylor, D. & Marsh, S. (1977). Implications of long term follow-up studies in epilepsy: with a note on the cause of death. In J. Penry (Ed.), *Epilepsy: The eighth international symposium.* New York: Raven Press.

Taylor, D., & Marsh, S. (1979). The influence of sex and side of operation on personality questionnaire responses after temporal lobectomy. In J. Gruzelier & P. Flor-Henry (Eds.), *Hemispheric asymmetries of function in psychopathology* (pp. 391–400). Amsterdam: Elsevier.

Trimble, M. (1983). Personality disturbances in epilepsy. *Neurology, 33,* 1332–1334.

Walker, A., & Blumer, D. (1977). Long term behavioral effects of temporal lobectomy for temporal lobe epilepsy. *McLean Hospital Journal,* June, 85–107.

Walker, A., & Blumer, D. (1984). Behavioral effects of temporal lobectomy for temporal lobe epilepsy. In D. Blumer (Ed.), *Psychiatric aspects of epilepsy* (pp. 295–323). Washington: American Psychiatric Press.

III

Treatment Approaches to Epilepsy

9

Medical Treatment of Epilepsy

GERALD C. McINTOSH

A variety of anticonvulsant drugs are currently available for the treatment of patients with epilepsy, and administration of anticonvulsant medications remains the primary method of therapy for control of seizures. The initial choice of anticonvulsant is usually based on the seizure classification, as these drugs are optimally administered based on their effectiveness for a specific seizure diagnosis (Macdonald & McLean, 1986).

By use of experimental models and clinical efficacy assessments, the specific utility of various anticonvulsants and their optimal dosage and administration have been fairly well characterized. The present clinical movement is in the direction of "monotherapy" as opposed to "polypharmacy" (Reynolds & Shorvan, 1981; Wilder, 1987). Anticonvulsant selection is facilitated by an improved understanding of the specifics of anticonvulsant drug effectiveness (Wilder, 1987). The mechanisms of action of individual anticonvulsant medications as applied to monotherapy of the epilepsies are reviewed in the following pages, as are initiation and cessation of anticonvulsant therapy.

Phenytoin, phenobarbital, primidone, valproic acid, ethosuximide, and carbamazepine are the major anticonvulsants reviewed. Supplemental use of benzodiazepine-type anticonvulsants is covered as well.

MECHANISMS OF ACTION

A correlation between seizure type and anticonvulsant mechanism of action is the focal point of a well-conceived understanding of medical treatment for epilepsy. Seizures of localized origin tend to be controlled better by different anticonvulsant

GERALD C. McINTOSH • Rehabilitation Department and Life Skills Rehabilitation Center, Poudre Valley Hospital, Fort Collins, Colorado 80524.

The Neuropsychology of Epilepsy, edited by Thomas L. Bennett. Plenum Press, New York, 1992.

drugs than do primary generalized seizures. In general, anticonvulsants work well either for control of partial and secondarily generalized seizures or for control of primary generalized seizures. This pattern of effectiveness can be best explained with an understanding of anticonvulsant mechanism of action based on experimental studies. Most anticonvulsants have some efficacy for all seizure types.

Phenytoin, carbamazepine, and to a lesser extent phenobarbital and primidone reduce sustained repetitive neuronal discharges by direct membrane actions. These drugs produce reduction in repetitive neuronal firing and block seizures provoked by electrical induction, so-called maximal electroshock seizures (MES), in experimental studies. Each is an effective anticonvulsant for the control of partial complex seizures, secondary generalized seizures, and also most generalized tonic–clonic seizures.

Clonazepam (a prototype for benzodiazepine anticonvulsants in this discussion) and ethosuximide do not suppress repetitive neural firing or effectively block MES. These drugs are not effective for control of partial complex, secondary generalized, or generalized tonic–clonic seizures. They do enhance γ-aminobutyric acid (GABA) responses and block seizures induced by injection of pentylentetrazole (PTZ), a chemical that lowers seizure threshold. Both of these anticonvulsants are effective, ethosuximide more so, for control of generalized absence seizures.

Valproic acid is effective for both generalized tonic–clonic seizures and generalized absence seizures and is somewhat less effective for partial complex seizures. This drug shows experimental efficacy by reduction of repetitive firing, blocking of MES seizures, and blocking of PTZ seizures. Valproic acid also seems to have some GABA enhancement characteristics.

Table 9.1 outlines this pattern of clinical effectiveness and associated cellular and synaptic effects. More details of the association between the mechanism of action and clinical efficacy are reviewed as each separate anticonvulsant is discussed in more detail later in this chapter.

INITIATION AND CESSATION OF ANTICONVULSANT THERAPY IN EPILEPSY TREATMENT

A great many individuals will come to medical attention after a first-ever seizure. About half of these will have an underlying brain or systemic disease process to which therapy can be directed, and most frequently that therapy includes appropriate anticonvulsant drugs. When the first-ever seizure is unprovoked, the therapeutic approach remains controversial (Hauser, 1986; Hart & Easton, 1986; Fromm, 1987; Fisher, 1987; Dasheiff, 1987). It is clear that the approach to therapy should be individualized, but several factors appear to be helpful to the decision-making process. These include the risk of further seizures, risk of complications from anticonvulsant therapy, and specific factors affecting these risks such as prior central nervous system insult, family history, and electroencephalographic (EEG) findings (Hauser, 1986). Treatment decisions may then be based on estimates of seizure recurrence, inferring the diagnosis of epilepsy, versus potential drug toxicity. Ideally

TABLE 9.1.   Anticonvulsant Mechanism of Action and Clinical Efficacy[a]

Anticonvulsant	GTC	PC	GA	RF	MES	GABA	PTZ
Phenytoin	++	++	−	++	++	−	−
Carbamazepine	++	++	−	++	++	−	−
Primidone	+	++	−	++	++	−	−
Phenobarbital	+	+	−	+	++	+	+
Valproic acid	++	+	++	++	++	+	++
Clonazepam	+	−	++	+	+	++	++
Ethosuximide	−	−	++	−	−	−	++

[a]GTC, efficacy against generalized tonic–clonic seizures; PC, efficacy against partial complex seizures; GA, efficacy against generalized absence seizures; RF, reduction of repetitive firing; MES, block of maximal electroshock seizures; GABA, enhamcement of GABA responses; PTZ, blocking of pentylenotetrazole seizures. Derived from Macdonald and McLean (1986).

the decision can be shared by the patient with the physician in the role of advisor. Unfortunately, there are no hard and fast rules to guide this decision-making process.

For the most part, the diagnosis of epilepsy involves a lifelong commitment to anticonvulsant therapy, but in fact some of the individuals who receive a diagnosis of epilepsy may expect to be seizure-free off medications. There seems to be little agreement on the potential predictions of successful medication withdrawal (Wallis, 1987). The presence of an abnormal EEG pattern and the occurrence of generalized seizures have been said to be relative predictive factors of poor chance for successful discontinuation of medication, especially in children. In a recent study, the presence of partial complex seizures with secondary generalization and persistance of EEG abnormality indicated a higher risk of seizure recurrence after anticonvulsant withdrawal (Callaghan, Garrett, & Goggin, 1988). Individual considerations, such as need for driving privileges, often sway the clinical decision. The patient should have a clear understanding of the consequences of an unexpected seizure prior to medication withdrawal. When relapses occur, then reinitiation with anticonvulsant monotherapy is the path of first choice.

MONOTHERAPY IN EPILEPSY TREATMENT

The treatment of many epileptic patients is often best accomplished with the use of one drug rather than with multiple drugs. Monotherapy frequently provides better seizure control with less drug toxicity or interactions. The use of multiple anticonvulsants has some historical base, as anticonvulsants tended to be added on when new drugs were introduced. The first major useful anticonvulsants, phenytoin and phenobarbital, were once believed, based on clinical trials, to have synergistic anticonvulsant activities, and that belief was held for many years. In fact, until quite recently a capsule combining these drugs was commercially available (Wilder, 1987). Within the last 15 years, research has focused on the pharmacokinetics of individual and combined anticonvulsants, and further clinical trials have demonstrated the ineffi-

ciency of polypharmacy (Reynolds & Shorvan, 1981). The key benefits of monotherapy are generally improved seizure control and lowered risk of medication-
induced toxicity, but drug selection for specific seizure type is the key factor
determining therapeutic success. The relationship between seizure type and drug
selection is discussed further as specific anticonvulsants are reviewed. The therapeutic range for an individual anticonvulsant is the serum concentration at which the drug
is therapeutic but not toxic in the majority of treated patients (Livingston, Berman, &
Pauli, 1975). Over the past 15 years or so the use of serum concentration to guide
epilepsy therapy has become the accepted therapeutic management technique. However, serum concentrations should only be used as general guidelines for epilepsy
therapy with anticonvulsant drugs, because some patients may require and tolerate
levels above the therapeutic range, and others may have their seizures well controlled
with levels below the therapeutic range.

Reviews of the basic pharmacology, therapeutic efficacy, and toxic potentials for
each anticonvulsant are presented in the next several sections.

PHENYTOIN

Phenytoin (Dilantin®) was initially investigated using animal models by Merritt
and Putnam (1938). After its introduction other hydantoins were developed but later
discarded as anticonvulsants because of either reduced efficacy or toxic side effects.
Today phenytoin is essentially the only drug within this group that remains in clinical
use. Phenytoin is effective in both generalized tonic–clonic seizures and all types of
partial seizures (Macdonald & McLean, 1986; Eadie & Tyrer, 1980). Doses of 5–7
mg/kg per day achieve serum concentrations of 10–20 μg/mL, considered the
therapeutic range for the drug, but since phenytoin is 90% protein bound, free serum
and CSF concentrations need then be 1–2 μg/mL to be in the effective range
(Livingstone et al., 1975). Experimentally, phenytoin is effective against MES
seizures but ineffective against PTZ seizures (Macdonald & McLean, 1986). The
mechanism of action reported for phenytoin involves direct membrane actions that
limit sustained rapid firing of action potentials. The exact mechanism of the phenytoin block on repetitive firing remains to be clearly demonstrated.

In a population of persons treated chronically with phenytoin, even if the dosage
is expressed on a body weight basis, there is wide scatter of serum levels in different
people for any particular phenytoin dose. These variations necessitate adjustments in
dosage for individuals based on periodic serum concentrations in order to achieve
optimal therapy (Eadie & Tyrer, 1980; Wilder, Buchanan, & Serrano, 1973). Plasma
phenytoin concentrations of 10–20 μg/mL offer the best chances of controlling the
types of seizures responsive to the drug with the minimal risk of causing overdosage
effects (Eadie & Tyrer, 1980).

As phenytoin levels rise, neurotoxic effects appear. Horizontal nystagmus tends
to appear when levels reach 20 μg/mL. Diplopia and ataxia with nystagmus are
consistently present with levels of 30 μg/mL, and at levels of 50 μg/mL, lethargy or

coma is typical (Wilder *et al.*, 1973). Rarely, phenytoin may cause dyskinesia, dystonia, or choreiform movements (Kooiker & Sumi, 1974). Peripheral nerve conduction is also slowed with phenytoin intoxication (Chokroverty & Sayed, 1975). The severity of gingival hyperplasia, which is a common cosmetic side effect, also correlates with increased but not necessarily toxic phenytoin levels (Little, Girgis, & Masotti, 1975). Other potential side effects include overgrowth of body hair on the trunk and limbs, coarsing of facial features, hypocalcemia and osteomalacia, folate deficiency with megaloblastic anemia, immunologic abnormalities, and decreased insulin release from the pancreas (Eadie & Tyrer, 1980). Idiosyncratic effects include skin rashes, leukopenia and erythroid aplasia, pseudolymphoma syndrome, and hepatitis (Eadie & Tyrer, 1980). Maternal phenytoin intake appears to be associated with a doubled risk of fetal dysmorphogenesis, but there is no rigid proof that phenytoin itself causes any specific dysmorphia in humans (Janz, 1975). For the present, most authors agree that fetal risk in continuing anticonvulsant therapy during pregnancy is less than maternal and fetal risks when treatment is discontinued (Janz, 1975).

CARBAMAZEPINE

Carbamazepine (Tegretol®) was approved for antiepileptic therapy in the United States in 1974 after over 10 years of usage in Europe for the treatment of epilepsy and trigeminal neuralgia (Blom, 1962). Carbamazepine is clinically effective against partial seizures and generalized tonic–clonic seizures but ineffective against generalized absence seizures (Cereghino, Brock, VanMeter, Penry, Smith, & White, 1974). The usual adult dosage is 10–20 mg/kg per day needed to achieve therapeutic serum levels of 4–12 μg/mL and CSF levels of 1–3 μg/mL. Carbamazepine, like phenytoin, inhibits MES seizures but is ineffective against PTZ seizures (Julien & Hollister, 1975).

The mechanism of action for the anticonvulsant activity of carbamazepine appears to be similar to that of phenytoin, and although it has been thoroughly studied, it is incompletely understood. Probably through direct membrane action carbamazepine inhibits repetitive firing in experimental settings, but further understanding of a more exact mechanism of action remains to be elucidated (McLean & Macdonald, 1984).

A great deal of variability has been noted in absorption and time to achieve peak plasma level (Cotter, Eadie, Hooper, Lander, Smith, & Tyrer, 1977). Elimination rates are also individually variable in humans (Cotter *et al.*, 1977). The therapeutic range for the drug is generally considered to be in the 4–12 μg/mL range (Schneider, 1975). Individual epileptics frequently tolerate serum concentrations greater than 12 μg/mL, and it may, at times, be worthwhile to try a higher dosage to achieve optimal seizure control, all the while observing for toxic side effects. At high therapeutic levels, sedation, nystagmus, blurred vision, and dysequilibrium are reported in approximately 50% of the patients (Schneider, 1975). Tolerance to the sedative side effects occurs with time, but they may be a major problem with initiation of treatment. Carbamazepine overdosage has been reported to increase seizure activity. Dermatological, hepatic, and blood dyscrasias occur as idiosyncratic effects, but serious hematological disorders are in fact rare (Livingstone, Pauli, & Pruce, 1978). Adverse effects on the developing fetus have recently been reported. Because cognitive and behavioral side effects are less for carbamazepine than for other anticonvulsants effective for posttraumatic seizures, it is currently the drug of choice in that clinical circumstance (Glenn, 1986).

VALPROIC ACID

Valproic acid (Depakene® and Depakote), which was identified as an anticonvulsant in 1963 (Meunier, Carraz, Meunier, Eymard, & Aimard, 1963), was released in the United States for clinical use in 1978. It is effective for control of generalized absence, myoclonic, and generalized motor seizures (Bruni & Wilder, 1979). Valproic acid is less effective for partial and partial complex seizures but may be effective an monotherapy or as adjunctive therapy, especially when partial seizures are secondarily generalized (Wilder, 1987). Relatively high doses, 30–60 mg per day, are necessary to achieve serum levels in a therapeutic range of 50–100 μg/mL. The CSF at these same levels varies from 3 to 30 μg/mL because of highly variable serum protein binding of the drug (Shuto & Nishigaki, 1970). Valproic acid is effective against both MES and PTZ seizures (Chapman, Keane, Meldrum, Simiand, & Vernieres, 1982).

The mechanism of action for valproic acid may involve changes in GABAergic synaptic activity (Chapman et al., 1982). At least the observable activity against PTZ seizures and the clinical efficacy against generalized absence seizures can be correlated with this activity (Simon & Penry, 1975). The action against MES seizures and generalized tonic–clonic epilepsy, which is probably associated with the experimental limitation of high-frequency repetitive firing of neurons as observed with valproic acid and other anticonvulsants, is less well defined for valproic acid by experimental study (Chapman et al., 1982; Simon & Penry, 1975).

Valproic acid is effective as sole therapy for primary generalized epilepsy and, alone or in conjunction with other anticonvulsants, as therapy for all varieties of partial and secondary generalized epilepsy (Wilder, 1987). The drug has a relatively rapid pattern of absorption and high protein binding, which necessitates high dosage relative to other anticonvulsant drugs in common usage. Characteristically, phenobarbital levels rise and phenytoin levels fall when valproic acid is added to a therapeutic seizure control program using those anticonvulsants in combination (Covanis, Gupta, & Jeavons, 1982). Clinically, this is quite important, as valproic acid continues to be used in conjunction with phenytoin and/or phenobarbital quite frequently in efforts to achieve better seizure control in difficult generalized motor, partial, and secondary generalized epilepsy (Covanis et al., 1982). Little change in carbamazepine levels is noted with addition of valproic acid (Covanis et al., 1982). Gastrointestinal symptoms caused by local irritation are the most common observed toxic side effects and at times are severe enough to lead to cessation of therapy. Sedation is the most common CNS effect, but at high doses tremor and ataxia are observed. Hematological and hepatotoxic effects have also been reported, and transient hair loss is seen not infrequently. Fetal dysmorphic effects have been identified in experimental animals, but such effects have not been conclusively demonstrated in humans.

ETHOSUXIMIDE

Ethosuximide (Zarontin®) remains the drug most commonly used for control of generalized absence seizures, although it is being displaced to an extent by valproic acid. Ethosuximide is generally not useful in the treatment of other seizure types (Brown, Dreifuss, Dyken, Goode, Perry, Porter, White, & White, 1975). The usual dosage of ethosuximide is 20–40 mg/kg per day, yielding therapeutic levels of 40–100 μg/mL in both blood and CSF. In experimental study the drug is effective against PTZ seizures but is ineffective against MES seizures. The mechanism of action for ethosuximide is unknown, as no definite membrane actions, neurotransmitter-related actions, or reduction of repetitive firing have been shown when the drug has been studied experimentally (Macdonald & McLean, 1986).

Local irritative gastrointestinal effects are common, and sedative-type side effects are frequently observed. Idiosyncratic effects are mainly dermatologic and rarely hematological.

PHENOBARBITAL

Phenobarbital was introduced as an anticonvulsant in 1912 by Hauptmann (1912). It is useful in the management of all types of seizures except generalized absence. Therapeutic serum levels are in the range of 10–40 μg/mL with CSF concentrations of 5–25 μg/mL (Eadie & Tyrer, 1980). In animal models phenobarbital is effective against both MES and PTZ seizures (Macdonald & McLean, 1986).

The mechanism of action for phenobarbital is complex and remains incompletely understood (Macdonald & McLean, 1986). At the postsynaptic level, barbituates enhance GABAergic inhibition and reduce glutamate and cholinergic excitation. Presynaptically, barbiturates reduce calcium entry and thereby block release of neurotransmitters. At the nerve cell membrane level they reduce sodium and potassium conductances and block repetitive firing. Most of these actions probably contribute to the clinical efficacy and toxic effects of the drugs, but current thinking is that the major anticonvulsant action is postsynaptic and therefore at the neurotransmitter level (Macdonald & McLean, 1986).

Individual variation in metabolism and drug tolerance are typical for phenobarbital (Eadie & Tyrer, 1980). Although it is generally a depressant on neural function, in some individuals, particularly children and the elderly, an irritable reaction or stimulant effect is noted. In general, metabolism is slow, with maximum drug levels after a single dose occurring at 6 to 18 h, followed by a clearance over several days. Drowsiness is the most common side effect but will pass gradually without reduction in dosage. Confusion, personality change, and blunting of intellectual functioning are also common. Dermatologic reactions and blood dyscrasias are the common idiosyncratic effects. Although there are reports of possible teratogenic effects, most authors do not consider phenobarbital itself to be dysmorphogenic (Janz, 1975). Barbiturate anticonvulsants including phenobarbital may cause a withdrawal syndrome including withdrawal seizures.

PRIMIDONE

Primidone (Mysoline®) is potentially useful in most epilepsies other than primary generalized absence seizures. The drug is metabolized to two active anticonvulsant compounds, phenylethylmalonamide (PEMA) and phenobarbital (Bourgeois, Dodson, & Ferandelli, 1983). Usual dosage is 10–25 mg/kg per day to achieve therapeutic serum levels of 5–20 μg/mL with CSF concentrations of 80% of total serum concentration. It is more effective against MES seizures than PTZ seizures and ineffective against PTZ seizures if metabolism to phenobarbital is blocked (Macdonald & McLean, 1986).

Uncertainty remains over whether primidone is an effective anticonvulsant alone of if its efficacy is attributable to its metabolites PEMA and phenobarbital (Macdonald & McLean, 1986). Experimental studies have demonstrated independent action of primidone alone against MES seizures but not against PTZ seizures. Phenobarbital is effective against both types of experimental seizures, and PEMA is a relatively ineffective drug unless administered at toxic doses. Through the combined actions of primidone and phenobarbital, involving the mechanisms of postsynaptic neurotransmitter action modification, presynaptic reduction of calcium entry to block neurotransmitter release, and reduction in sodium and potassium conductances to block repetitive firing, the drug has complex actions responsible for it efficacy. More specific mechanisms of action remain uncertain (Macdonald & McLean, 1986).

Because of the biotransformation pattern and mixed mechanism of action of primidone as well as individual variabilities, dosage and serum levels need to be followed closely when primidone is used clinically (Eadie & Tyrer, 1980). Since primidone is metabolized to PEMA and phenobarbital, there is an initial effect and peak level of primidone, followed later by a gradual elevation of phenobarbital levels and effects. A steady state can be reached after several days. Mainly for convenience but also because it reflects clinical efficacy, the usual practice is to follow primidone levels and to establish a therapeutic concentration in the range of 8–12 μg/mL. No definite relationship between drug level and dosage can be predicted for individual patients.

Interpretation of toxic symptoms is also difficult because of the complex metabolism. Sedative side effects are particularly troublesome, even at subtherapeutic levels of primidone, especially when therapy is being initiated. Other potential dose-related side effects include dizziness, ataxia, nystagmus, diplopia, asterixis, glossitis, and folic acid deficiency producing megaloblastic erythrocytes. Possible idiosyncratic reactions include rashes, blood dyscrasias, lupus-like syndrome, and lymphadenopathy. Potential fetal toxicity is as might be expected for phenobarbital (Janz, 1975). Withdrawal syndromes and seizures may occur if primidone therapy is ceased abruptly.

BENZODIAZEPINES

Several benzodiazepines are in use as secondary anticonvulsants, but diazepam (Valium®) and clonazepam (Klonopin®) are the only drugs in this group to be used extensively in epilepsy treatment at the present time (Browne & Penry, 1973). Diazepam is used primarily in the acute control of status epilepticus but has been reported to be effective against a variety of epileptic disorders, including myoclonic, atonic, absence, photosensitive, and alcohol-withdrawal seizures. Clonazepam is used for myoclonic seizures, atonic seizures, infantile spasms, and as adjunctive treatment for absence seizures. Both of these drugs are effective against PTZ seizures but block MES seizures only in toxic doses (Macdonald & McLean, 1986).

Benzodiazepines appear to act at the membrane level and also alter synaptic transmission by enhancing inhibition (Vyskocil, 1977; Macdonald & McLean, 1986). The inhibition of synaptic transmission is mainly related to GABA enhancement (Skerritt & MacDonald, 1984). An effect on sodium, potassium, and chloride conductances in neuronal cell membranes reduces repetitive firing as well (Vyskocil, 1977).

Diazepam tolerance usually makes any attempts at long-term oral anticonvulsant treatment unrewarding. Clonazepam, on the other hand, remains a commonly used anticonvulsant for a variety of seizure types, although rarely a first-line drug except in the instance of myoclonic seizures. Dose-dependent toxic effects are usually sedative, and idiosyncratic responses are rare (Edwards, 1974). Withdrawal syndromes may occur when benzodiazepines are abruptly discontinued (Vyas & Carney, 1975).

ANTICONVULSANTS AND COGNITIVE FUNCTION

A variety of cognitive impairments have been described in individuals with epilepsy, including memory problems, reduced attention, and mental slowness (Delaney, Rosen, Mattson, & Novelly, 1980; Stores, Hart, & Piran, 1978; Addy, 1987). These cognitive disorders have been thought to reflect structural brain damage, secondary seizure effects, "subclinical" seizure activity, anticonvulsant effects, or any combination of these mechanisms (Thompson & Trimble, 1982). The variations and discrepancies in reports of the cognitive effects of anticonvulsants seem to be related to methodological differences including the type of psychological testing employed, the population studied, and dosage and duration of treatment (Dikmen, 1980; Trimble & Reynolds, 1976; Thompson & Trimble, 1982).

Any epileptic population has an inherent heterogeneity of cognitive and behavioral characteristics, which has to be taken into account in analyzing the potential effects of various anticonvulsants on performance in cognitive assessments. Recent studies have identified differences in the relative effects of these drugs (Thompson & Trimble, 1982; Vining, 1987). Studies involving nonepileptic volunteers have been helpful because more rigorous study design can be organized than in patient sample studies. These studies have demonstrated a measurable decline in test performance with exposure to most of the major anticonvulsants (Thompson & Trimble, 1982; Vining, 1987). There are, however, differences between drugs that were readily apparent, and, in general, higher dosage of any anticonvulsant produces greater severity of cognitive disturbance (Vining, 1987). Since an epileptic takes anticonvulsant medications for longer time periods, and these drugs could produce differing consequences in abnormal versus normal brain, studies in nonepileptics have been questioned. Two axioms have developed from clinical studies with epileptic and nonepileptic populations. First, a reduction in polypharmacy toward monotherapy has a beneficial effect on the cognitive functions. Secondly, both carbamazepine and valproic acid are less detrimental to cognition in comparison to other anticonvulsants (Vining, 1987). The topic of anticonvulsants and their effects on cognition is discussed in greater detail in Chapter 5.

SUMMARY

The major anticonvulsants currently used in the treatment of epilepsy, their mechanism of action, and efficacy by seizure type have been discussed above. Proper selection of drug and guidelines for initiation and cessation of anticonvulsant drug therapy have also been reviewed. Anticonvulsant drugs remain the mainstay of epilepsy treatment. Efforts to develop new anticonvulsants continue with perhaps improved efficacy and reduced side effects on the horizon.

REFERENCES

Addy, D. P. (1987). Cognitive function in children with epilepsy. *Developmental Medicine and Child Neurology, 29*, 394–404.

Blom, S. (1962). Trigeminal neuralgia: Its treatment with a new anticonvulsant drug. *Lancet, 1*, 839–840.

Bourgeois, B. F. D., Dodson, E., & Ferandelli, J. A. (1983). Primidone, phenobarbital and PEMA: 1. Seizure protection, neurotoxicity and therapeutic index of individual compounds in mice. *Neurology, 33*, 283–290.

Browne, T. R., & Penry, J. K. (1973). Benzodiazepines in the treatment of epilepsy: A review. *Epilepsia, 14*, 277–310.

Browne, T. R., Dreifuss, F. E., Dyken, P. R., Goode, D. J., Perry, J. R., Porter, R. J., White, B. G., & White, P. T. (1975). Ethosuximide in the treatment of absence (petit mal) seizures. *Neurology, 25*, 515–524.

Bruni, J., & Wilder, B. J. (1979). Valproic acid—review of a new antiepileptic drug. *Archives of Neurology, 36*, 393–398.

Callaghan, N., Garrett, A., & Goggin, T. (1988). Withdrawal of anticonvulsant drugs in patients free of seizures for two years. *New England Journal of Medicine, 318*, 942–946.

Cereghino, J. J., Brock, J. T., VanMeter, J. C., Penry, J. K., Smith, L. D., & White, B. G. (1974). Carbamazepine for epilepsy. A controlled prospective evaluation. *Neurology, 24*, 401–410.

Chapman, A., Keane, P. E., Meldrum, B. S., Simiand, J., & Vernieres, J. C. (1982). Mechanisms of anticonvulsant action of valproate. *Progress in Neurobiology, 19*, 315–359.

Chokroverty, S., & Sayed, Z. A. (1975). Motor nerve conduction study in patients on diphenylhydantoin therapy. *Journal of Neurology, Neurosurgery and Psychiatry, 38*, 1235–1239.

Cotter, L. M., Eadie, M. J., Hooper, W. D., Lander, C. M., Smith, G. A., & Tyrer, J. H. (1977). The pharmokinetics of carbamazepine. *European Journal of Clinical Pharmacology, 12*, 451–456.

Covanis, A., Gupta, A. K., & Jeavons, P. M. (1982). Sodium valproate: Monotherapy and polytherapy. *Epilepsia, 23*, 693–720.

Dasheiff, R. (1987). First seizure management—reconsidered response III. *Archives of Neurology, 44*, 1190–1191.

Delaney, R. C., Rosen, R. J., Mattson, R. H., & Novelly, R. A. (1980). Memory function in focal epilepsy. A comparison of non-surgical unilateral temporal lobe and frontal lobe samples. *Cortex, 16*, 103–117.

Dikmen, S. (1980). Neuropsychological aspects of epilepsy. In *A multidisciplinary handbook of epilepsy* (pp. 36–73). Springfield, IL: Charles C. Thomas.

Eadie, M. J., & Tyrer, J. H. (1980). *Anticonvulsant therapy: Pharmacological basis and practice.* New York: Churchill Livingston.

Edwards, V. E. (1974). Side effects of clonazepan therapy. *Proceedings of the Australian Association of Neurologists, 11*, 199–202.

Fisher, R. S. (1987). First seizure management—reconsidered response II. *Archives of Neurology, 44*, 1189–1190.

Fromm, G. H. (1987) First seizure management—reconsidered response I. *Archives of Neurology, 44*, 1189.

Glenn, M. B. (1986) Anticonvulsants for prophylaxis of post-traumatic seizures. *Journal of Head Trauma Rehabilitation, 1*, 73–74.

Hart, R. G., & Easton, J. D. (1986). Seizure recurrence after a first unprovoked seizure. *Archives of Neurology, 43*, 1289–1290.

Hauptmann, A. (1912). Luminal bei Epilepsie. *Munchener Medizinischer Wochenschrift, 59*, 1907–1909.

Hauser, W. A. (1986). Should people be treated after a first seizure. *Archives of Neurology, 43*, 1287–1288.

Janz, D. (1975). The teratogenic risk of anti-epileptic drugs. *Epilepsia, 16*, 159–169.

Julien, R. M., & Hollister, R. D. (1975). Carbamazepine mechanism of action. *Advances in Neurology, 11*, 263–276.

Kooiker, J. C., & Sumi, S. M. (1974). Movement disorder as a manifestation of diphenylhydantoin intoxication. *Neurology, 24*, 68–71.

Little, T. M., Girgis, S. S., & Masotti, R. E. (1975). Diphenylhydantoin induced gingival hyperplasia: Its response to change in drug dosage. *Developmental Medicine and Child Neurology, 17*, 421–424.

Livingston, S., Berman, W., & Pauli, L. L. (1975). Anticonvulsant drug blood levels. Practical applications based on 12 years' experience. *Journal of the American Medical Association, 232*, 60–62.

Livingston, S., Pauli, L. L., & Pruce, I. (1978). No proven relationship of carbamazepine therapy to blood dyscrasias. *Neurology, 28*, 101.

Macdonald, R. L., & McLean, M. J. (1986). Anticonvulsant drugs: Mechanism of action. *Advances in Neurology, 44*, 713–736.

McLean, M. J., & Macdonald, R. L. (1984). Limitation of high frequency repetitive firing of cultured mouse neurons by anticonvulsant drugs. *Neurology, 34* (Supplement 1), 288.

Merritt, H. H., & Putnam, T. J. (1938). A new series of anticonvulsant drugs tested by experiments on animals. *Archives of Neurology and Psychiatry*, *39*, 1003–1015.

Meunier, G., Carraz, G., Meunier, Y., Eymard, P., & Aimard, M. (1963). Proprietes pharmacodynamiques de l'acide *n*-propylacetique. *Therapie*, *18*, 435–438.

Reynolds, E. H., & Shorvan, S. D. (1981). Monotherapy or polytherapy for epilepsy. *Epilepsia*, *22*, 1–10.

Shuto, N., & Nishigaki, T. (1970) The pharmacological studies on sodium dipropylacetate: Anticonvulsant activities and general pharmacological actions. *Pharmacokinetics*, *4*, 937–949.

Simon, D., & Penry, J. K. (1975). Sodium di-*n*-propylacetate (DPA) in the treatment of epilepsy: A review. *Epilepsy*, *16*, 549–573.

Skerritt, J. H., & MacDonald, R. L. (1984). Diazepam enhances the action but not the binding of the GABA analog THIP. *Brain Research*, *297*, 181–186.

Stores, G., Hart, J., & Piran, N. (1978). Inattentiveness in school children with epilepsy. *Epilepsia*, *19*, 169–175.

Thompson, P. J., & Trimble, M. R. (1982). Anticonvulsant drugs and cognitive functions. *Epilepsia*, *23*, 531–544.

Trimble, M. R., & Reynolds, E. H. (1976). Anticonvulsant drugs and mental symptoms: A review. *Psychology and Medicine*, *6*, 169–178.

Vining, E. P. G. (1987). Cognitive dysfunction associated with antiepileptic drug therapy. *Epilepsia*, *28* (Supplement 2), 518–522.

Vyas, F., & Carney, M. W. P. (1975). Diazepan withdrawal fits. *British Medical Journal*, *4*, 44.

Vyskocil, F. (1977). Diazepan blockade of repetitive action potentials in skeletal muscle fibers. A model of its membrane action. *Brain Research*, *133*, 315–328.

Wallis, W. E. (1987). Withdrawal of anticonvulsant drugs in seizure-free epileptic patients. *Clinical Neuropharmacology*, *10*, 423–433.

Wilder, B. J. (1987). Treatment considerations in anticonvulsant monotherapy. *Epilepsia*, *28* (Supplement 2), S1–S7.

Wilder, B. J., Buchanan, R. A., & Serrano, E. E. (1973). Correlation of acute diphenylhydantoin in toxication with plasma levels and metabolite excretion. *Neurology*, *23*, 1329–1322.

10

Neuropsychological Prediction and Outcome Measures in Relation to EEG Feedback Training for the Treatment of Epilepsy

DELEE LANTZ and M. B. STERMAN

Neuropsychological tests have been of value in assessing individuals with epilepsy for a variety of purposes. In addition to their use in determining the type and extent of neuropsychological impairment relative to nonepileptic controls (e.g., Dodrill, 1978), they have been used to assess and select candidates for specific interventions and to evaluate changes in functioning following those interventions. Tests have been used to assess patients prior to surgical treatment of seizures and to evaluate changes in cognitive and psychosocial functioning following surgery (Horowitz & Cohen, 1968; Lieb, Rausch, Engel, Brown, & Crandall, 1982; Meier & French, 1965, 1966; Milner, 1975; Novelly, Augustine, Mattson, Glaser, Williamson, Spencer, & Spencer, 1984; Rausch, McCreary, & Crandall, 1977; Wannamaker & Matthews, 1976). They have also been used to evaluate the effects of anticonvulsant therapy on functioning (see reviews by Dodrill, 1981; Trimble & Thompson, 1983).

In the work reviewed here, a battery of neuropsychological tests was used for these same purposes to assess individuals with epilepsy undergoing an alternative intervention, EEG feedback training (Lantz & Sterman, 1988, 1989). This technique

DELEE LANTZ and M. B. STERMAN • Departments of Anatomy and Psychiatry, U.C.L.A. School of Medicine, Los Angeles, California 90024, and Neuropsychology Research, Veterans Administration Medical Center, Sepulveda, California 91343.

The Neuropsychology of Epilepsy, edited by Thomas L. Bennett. Plenum Press, New York, 1992.

is directed to EEG normalization using operant conditioning of the EEG and has been explored in several laboratories over the past decade (Kuhlman, 1978; Lantz & Sterman, 1988, Lubar, Shabsin, Natelson, Holder, Whitsett, Pamplin, & Krulikowski, 1981; Sterman, 1982; Sterman & Friar, 1972; Sterman, Macdonald, & Stone, 1974; Sterman & Shouse, 1980; Wyler, Robbins, & Dodrill, 1979). Cognitive, motor, and psychosocial tests were administered to 24 subjects for the purposes of (1) describing a sample of drug-refractory individuals with chronic, frequent, and intractable seizures; (2) determining whether individuals most and least likely to benefit from EEG training can be identified in advance of training; (3) evaluating changes in functioning that result from this training; (4) determining whether there are selective changes in lateralized memory tasks predictable by the side of epileptogenic lesions; and (5) determining whether observed changes are specific effects dependent on learning the EEG-training task and on seizure reduction or whether they are nonspecific effects of participating in a study.

METHODS AND STUDY GROUPS

The subjects in these studies were 24 chronic, drug-refractory patients with epilepsy participating in an EEG feedback training study (Sterman & Lantz, 1981). All had well-documented seizure disorders involving motor symptomatology, the majority having been monitored by continuous EEG and video recording during hospitalizations (see Table 10.1 for group characteristics). Motor symptoms during seizures were a prerequisite for inclusion in the study, since the model on which EEG normalization training is based focuses on sensorimotor system mechanisms and motor deficits (Sterman, 1977). The side and site of the epileptogenic focus were determined by serial clinical and all-night sleep EEGs, computerized tomography scans and clinical evaluation in all subjects, and by depth electrode recordings in four subjects. All subjects had seizure disorders that were uncontrolled by medications. Drug regimens remained constant throughout the study. To monitor drug compliance, anticonvulsant serum levels were obtained at the outset and at 6-week intervals throughout the study. Individuals with progressive neurological disease, significant psychopathology, or a history of poor medical compliance were excluded.

Subjects were matched as closely as possible for age and seizure characteristics and assigned to one of three groups: a tabulation control group, a non-contingent-training control group, and a contingent-training-only group. Figure 10.1 shows the design of the study and indicates when neuropsychological tests were administered. Following a 6-week baseline period during which all subjects tabulated seizures, the contingent-training-only group began EEG feedback training. Contingent training consisted of feedback for bipolar EEG components of left sensorimotor cortex, with electrodes placed at C1 and C5. Reward was given for increasing 11–15 Hz activity while suppressing 0–5 Hz, 20–25 Hz, and high-voltage transients (50 μV or above). Feedback was in the form of an electronic soccer game, with 11–15 Hz represented by a lighted ball moving up the field with increases in amplitude. The EEG activity at

TABLE 10.1.   Description of the Sample

Variable	Mean, range, number	Variable	Mean, range, number
1. Sex		6. Side	
Male	15	Right	7
Female	9	Left	12
2. Age, years (mean)	28.37	Bilateral	5
Range	15–53	7. Age at onset, years (mean)	12.57
3. Primary seizure type		Range	½–50
Complex partial	17	8. Duration, years (mean)	15.1
Genralized tonic–clonic	4	Range	3–38
Elementaary partial	3	9. Anticonvulsants (number of subjects)	
4. Seizure frequency per month		Carbamazepine	14
(mean)	21.2	Phenytoin	13
Range	3–70	Sodium valproate	13
5. Focus		Phenobarbital	5
Generalized	2	Primidone	4
Temporal	12	Ethosuximide	3
Frontotemporal	8	Other	5
Temporal–parietal	1	10. Number of anticonvulsants taken	1.38
Central parietal	1	(mean)	
		Range	1–4

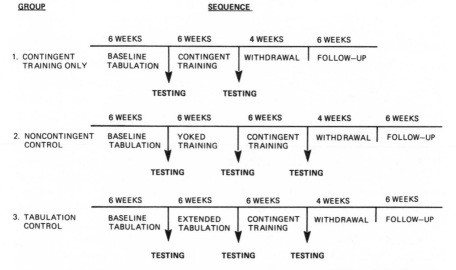

FIGURE 10.1. Experimental design, indicating when test battery was administered to each group.

0–5 and 20–25 Hz, as well as high-voltage transients, was represented as lighted "goalies," which were to be kept deactivated. A goal could be achieved only by increasing the incidence and/or amplitude of 11–15 Hz activity to a criterion level (100% of the subject's baseline level) and by decreasing amplitude in 0–5 and 20–25 Hz to criterion (50% below the subject's baseline level). If that pattern was maintained for at least 0.5 s, the ball entered the goal box, a tone sounded, and a score was registered on the scoreboard for that quarter. Each quarter was 7 min, with a 1-min rest between quarters. Subjects received 30-min training sessions three times a week for 6 weeks. They were withdrawn from training over the next 4 weeks through a gradual reduction of training sessions. They then completed 6 weeks of follow-up seizure tabulation.

The noncontingent control group began EEG feedback "training" sessions following the baseline tabulation period. Each subject in this group was yoked to a contingent subject and received the feedback display and rewards generated by the yoked contingent partner via tape-recorded EEG data. Noncontingent subjects also came for 30-min sessions three times a week for 6 weeks and were unaware of the noncontingent nature of their rewards.

The tabulation control group continued tabulating seizures during a second 6-week period and did not come to the laboratory. Following the 6-week control period, both the noncontingent control group and the tabulation control group received 6 weeks of contingent feedback training followed by 4 weeks of withdrawal training and 6 weeks of follow-up seizure tabulation.

Neuropsychological tests were administered following baseline seizure tabulation, control condition (control subjects only), and contingent training. Thus, control subjects were tested three times, whereas contingent-training-only subjects were tested twice.

A subset of the psychosocial, cognitive, and motor tests of the Neuropsychological Battery for Epilepsy (Dodrill, 1978) was employed and consisted of the following: the Minnesota Multiphasic Personality Inventory (MMPI), Wonderlic Personnel Test, Wechsler Memory Scale: Logical Memory and Visual Reproduction, Seashore Tonal Memory Test, Fingertip Number Writing Perception, Finger Tapping, Name Writing, and the first half of the Stroop Color–Word Test. This particular subset was selected with the goal of sampling a range of performances and minimizing test administration time while maximizing discrimination relative to nonepileptic groups and, hence, sensitivity to epilepsy-related variables. Thus, the Halstead Category test, for instance, with the longest administration time and the lowest discriminability index in the full battery, was eliminated. In addition to the tests listed above, four scales of the Washington Psychosocial Seizure Inventory (WPSI) and a Word List Recall Test using the common nouns of the Buschke Memory Test were given.

The 71-item Mini-Mult form of the MMPI was chosen over the longer forms because of the considerable savings in time and the difficulty with sustained attention experienced by these subjects. The Wonderlic was used in place of a full-scale intelligence test on the basis of Dodrill's finding that this 12-min test can be used to estimate the WAIS Full-Scale IQ of persons with epilepsy with minimal error (Dodrill, 1980).

Test administration required 90–120 min exclusive of the MMPI and the WPSI, which took approximately 30 additional minutes of self-administration. Tests were administered and scored by psychologists who were not connected with the laboratory and who were blind to the subject's group assignment and condition just completed. Alternate forms of the tests were used, where available, for repeated administrations and were given in a counterbalanced order.

BASELINE DESCRIPTIVE RESULTS

Normative data for most of the test battery employed are available from a control group of 50 nonepileptic subjects who were matched for age, sex, education, and occupational status with the subjects with epilepsy serving as the standardization group for the battery (Dodrill, 1978). Scores across tests could, therefore, be compared with a single, appropriate nonepileptic control group as well as with another group of subjects with epilepsy. This comparison indicated clearly that the epileptic group performed significantly more poorly than nonepileptic controls on all measures except Name Writing, as determined by t tests ($ps < .025$). There were few significant differences between this sample and the sample of epileptic subjects comprising the standardization group. The mean percentage of tests outside of normal limits was 69.58%.

Scores on the two psychosocial tests, the WPSI and the MMPI, were elevated beyond normal range in our group. Scores on the WPSI scales used fell between 3.0 and 3.5 of the Professional Rating categories, indicating moderately severe adjustment problems. A comparison of the MMPI mean profiles of 500 patients with epilepsy given the Long Form (unpublished data provided by C. B. Dodrill) is of special interest, since it bears on the question of the usefulness of the much shorter Mini-Mult. The two profiles are presented together in Fig. 10.2 (the Mini-Mult eliminates scales 5 and 0). With the exception of scale 7, which for the Dodrill sample is somewhat higher relative to the other scales than it was for our sample, the profiles are very similar. A two-point code of 2–8/8–2 with secondary peaks of 4–7/7–4 describes both profiles. Clinical scales were more elevated for our sample. We interpret this difference as indicative of the homogeneity of our sample with respect to chronicity and intractability as compared to the Dodrill sample.

In summary, our epileptic subject population showed significant deficits in a wide variety of functioning as measured by psychosocial, cognitive, and motor tests.

PREDICTIVE RESULTS

A statistically significant reduction in seizures did not occur following control conditions but did occur following the contingent training condition ($t = 3.44$; $p < .005$). These are grouped results, however, and individual responses ranged from 0% to 100% reduction. Median seizure reduction was 61%. One of the purposes of neuropsychological testing was to determine whether baseline, pretraining tests can

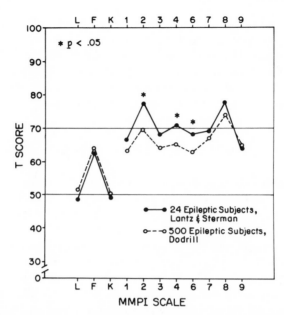

FIGURE 10.2. Comparison of baseline Mini-Mult MMPI scores for 24 subjects in the present study with Long Form MMPI scores for a larger independent sample of subjects with epilepsy (unpublished data provided by C. B. Dodrill).

be helpful in selecting subjects who are most likely to benefit from EEG feedback training. Means for baseline scores were therefore computed separately for the 12 subjects who were subsequently above the group median in seizure reduction at the end of EEG training and for the 12 subjects who were subsequently below the group median. It is important to emphasize that seizure reduction was strongly associated with acquisition of the EEG training task. Acquisition was measured by the percentage change in rewards received (that is, number of times criterion training goals were achieved) between the first 2 weeks of training and the last 2 weeks of training. The group above the median in seizure reduction showed a 91.08% improvement in performance on the EEG task in significant contrast to the group below the median, which showed a 25.5% improvement ($t = 2/25$; $p < .025$). There was even a modest but significant dose-specific response to training: the rank-order correlation between training acquisition and reduction in seizures was 0.46 ($p < .05$).

There were no significant differences in age, sex, education, or seizure characteristics (type, side, site, frequency, duration, or age at onset) between the two outcome groups. Means and ranges were very similar. The number of subjects taking each kind of anticonvulsant medication was also similar; however, subjects below the median were more likely to be taking more medications in combination ($\chi^2 = 6.04$; $p < .02$).

The MMPI and WPSI profiles for the two outcome groups are shown in Figs.

10.3 and 10.4. To determine whether overall profile elevations were different, Hotelling's T^2, a multivariate analogue of the t-tests, was used across the MMPI validity scales, MMPI clinical scales, and WPSI scales. Results indicated significantly lower, more normal, overall profiles for the subjects above the median seizure reduction level on the MMPI clinical scales and the WPSI ($T^2 = 30.56$ and $T^2 = 15.89$; $ps < .05$). The MMPI validity scale profiles were not significantly different between these groups, indicating that a difference in test-taking attitude does not account for the difference in the MMPI clinical scales. The number of MMPI T scores greater than 70 was also significantly lower in the better-outcome group ($t = 1.75$; $p < .05$), as was the number of critical items checked on the WPSI ($t = 2.44$; $p < .02$).

Few of the other tests discriminated between the two groups (see Table 10.2 for baseline scores); however, subjects above the median in seizure reduction performed significantly better at the outset on the Wonderlic, a test of problem-solving ability highly correlated with the WAIS Full-Scale IQ score ($t = 1.76$; $p < .05$). Subjects below the median performed significantly better on the tests with the largest motor component: Finger Tapping, Dominant Hand, Nondominant Hand, and Total scores; and Name Writing, Dominant Hand, and Total score (smallest $t = 2.82$; smallest $p < .005$). The mean percentage of tests outside of normal limits was nearly identical: 70% for more-successful subjects and 69.17% for less-successful subjects.

To summarize, subjects showing the greatest seizure reduction were more intact psychologically, performed better on the test most correlated with IQ values, and

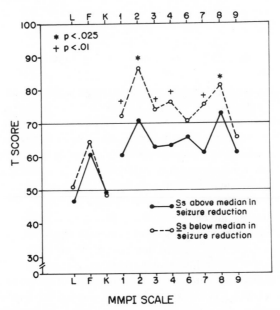

FIGURE 10.3. Baseline MMPI scores for subjects above and below the median in seizure reduction following EEG feedback training.

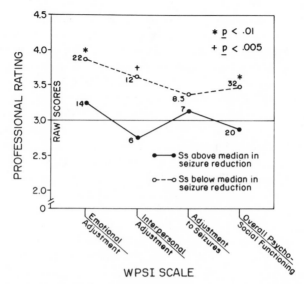

FIGURE 10.4. Baseline Washington Psychosocial Seizure Inventory scores for subjects above and below the median in seizure reduction following EEG feedback training.

showed greater deficit in motor performance at baseline testing than subjects showing less seizure reduction. Other cognitive tests did not differentiate the two groups.

CHANGES IN TEST PERFORMANCE FOLLOWING TRAINING

The third objective of this study was to determine whether there were changes in test performance following EEG feedback training for normalization. To determine this, and also to assess the effects of sex and success of training on changes in test performance, three-way analyses of variance (ANOVAs) were performed on all tests. Sex (males versus females), outcome (above median in seizure reduction versus below median), and repeated measures (baseline versus posttraining test scores) were thus examined individually (main effects) and in combination (interaction effects). There were few main effects on the cognitive and motor tasks. The ANOVA result of greatest interest was the interaction between outcome and repeated measures. Findings here indicated that the more successfully trained subjects improved on posttraining testing whereas the less successfully trained subjects did not, although these groups did not differ at baseline testing. This interaction was significant for the Wonderlic, WMS, Visual Reproduction, Stroop II (Time and Errors), Stroop II − I (Time and Errors), Word List Recall, Fingertip Writing Perception, Nondominant Hand, and percentage of tests within normal limits ($Fs = 4.50$ to 15.27; $ps < .05$ to $.0009$).

TABLE 10.2. Means and Standard Deviations of Test Scores for Subjects above or below the Median in Seizure Reduction

Test	Subjects above the median in seizure reduction (n = 12)					Subjects below the median in seizure reduction (n = 12)				
	Baseline		Posttraining			Baseline		Posttraining		
	Mean	(S.D.)	Mean	(S.D.)	t^a	Mean	(S.D.)	Mean	(S.D.)	t^a
Wonderlic (raw score)	15.75	(7.34)	17.42	(9.02)	-1.89[b]	11.09	(5.84)	13.27	(8.82)	-1.76[b]
Logical Memory, average	7.50	(4.31)	8.25	(3.23)		6.50	(3.87)	6.17	(3.40)	
Visual Reproduction	10.04	(2.73)	11.37	(1.89)	-2.33[c]	9.95	(2.86)	10.33	(2.96)	-0.35
Seashore Tonal Memory Test	16.83	(6.73)	18.58	(7.67)		14.83	(5.52)	16.41	(7.43)	
Stroop I, time	71.83	(32.44)	77.33	(31.38)		69.42	(21.15)	72.25	(21.73)	
Stroop I, errors	1.08	(1.16)	1.17	(1.70)		1.08	(1.08)	1.92	(1.31)	
Stroop II, time	171.92	(79.51)	160.17	(80.29)	1.43	140.58	(45.37)	156.75	(54.09)	-1.79
Stroop II, errors	7.42	(4.60)	4.25	(4.27)	2.36[c]	5.00	(4.35)	5.92	(3.48)	-0.91
Stroop II − I, time	100.08	(63.12)	82.83	(60.68)	2.32[c]	71.17	(42.15)	84.50	(51.37)	-1.29
Stroop II − I, errors	6.41	(4.66)	3.08	(4.91)	2.26[c]	3.91	(4.21)	4.00	(3.16)	-0.08
Word List Recall	6.00	(1.24)	6.75	(1.14)	-2.60[c]	7.00	(1.28)	5.58	(2.15)	-2.28[c]
Name Writing, dom. hand (let/s)	1.43	(0.26)	1.58	(0.27)	-2.39[c]	1.83	(0.37)	1.93	(0.53)	-1.27
Name Writing, nondom. hand	0.70	(0.18)	0.66	(0.11)		0.67	(0.13)	0.61	(0.14)	
Name Writing, average	1.07	(0.18)	1.12	(0.13)		1.21	(0.20)	1.23	(0.30)	
Fingertip Writing, dom. hand, errors	2.90	(2.88)	3.50	(2.76)		4.27	(3.13)	4.63	(3.96)	
Fingertip Writing, nondom. hand	3.00	(2.30)	1.92	(2.10)	2.40[c]	3.90	(2.33)	4.30	(3.50)	-0.33
Fingertip Writing, total	5.90	(5.17)	5.70	(5.42)		8.10	(4.98)	8.80	(7.28)	
Finger Tapping, dom. hand (taps/10 s)	43.25	(6.01)	42.75	(6.70)		47.52	(4.01)	49.01	(5.50)	
Finger Tapping, nondom. hand	38.43	(2.98)	38.58	(3.72)		45.56	(6.54)	44.42	(8.83)	
Finger Tapping, total	81.68	(7.68)	81.33	(10.17)		93.11	(9.20)	93.87	(13.53)	
Percentage of tests outside normal limits	70.00	(29.23)	60.83	(23.91)	2.11[b]	69.17	(19.75)	65.83	(24.29)	1.30

^{a} t-Tests applied where significant analysis of variance repeated-measures effects were found.
^{b} $p < .05$.
^{c} $p < .025$.

Table 10.2 shows the *t*-test outcomes between baseline and posttraining comparisons for subjects above and below the median on all tests with significant repeated measures effects. Subjects above the median in seizure reduction improved significantly on 9 of these 10 tests, and subjects below the median improved on only one. Other ANOVA interaction effects were not significant.

To determine whether there were changes in the profile elevations of the MMPI and the WPSI following EEG training, Hotelling T^2s were used. These analyses revealed that posttraining profiles for subjects both above and below the median in seizure reduction were significantly less elevated (less abnormal) than baseline profiles for the MMPI clinical scales (T^2s = 30.45 and 15.89; ps < .05) but not for the validity scales or the WPSA. However, the MMPI improvement was greater for subjects above the median than for subjects below the median (T^2 = 30.56; p < .05). Results for the MMPI, then, differ from results for the cognitive and motor tests, where improvement was seen only among successful subjects.

It was important to determine whether the changes in test scores were actually a result of EEG normalization training or a consequence of the nonspecific effects of being a participant in the study. This was assessed by examining the changes following the control period, when no significant seizure change had occurred in either the tabulation or the yoked-control condition. Since there were no significant differences in change scores between the two control groups, their results were combined. Test scores for these 16 subjects were analyzed as a group and again separately for subjects subsequently above and below the seizure reduction median following contingent training. These postcontrol condition scores were compared with baseline and posttraining test scores. Only if greater change occurred following normalization training than following the control period can we assume that EEG training is specifically associated with improved performance. This, in fact, is the case for the cognitive and motor tests. There was only one instance of significantly improved performance (on the Stroop II − I, Errors, t = 2.83; p < .01) following control conditions, and this was found only for subjects subsequently above the median in seizure reduction. When control-condition and post-contingent-training scores were compared, however, improvements were found on nine measures for subjects above the median (smallest t = 1.84; smallest p < .05). Control subjects below the median improved only on the Seashore Tonal Memory Test (t = 2.35, p < .05).

A different pattern of change was observed for the MMPI. The overall clinical profile was significantly less elevated after the control condition for the eventually more successful subjects (T^2 = 1361.14; p < .004). No further significant change occurred following the contingent-training condition for these subjects. For the less-successful control subjects, the overall profiles were not significantly different from baseline after either the control or the training condition. No change in the WPSI was found following either the control period or contingent training.

It appears that for cognitive and motor tests the improved performance for successful subjects following EEG training was not a function of the nonspecific effects of simply participating in a study, since scores did not improve following control conditions. Improvement required contingent normalization training and seizure reduction. The MMPI changes, on the other hand, seem to reflect less specific and less consistent effects. Neither normalization training nor considerable seizure relief was a prerequisite for MMPI improvement.

SELECTIVE CHANGES PREDICTABLE BY SIDE OF LESION

Selective changes in cognitive functions have been found to occur in patients following unilateral surgical resection of temporal lobe tissues. It was of interest, therefore, to evaluate the possibility of similar changes following the far more benign and noninvasive EEG feedback treatment. Memory performance was chosen for analysis because there is compelling evidence for a specialization of the two temporal lobes for different kinds of memory, the left for verbal material and the right for visual and other nonverbal material (Delaney, Rosen, Mattson, & Novelly, 1980; Ladavas, Umilta, & Provinciali, 1979; Milner, 1968; Mungas, Ehlers, Walton, & McCutchen, 1985; Novelly et al., 1984; Novelly, Lifrak, & Spencer, 1985; Trimble & Thompson, 1983). Since memory for both types of material was impaired in the subjects in this study, we asked if memory function might improve differentially in subjects with unilateral left versus right temporal lobe lesions after successful EEG normalization training.

Twenty of the 24 subjects had confirmed unilateral lesions. All 20 were right-handed and presumed to be left hemisphere dominant for language. Unilateral focal abnormalities in all cases involved the temporal lobe, although not necessarily exclusively. The results of the four memory tests included in the battery were analyzed separately for these 20 subjects. These tests were the Wechsler Memory Scale Logical Memory, WMS Visual Reproduction, Seashore Tonal Memory Test, and the Buschke Word List Recall Test, all of which have well-documented lateralized temporal lobe involvement.

The previous analyses of all 24 subjects clearly indicated that test performance improved only for more successfully trained subjects and not for less successfully trained subjects. Therefore, the analysis of memory performance focused on the more successfully trained subjects with unilateral temporal lobe lesions. However, because of the smaller number of subjects in this analysis, further divided into right and left hemisphere groups, a less stringent criterion of "more successfully trained" was employed. With a criterion of 50% or greater reduction in reported seizures, 10 subjects with left temporal lobe lesions and 5 subjects with right temporal lobe lesions were identified. Results from these more successfully trained subjects with unilateral lesions were compared with results from four successfully trained subjects with generalized or bilateral lesions and five less successfully trained subjects with unilateral lesions.

Comparisons between baseline and posttraining scores (Fig. 10.5) revealed that

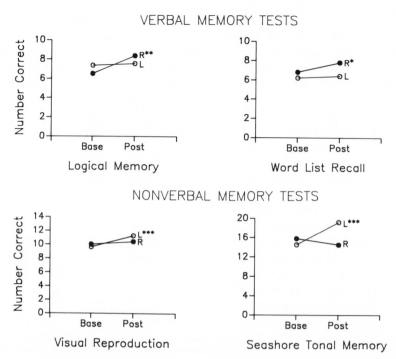

FIGURE 10.5. Baseline and posttraining scores on memory tests specific to left hemisphere (verbal memory) and right hemisphere (nonverbal memory). Asterisks indicate probability of significant differences: *$p < .10$; **$p < .05$; ***$p < .005$.

the successfully trained subjects with left hemisphere lesions improved significantly on the Wechsler Memory Scale Visual Reproduction and the Seashore Tonal Memory Test (ts = 4.04 and 3.69; ps < .005). These tests involve predominantly right hemisphere processing. Scores remained unchanged for the Wechsler Memory Scale Logical Memory and Buschke Word List Recall Test, tests involving predominantly left hemisphere processing. The opposite pattern of change was found for the subjects with right hemisphere lesions (ts = 2.18 and 1.82; ps < .05 and .10), although for this smaller group of five subjects a statistical trend rather than full significance was found for one of the tests. No significant changes from baseline occurred following control conditions. Further, no consistent pattern of change was found on any test for the four most successful subjects with generalized or bilateral lesions. Although the small number of less successfully trained subjects with unilateral lesions (three left hemisphere and two right hemisphere) precluded statistical analysis, no consistent pattern of change was observed in these groups as well.

In summary, although not significantly different at base line, subjects with right and left unilateral epileptogenic temporal lobe lesions improved differentially after training in ways that implicate specific hemispheric laterality effects.

DISCUSSION

Patient Characteristics

The patients in this study were shown to suffer deficits at the outset in a wide variety of cognitive, motor, and psychosocial functioning as compared to a non-epileptic control group. These findings are similar to the findings of Dodrill (1978), Dodrill, Breyer, Diamond, Dubinsky, & Geary, (1984), Matthews and Klove (1967, 1968), and Wannamaker and Matthews (1976).

Outcome Prediction

The same baseline tests were used in an attempt to differentiate eventually more successful subjects from less successful subjects. Successful subjects scored higher on the Wonderlic, a test yielding a WAIS Full-Scale IQ estimate. Other cognitive tests did not differentiate the two groups. In an EEG feedback study involving training over the area of focal abnormality and using the complete Neuropsychological Battery for Epilepsy, Wyler et al. (1979) found no prestudy differences between successful and unsuccessful subjects on cognitive tests, including the Wonderlic. However, Leib et al. (1982) and Wannamaker and Matthews (1976) found that the reduction in seizure frequency following surgery was more likely to occur in patients with higher presurgery IQ scores. It should be noted that the association between higher Wonderlic scores and greater seizure reduction found in this study was by no means absolute, since there were remarkable exceptions in individual subjects. However, it may be that more normal intellectual functioning, either directly or indirectly through association with greater cerebral intactness, is an advantage to individuals engaging in a learning experience such as EEG feedback training.

The finding that subsequently more successful subjects did far worse than less successful subjects in all baseline tests involving strong motor components is puzzling until it is related to the model underlying EEG normalization training. This model is based on animal studies that have focused on sensorimotor system mechanisms (Sterman, 1973; Sterman & Bowersox, 1981). It predicts motor deficits from thalamocortical dysfunction in some types of epilepsy and requires this condition for appropriate application of sensorimotor EEG feedback training. Further, one of the initial findings with the application of these methods in human epilepsy was a more favorable therapeutic response in seizure disorders involving primary motor components (Sterman et al., 1974). Therefore, a prerequisite for the effective application of this therapy might be evidence for such motor deficits. The type and level of medications known to affect motor performance (e.g., phenytoin, phenobarbital) were similar in the two outcome groups and do not explain the motor inferiority of the subjects who ultimately showed the best clinical response.

The two psychosocial tests—the MMPI and the WPSI—were found to be quite sensitive in predicting clinical response. Wyler et al. (1979) also found consistent statistical trends indicating that subjects who benefited from EEG training had more normal MMPI profiles at the outset than subjects who did not benefit from this training. Thus, better emotional and psychosocial adjustment may be more important prerequisites for successful EEG normalization training than level of cognitive functioning, at least in individuals of normal or near-normal intelligence.

The shortest version of the MMPI, the 71-item Mini-Mult, was used in this study and was one of the most powerful predictive tests in the entire battery. It has been noted that the Mini-Mult correlates more highly with the Long Form of the MMPI when populations are more extreme (Harford, Lubetkin, & Alpert, 1972; Kincannon, 1968; Lacks, 1970). The extreme elevations of this sample may be responsible for the close correspondence to the profile obtained for another sample given the Long Form. Aside from the question of validity compared to the longer forms, the Mini-Mult was itself a good discriminator of subjects more or less likely to benefit from training and was sensitive to changes following training. Further, individuals with intractable epilepsy, whose difficulties with attention, concentration, and self-esteem can often make the longer versions a frustrating and demoralizing experience, are good candidates for the application of this abbreviated evaluation tool.

No seizure variables (type, side, site, duration, frequency, or age of onset) predicted outcome of training, but one medication variable did. Subjects with poorer outcomes were more likely to be taking more medications in combination. Reynolds (1983) and Trimble and Thompson (1983) have argued that polytherapy has detrimental effects on many areas of functioning. A greater inability to benefit from EEG normalization training may be another case in point. It is possible, also, that the subjects on more medications were inflicted with more severe seizure disorders and that it was this, and not polytherapy *per se*, that led to both lower intellectual functioning and poorer outcomes. However, Reynolds (1983) has argued that polytherapy is often not a function of degree of severity, and Thompson and Trimble (1983) have demonstrated that when the number of medications is reduced, significant improvement on a variety of cognitive functions is seen. Thus, polytherapy itself may indeed directly affect ability to benefit from EEG training.

Posttraining Changes in Test Performance

Comparisons of cognitive and motor test scores before and after training revealed improvement on a number of measures among subjects who were above the median in seizure reduction but on only one measure among subjects below the median. Posttraining improvement was apparently not a function of the nonspecific effects of participating in the study, since scores did not improve following control periods. The practice effects of repeated testing also provided no alternative explanation, since neither control subjects above or below the median profit from a second test administration (postcontrol), and control subjects below the median do not profit from even a third administration (posttraining). Participation in contingent EEG normalization training is required, and that participation must be accompanied by response acquisition and associated significant seizure reduction.

The posttraining changes in test scores for successful subjects observed here are at variance with the findings reported by Wyler *et al.* (1979). Using a subset of their baseline battery for posttraining test administration, Wyler *et al.* found improvement only on the Wonderlic for subjects who benefited from EEG feedback training. This study differed from the present series, however, in a number of significant ways. In particular, these investigators provided EEG feedback reward for 18-Hz activity recorded over the cortical site of maximal focal abnormality, in contrast to our paradigm, which provided reward for 11–15 Hz activity recorded from the left sensorimotor (central) cortex. Half of the subjects in the Wyler *et al.* study received training for only 3 weeks, which may have been too brief a period for changes in cognitive functioning to occur. Further, aside from the Wonderlic, the subsets used for posttraining testing in that study and the present one had only two tests in common. Definitions of "successful" and "unsuccessful" subjects were also different. Wyler *et al.* used a statistically significant decrease in seizures following training as their criterion. Statistical significance may not have been the equivalent of clinical significance in all subjects, in which case improved functioning would not be expected. Moreover, the Wyler *et al.* study did not report whether seizure reduction was associated with actual acquisition of the conditioned EEG response or with another independent measure of change in the EEG. Successful subjects may have been successful for reasons other than significant alteration of cortical activity, and those reasons may have had less effect on intellectual functioning. Success in the present study was highly associated with acquisition of the training task.

Improvement in psychological functioning, as measured by the MMPI, was observed in both outcome groups, although this improvement was greater in the more successful group. Moreover, improvement was as likely to be seen after the control period, when seizures had not significantly decreased, as after EEG training. Thus, we cannot conclude that either EEG normalization training or seizure reduction is necessary for improvement in psychological status. Nonspecific aspects of participating in a treatment protocol apparently affected both groups of subjects.

Selective Changes Predictable by Side of Lesion

At base line, the right and left hemisphere groups did not differ significantly on any of the four memory tests, all of which tested immediate recall of material. This is consistent with numerous findings indicating that differences between groups with right and left temporal lobe lesions are not usually found on tests of immediate recall but are detected on delayed recall (Milner, 1968, 1975; Mungas *et al.*, 1985; Russell, 1975; Trimble & Thompson, 1983). However, following EEG training, differential improvements occurred. Subjects with left temporal lobe foci improved on memory tests involving the right temporal lobe. Subjects with right temporal lobe foci improved on memory tests involving the left temporal lobe. That is, memory improvement was seen in both groups in types of memory associated specifically with the hemisphere contralateral to their lesions. Improvement was not seen in either group in types of memory specific to the impaired hemisphere. Althrough the number of subjects in these groups was relatively small, a clear and consistent pattern of change emerged that suggests differential lateralized improvements predictable by the side of the lesion.

In a study of patients who had undergone temporal lobectomy, Novelly *et al.* (1984) found improvement on memory tasks related to the nonresected side in their "good-outcome group." That is, improvement was on the side contralateral to the seizure focus. However, they also found an enduring memory impairment on memory tasks related to the resected side, as have other postsurgical studies (Blakemore & Falconer, 1967; Milner, 1967, 1968, 1975). Since, unlike surgery, EEG feedback training does not involve the removal of tissue, it is not surprising that the present study did not find corresponding decrements. We would argue, as did Novelly *et al.* (1984), that the improvement seen in performance specific to the unimpaired temporal lobe probably occurred as a result of a reduction in disruptive discharge originating from the impaired temporal lobe. Interictal decreases in abnormal electrical activity have been found in both hemispheres following EEG feedback training (Sterman & Shouse, 1980). Also, fewer disruptions in the form of seizures occur in the more successfully trained subjects displaying this selective improvement. However, the epileptogenic tissue underlying the abnormal activity is still present in the affected hemisphere and apparently continues to impair performance in that hemisphere.

Specific versus Nonspecific Changes

It is important to try to determine whether improvement in neuropsychological functioning following any intervention is brought about by the specific intervention or by more general and nonspecific aspects of the total situation. If the latter is true, no claim can be made for the efficacy of the treatment *per se*. Given this conclusion, there may be more cost-effective, shorter, and, in the case of surgery and medication, less risky ways to bring about the same results. Simple participation in a study, such as the one described here, can bring about enhanced alertness and attention; increased activity level, social interactions, and self-esteem; lower social isolation and depression; and renewed optimism. All of these things can affect neuropsychological functioning. We must evaluate the improvements seen in this study of EEG normalization training from this perspective.

Improved MMPI profiles seem to have been a function of the nonspecific benefits of participation. Subjects below the median in seizure reduction, with little change in EEG performance, showed these improvements, as did subjects above the median. Furthermore, improvement was as likely to occur after control conditions as after contingent EEG training. All other documented improvements, however, appear to be specific to the influence of EEG training. They were observed only in the subjects above the median in seizure reduction who showed strong acquisition of the rewarded EEG training response, and only following the contingent training condition. Analysis of lateralized memory improvements provided evidence that argues even more strongly for a specific training effect. These improvements occurred in a differential manner in individuals with unilateral right and left temporal lobe lesions. The specific and selective nature of this improvement, the fact that successful subjects with general or bilateral lesions showed no consistent pattern of improvement on these memory measures, and the lack of improvement following control conditions strongly mitigate against nonspecific interpretations. Alteration of the underlying neural substrate for epileptogenic discharge, brought about by EEG normalization training, seems to provide the best explanation for the improved neuropsychological functioning observed.

SUMMARY

In summary, the neuropsychological test results obtained from subjects receiving EEG feedback training directed to normalization suggested the following. (1) Individuals with severe seizure disorders show impairment in a wide variety of cognitive, motor, and psychosocial functioning. (2) Individuals with higher baseline scores on the Wonderlic (a test highly correlated with the WAIS Full-Scale IQ score), the MMPI, and the WPSI, and lower baseline scores on motor tests are more likely to benefit clinically from this training. Fewer medications were also associated with more successful outcomes. (3) Improvement on numerous cognitive, motor, and psychosocial measures occurred exclusively in subjects who were more successful in acquiring the trained response and reducing seizures. (4) Successfully trained subjects with unilateral temporal lobe lesions improved selectively on types of memory specific to the hemisphere contralateral to their lesions. (5) All improvements, except those seen on MMPI profiles, appeared to be specific effects of EEG normalization training. They occurred only following contingent EEG training, not following control conditions, and only in subjects above the median in seizure reduction, with memory changes occurring in a differential manner depending on the side of the epileptogenic focus.

REFERENCES

Blakemore, C. B., & Falconer, M. A. (1967). Long term effects of anterior temporal lobectomy on certain cognitive functions. *Journal of Neurology Neurosurgery and Psychiatry*, *30*, 364–367.

Delaney, R., Rosen, A., Mattson, R., & Novelly, R. (1980). Memory function in focal epilepsy: A comparison of nonsurgical, unilateral temporal lobe and frontal lobe samples. *Cortex*, *16*, 103–117.

Dodrill, C. B. (1978). A neuropsychological battery for epilepsy. *Epilepsia*, *19*, 611–623.

Dodrill, C. B. (1980). Rapid evaluation of intelligence in adults with epilepsy. *Epilepsia*, *21*, 359–367.

Dodrill, C. B. (1981). Neuropsychology of epilepsy. In S. B. Filskov & T. J. Ball (Eds.), *Handbook of clinical neuropsychology* (pp. 366–395). New York: John Wiley & Sons.

Dodrill, C. B., Breyer, D. N., Diamond, M. B., Dubinsky, B. L., & Geary, B. (1984). Psychosocial problems among adults with epilepsy. *Epilepsia*, *25*, 168–175.

Harford, T., Lubetkin, B., & Alpert, B. (1972). Comparison of the standard MMPI and the Mini-Mult in a psychiatric out-patient clinic. *Journal of Consulting and Clinical Psychology*, *39*, 243–245.

Horowitz, M. J., & Cohen, F. M. (1968). Temporal lobe epilepsy—effect of lobectomy on psychosocial functioning. *Epilepsia*, *9*, 23–41.

Kincannon, J. C. (1968). Prediction of the standard MMPI scale scores from 71 items: The Mini-Mult. *Journal of Consulting and Clinical Psychology*, *32*, 319–325.

Kuhlman, W. N. (1978). EEG feedback training: Enhancement of somatosensory cortical activity. *Electroencephalogry and Clinical Neurophysiology, 45,* 290–294.

Lacks, P. B. (1970). Further investigation of the Mini-Mult. *Journal of Consulting Clinical Psychology, 35,* 126–127.

Ladavas, E., Umilta, C., & Provinciali, L. (1979). Hemisphere-dependent cognitive performances in epileptic patients. *Epilepsia, 20,* 493–502.

Lantz, D., & Sterman, M. B. (1988). Neuropsychological assessment of subjects with uncontrolled epilepsy: Effects of EEG training. *Epilepsia, 29,* 163–171.

Leib, J. P., Rausch, R., Engel, J., Brown, W. J., & Crandall, P. (1982). Changes in intelligence following temporal lobectomy: Relationship to EEG activity, seizure relief and pathology. *Epilepsia, 23,* 1–13.

Lubar, J. F., Shabsin, H., Natelson, S. E., Holder, G. S., Whitsett, S. F., Pamplin, W. E., & Krulikowski, D. (1981). EEG operant conditioning in intractable epilepsy. *Archives of Neurology, 38,* 700–704.

Matthews, C. G., & Klove, H. (1967). Differential psychological performances in major motor, psychomotor and mixed seizure classifications of known and unknown etiology. *Epilepsia, 8,* 117–128.

Matthews, C. G., & Klove, H. (1968). MMPI performances in major motor and mixed seizure classifications of known and unknown etiology. *Epilepsia, 9,* 43–53.

Meier, M. J., & French, L. A. (1965). Changes in MMPI scale scores and an index of psychopathology following unilateral temporal lobectomy for epilepsy. *Epilepsia, 6,* 263–273.

Meier, M. J., & French, L. A. (1966). Longitudinal assessment of intellectual functioning following unilateral temporal lobectomy. *Journal of Clinical Psychology, 22,* 22–27.

Milner, B. (1967). Brain mechanisms suggested by studies of temporal lobes. In F. L. Darley (Ed.), *Brain mechanisms underlying speech and language* (p. 122). New York: Grune & Stratton.

Milner, B. (1968). Visual recognition and recall after right temporal excision in man. *Neuropsychologia, 6,* 191–210.

Milner, B. (1975). Psychological aspects of focal epilepsy and its neurosurgical mangement. In D. P. Purpura, J. K. Penry, & R. D. Walter (Eds.), *Advances in neurology* (pp. 299–322). New York: Raven Press.

Mungas, D., Ehlers, C., Walton, N., & McCutchen, C. (1985). Verbal learning differences in epileptic patients with left and right temporal lobe foci. *Epilepsia, 26,* 340–345.

Novelly, R. A., Augustine, E. A., Mattson, R. H., Glaser, G. H., Williamson, P. D., Spencer, D. D., & Spencer, S. S. (1984). Selective memory improvement and impairment in temporal lobectomy for epilepsy. *Annuals of Neurology, 15,* 64–67.

Novelly, R. A., Lifrak, M. D., & Spencer, D. (1985). Side and site of focal lesion associated with intracarotid amytal memory impairment. *Epilepsia, 26,* 547.

Rausch, R., McCreary, C., & Crandall, P. H. (1977). Psychosocial functioning following successful surgical relief from seizures. Evidence of prediction from preoperative personality characteristics. *Journal of Psychosomatic Research, 21,* 141–146.

Reynolds, E. H. (1983). Mental effects of antiepileptic medication: A review. *Epilepsia, 24,* S285–S295.

Russell, E. (1975). A multiple scoring method for the assessment of complex memory functions. *Journal of Consulting and Clinical Psychology, 43,* 800–809.

Sterman, M. B. (1973). Neurophysiologic and clinical studies of sensorimotor EEG biofeedback training. *Seminars in Psychiatry, 5,* 507–525.

Sterman, M. B. (1982). EEG feedback in the treatment of epilepsy: An overview circa 1980. In L. White & B. Tursky (Eds.), *Clinical biofeedback: Efficacy and mechanisms* (pp. 311–330). New York: Guilford Press.

Sterman, M. B., & Shouse, M. N. (1980). Quantitative analysis of training, sleep EEG and clinical response to EEG operant conditioning in epileptics. *Electroencephalogry and Clinical Neurophysiology, 49,* 558–576.

Sterman, M. B., & Bowersox, S. S. (1981). Sensorimotor EEG rhythmic activity: A functional gate mechanism. *Sleep, 4,* 408–422.

Sterman, M. B., & Lantz, D. (1981). Effects of sensorimotor EEG normalization feedback training on seizure rate in poorly controlled epileptics. Society proceedings. *Electroencephalogry and Clinical Neurophysiology, 51*, 23P.

Sterman, M. B., Macdonald, L. R., & Stone, R. K. (1974). Biofeedback training of the sensorimotor EEG rhythm in man: Effects on epilepsy. *Epilepsia, 15*, 395–416.

Thompson, P. J., & Trimble, M. R. (1983). The effects of anticonvulsant drugs on cognitive function: Relation to serum level. *Journal of Neurology, Neurosurgery and Psychiatry, 46*, 277–333.

Trimble, M. P., & Thompson, P. J. (1983). Anticonvulsant drugs, cognitive function and behavior. *Epilepsia, 24*, S55–S63.

Wannamaker, B. B., & Matthews, C. G. (1976). Prognostic implications of neuropsychological test performance for surgical treatment of epilepsy. *Journal of Nervous and Mental Disease, 163*, 29–34.

Wyler, A. R., Robbins, C. A., & Dodrill, C. B. (1979). EEG operant conditioning for control of epilepsy. *Epilepsia, 20*, 279–286.

11

Criteria and Validity Issues in Wada Assessment

DAVID W. LORING, KIMFORD J. MEADOR, and GREGORY P. LEE

The administration of sodium amobarbital (Sodium Amytal®) via the carotid artery was introduced by Juhn Wada in 1949 as a technique to determine cerebral language laterality, and this technique has subsequently become known as the Wada test (Wada, 1949). Wada testing has become an indispensable part of the preoperative evaluation in patients who are candidates for epilepsy surgery and was designed to determine cerebral language laterality. More recently, the procedure has become one of the techniques used by neuropsychologists to establish risk for the development of post-surgical anterograde amnesia. However, Wada testing is not standardized and varies between centers, reflecting the training as well as the theoretical assumptions of the examiners. Medication dosage also differs, but at most centers, the procedure involves injection of 100–200 mg sodium amobarbital into a single carotid artery following a transfemoral approach. Sodium amobarbital is presumed to pharmacologically inactivate the distribution of the anterior and middle cerebral arteries for several minutes, although individual variability in cerebral vasculature exists (e.g., cross flow, posterior cerebral artery filling). During the period of hemispheric anesthesia, the patient undergoes language and memory evaluation. This chapter focuses primarily on recent work at the Medical College of Georgia that challenges some of the commonly held assumptions derived from Wada testing and also highlights methodological issues and limitations of this technique that should be considered when making individual patient inferences.

DAVID W. LORING • Section of Behavioral Neurology, Department of Neurology, Medical College of Georgia, Augusta, Georgia 30912–3275.   KIMFORD J. MEADOR • Section of Behavioral Neurology, Department of Neurology, Medical College of Georgia, Augusta, Georgia 30912–3200. GREGORY P. LEE • Department of Psychiatry, and Section of Neurosurgery, Department of Surgery, Medical College of Georgia, Augusta, Georgia 30912–4010.

The Neuropsychology of Epilepsy, edited by Thomas L. Bennett. Plenum Press, New York, 1992.

LANGUAGE TESTING

The first systematic application of Wada testing to establish cerebral language laterality during the preoperative evaluation for epilepsy surgery was conducted at the Montreal Neurological Institute (Wada & Rasmussen, 1960). Twenty patients received 150–200 mg sodium amobarbital injections using a common carotid artery approach without complication, thereby establishing both the technical and practical applicability. Surgery was performed on 17 patients, all of whom appeared correctly classified based on the presence or absence of immediate postoperative aphasia.

Branch, Milner, and Rasmussen (1964) reported language findings in 123 patients who underwent Wada assessment. Four patients had unsatisfactory studies, and only 97 of the remaining 119 patients underwent bilateral testing. The language assessment included object naming, counting, and recitation of the days of the week both forward and in reverse serial order. Ninety percent of right-handed patients were left cerebral language dominant. Of patients sustaining left cerebral injury before age 5, 22% of patients were left cerebral dominant, 67% were right hemisphere language dominant, and 11% had bilateral speech. This sharply contrasted with patients without early left hemisphere injury, 64% of whom were left cerebral language dominant, 20% were right cerebral language dominant, and 16% exhibited bilateral language representation.

This report empirically confirmed that age of cerebral insult was an important factor potentially affecting cerebral language lateralization. However, it is also important because it described a patient who was determined to be right cerebral language dominant by Wada testing but suffered a mild but definite aphasia following left hemisphere resection involving Broca's area. The postoperative aphasia illustrates that the Wada testing procedure used in this patient series failed to indicated the presence of additional left hemisphere language representation. As is well known to psychologists, absence of evidence is not evidence of absence, and the sensitivity of Wada testing depends on many factors including the method of language assessment during hemispheric anesthesia.

In the largest and most commonly cited patient series, Rasmussen and Milner (1977) reported that 96% of dextral patients without evidence of early left hemisphere damage were left cerebral language dominant; all remaining right-handed patients were right cerebral language dominant. In contrast, language in left- or mixed-handed patients without early injury was less strongly lateralized to the left hemisphere, with only 70% displaying left language cerebral dominance. The remaining patients were divided equally between bilateral speech and right cerebral dominance (15% each). As Woods, Dodrill, and Ojemann (1988) note, results of these early series are frequently cited without reservation and generalized as representative of the population at large. However, the procedure at the Montreal Neurological Institute is performed only on nondextral patients (i.e., left-handed or ambidextrous) or for dextral patients when some clinical doubt regarding language representation exists. Jones-Gotman (1990) reported that only 35–45% of the patients at the Montreal Neurological Institute who are candidates for epilepsy surgery undergo Wada evaluation. Consequently, these figures are not necessarily even representative of patients with intractable epilepsy.

The incidence of cerebral language dominance varies depending on the institution performing the assessment. For example, Hommes and Panhuysen (1970) reported some right cerebral language representation in 9/11 depressed patients. Similarly, aphasic errors were present following both left and right hemisphere injections in 14/23 patients assessed by Oxbury and Oxbury (1984). In an international survey of epilepsy surgery centers, Snyder, Novelly, and Harris (1990) found that the incidence of bilateral speech ranged from 0% to 60%. These data confirm that variables such as criteria for patient inclusion, variation in language assessments employed by various epilepsy surgery centers, as well as a relatively low base rate of non-left cerebral language dominance are contributing to variability in the reported language representation.

The Wada procedure developed at the Medical College of Georgia (MCG) was designed to assess four linguistic areas (Loring, Meador, Lee, Murro, Flanigin, Smith, Gallagher, & King, 1990d). The language tasks include overlearned verbal sequences, comprehension, confrontation naming, and repetition. The procedure at MCG is performed immediately following the arteriogram, and both left and right amobarbital injections are performed on the same day separated by at least 30 min. We have chosen this method to minimize the number of femoral punctures. At the beginning of the procedure, the patient is supine with his or her hands held straight up with the palms turned rostrally and the fingers spread. The patient begins counting repeatedly from 1 to 20 employing a normal cadence. An initial injection of 100 mg sodium amobarbital (5% solution) is administered by hand over a 4-s interval. Incremental injections of 50 mg are administered up to a maximum of 200 mg total necessary to produce a contralateral hemiplegia.

After amobarbital administration, an expressive language score (0–4) is given based on disruption of the patient's counting ability. A score of 0 reflects normal cadence, slowed cadence, or a brief pause lasting less than 20 s. Because of the acute medication effects, there are instances in which a patient will stop counting briefly. However, if the patient is able to resume counting following prompting by the examiner, no language impairment is inferred. If no resumption occurs, patients are asked repeatedly to start again at "1"; since this portion of the sequence tends to be more overlearned, it is more resistant to sedative effects. Occasionally, two varieties of counting perseveration may be present. For example, patients may continue to count beyond the number "20." Alternatively, patients may resume counting despite repeated urging by the examiner to stop. Both types of counting perseveration errors are scored as 1. Sequencing errors, which are scored 2, would include responses such as "14, 15, 17, 18, 15." Some patients may perseverate on a single number and give responses such as "9–9–9–9–9," which is scored 3. More common for left cerebral injections, however, is a complete speech arrest that lasts several minutes before spontaneous language output or comprehension is resumed, and this pattern is scored 4.

Comprehension is assessed initially by having the patient execute simple commands including a midline command such as "stick out your tongue," although performance on this task is not formally scored. Approximately 1 min later, formal comprehension is assessed by presenting a modified token test and instructing the patient to execute commands of decreasing syntactic complexity. The most difficult item is a two-stage command involving inverted syntax (e.g., "point to the red circle after the green square"). The simplest command receiving credit is a simple single-stage command. Comprehension is assessed on a 0 to 3 point scale.

We require return of minimal language function (e.g., following a midline command or the presence of spontaneous vocalization) before proceeding with additional testing. After some language function is present, two real objects are presented, and the subject is asked to name them and is scored on a pass–fail basis. Following object naming, a nursery rhyme is read to the patient, and repetition is scored on a 0–3 rating scale. For all four language categories, 0 reflects normal language function. In addition to the rating assessment, paraphasic responses are noted, so that inferences of language representation are based on both negative (i.e., complete inability to perform tasks) as well as positive (i.e., presence of paraphasic errors) findings.

Language classification is based on the patient's performance on all four language tests. Since patient-to-patient variability exists regarding the behavioral effects of medication, we have adopted a conservative criterion to classify language. For language impairment to be inferred, as distinct from abulia or confusion, one of two error patterns must be displayed by the patient. In the first pattern, impairment scores greater than 0 must be present in at least two categories, with one of the scores being greater than 1. In the other error pattern, language representation is inferred if at least three of the four language categories are mildly impaired. Using this quantitative approach, we have examined both absolute language representation, in which language impairment was either present or absent in each hemisphere independently of the presence of language in the other hemisphere, and a relative language classification, in which a patient with bilateral language could be considered either left or right cerebral language dominant despite the presence of contralateral language function if greater language impairment was observed following a single injection.

To determine language laterality, we sum the language ratings for each patient and compute laterality ratios (i.e., $L - R/L + R$). With this formula, patients who fail linguistic tasks following left hemisphere injection only receive a language asymmetry score of $+1.0$, and conversely, patients with errors only following right hemisphere injection receive a rating of -1.0. When patients display laterality ratios either greater than .15 or less than $-.15$, the patient is considered to have bilateral language representation without a side of greater language representation. By using this technique, comparisons can be made between using a classification system in which patients were grouped according to the side of greater language impairment (e.g., $L > R$ classified as left) and one in which this patient is considered as simply having bilateral language, since some linguistic impairment was found after each injection.

We investigated language lateralization in 103 patients who were candidates for epilepsy surgery at the time of the evaluation (Loring *et al.*, 1990d). To ensure relative homogeneity in our patient sample, we developed inclusion criteria that required each patient to have bilaterally adequate intracarotid amobarbital studies. In addition, evidence of radiologic lesions in areas other than mesial temporal lobe was an exclusionary criterion. In this patient sample, which is presented in Table 11.1, 79 patients displayed exclusive left hemisphere language representation, two patients displayed exclusive right hemisphere language representation, and 22 patients displayed language representation to some degree in each cerebral hemisphere. In patients with evidence of bilateral language, three patterns of language asymmetries were discernable. Seventeen of 22 (77%) displayed asymmetric language representation by the above criteria (13 $L > R$, 4 $R > L$). No relative language dominance ($L = R$) was present in the remaining five patients.

Over the entire patient sample, 80% of right-handed patients had exclusive left hemisphere language representation, 19% had bilateral language, and only a single patient (1%) had language impairment following only the right hemisphere injection. Of the 12 nondextral patients, six had exclusive left hemisphere language, one had exclusive right hemisphere language, and five displayed bilateral language representation. When relative dominance was examined, 91% of the dextral patients were left cerebral language dominant, 4% were right cerebral language dominant, and 4% displayed mixed cerebral language dominance (one each in the latter two categories). Of the 12 nondextral patients, nine were left cerebral language dominant, two were right cerebral language dominant, and one patient displayed mixed language.

These data provide evidence that exclusive right hemisphere cerebral language dominance with no left cerebral language representation occurs rarely. A single dextral patient with no evidence of early injury displayed exclusive right cerebral language in this patient series. In addition, in our nondextral group, only one patient displayed exclusive right hemisphere language, and his seizures began at age 3, which raises the possibility of early brain injury. Across our entire patient series, 21% of the patients had bilateral cerebral language representation, and only 2% displayed exclusive right hemisphere language.

Our Wada data also are consistent with the doctrine that left- or mixed-handedness is a marker of mixed cerebral language dominance. For example, among nondextral patients, right cerebral language dominance has been estimated to be as high as 40% (Roberts, 1969). In an autopsy study, Gloning (1977) examined the incidence of aphasia in patients with structural lesions and found that 80% of dextral

TABLE 11.1.   Incidence of Language Representation
from the Loring et al. (1990b) Patient Series
for Both Exclusive Representation
and Relative Dominance Criteria ($n = 103$)

	Left	Bilateral	Right
Exclusive representation	79 (77%)	22 (21%)	2 (2%)
Relative dominance	92 (89%)	5 (5%)	6 (6%)

patients with lesions of the left cerebral hemisphere had some degree of aphasia, whereas no right-handed patients who had right hemisphere lesions had impaired language function. In contrast, the presence of aphasia was approximately 80% in nondextral patients regardless of the side of hemispheric involvement. Bilaterality of language also is suggested by reports of more complete recovery from aphasia in nondextral as compared to dextral patients (Luria, 1979). In our patient series, the proportion of nondextrals was significantly higher in mixed and right cerebral language dominant patients than in the exclusive left hemisphere language representation group.

Our data further suggest that a continuum of language representation exists extending from exclusively left, greater left than right, mixed, greater right than left, to exclusively right. A language laterality continuum from left to right should be predicted given the relationship of handedness to cerebral language dominance. For example, patients commonly are rated in the degrees of handedness on a continuum from strongly dextral, moderately dextral mixed, to moderately sinistral, and strongly sinistral. Thus, one should not expect language laterality to be primarily discrete when handedness is continuous. Consequently, we believe that the previously reported high incidence of right hemisphere speech language dominance likely reflects an artifact of dichotomizing a continuous variable. Our results indicate that when language functioning is not solely under the left cerebral influence for whatever reasons (such as handedness or early brain injury), some degree of bilaterality is the rule rather than the exception.

Although our Wada testing has been validated primarily on patients undergoing left temporal lobectomy, two right-handed patients in this series who presented with bilateral language (one $L > R$, one $R > L$) underwent subsequent right temporal lobectomy. Results of the Wada evaluation revealed a combination of paraphasic errors, impaired comprehension, and counting/sequencing errors that raised the possibility of right cerebral language dominance. Functional cortical mapping at the time of surgery revealed a combination of posterior frontal and/or perisylvian regions that produced speech arrest when they were stimulated electrically by the operating surgeon. Similar results were reported by Rosenbaum, DeToledo, Smith, Kramer, Stanulis, and Kennedy (1989) in patients with right seizure onset and right cerebral language dominance. Further, formal language assessment was conducted in one of our patients during the initial week following surgery, and significant paraphasic responses were noted (Loring, Meador, Lee, Flanigin, King, & Smith, 1990c). These reports illustrate that language dominance should be established in all patients who are candidates for epilepsy surgery, even if they are right-handed and their seizures originate from the right temporal lobe.

MEMORY TESTING

Temporal lobe structures are thought to be important in the acquisition and consolidation of new material into memory. The well-known patient H.M. became amnestic following bitemporal resection that included hippocampus. In addition, patients undergoing unilateral temporal lobectomy are felt to be at risk for postsurgical amnesia if sufficient hippocampal dysfunction is present contralateral to the temporal lobectomy. In most cases, removal of the anterior hippocampus during temporal lobectomy poses no significant risk to memory function because the hippocampus is moderately to severely gliotic and is consequently dysfunctional. Therefore, recent memory function may be assumed by other brain structures, although memory performance is not necessarily at the level that one would expect without the presence of the hippocampal lesion. A serious memory impairment may be created following unilateral temporal lobectomy, however, if there is significant hippocampal dysfunction contralateral to surgery. After observing severe memory impairment in two patients following unilateral temporal lobectomy, Penfield and Milner (1958) postulated that occult contralateral dysfunction was present. This postulation was confirmed by Penfield and Mathieson (1974), who reported that at autopsy one of these patients had extensive atrophy of the nonresected hippocampus. Consequently, the ability to predict patients with significant contralateral dysfunction became an important goal of the preoperative evaluation for temporal lobectomy.

The Wada test has evolved into the primary procedure used by many centers to identify patients thought to be at risk for postsurgical amnesia. The rationale underlying memory testing during the period of hemispheric anesthesia is that the injection creates a state of temporary dysfunction ipsilateral to the side of surgery that models the effects of surgery on recent memory. If the patient is unable to remember a sufficient number of stimulus items presented to him or her, the patient is felt to be at risk for postsurgical anterograde amnesia. Depending on the philosophical orientation of the center performing the assessment, the patient may either be rejected for surgery or undergo a more limited resection that excludes hippocampus. Because there have been no reports of significant memory failure after inclusion of the memory component into this procedure by the Montreal Neurological Institute, it has been adopted widely and is an accepted practice in the preoperative workup for epilepsy surgery.

However, the clinical constraints placed on Wada memory testing have prevented this technique from being adequately validated. Since memory data from the Wada procedure are used to determine surgical candidacy for hippocampal resection, the dependent variable is confounded with the predictor variable requiring validation. Without performing a consecutive series of patients on whom a decision to involve hippocampus is not based on the Wada, one cannot determine the statistical or predictive efficacy of this procedure for identifying risk for postresection amnesia. Even though there may have been no cases of amnesia after implementation of this technique, causal linkage cannot be inferred. This is analogous to saying that since nuclear weapons have not been used in war since the Dodgers moved from Brooklyn to Los Angeles, then having the Dodgers in California prevents nuclear war. Rival explanations that are equally able to account for the absence of postresection amnesia include advancements in preoperative patient evaluation such as intracranial depth electrode implantation, more sophisticated neuropsychological assessment, and brain-imaging techniques including CT and MR scanning. These methods can better define the areas of seizure onset and lateralized dysfunction and, therefore, are also used to exclude inappropriate surgical candidates.

A more direct approach examining the sensitivity of Wada memory testing to contralateral hippocampal dysfunction is to evaluate memory performance when the perfused hemisphere is contralateral to the seizure focus. If Wada memory testing is sensitive to temporal lobe dysfunction contralateral to surgery, memory impairment should occur reliably following injection contralateral to the seizure focus, since resection of the contralateral temporal lobe would create a state of bilateral dysfunction and, presumably, anterograde amnesia. However, Rausch, Babb, Engel, and Crandall (1989) reported that 11 of 30 patients displayed adequate memory test following injection contralateral to the lesion and eventual resection. Similarly, Jones-Gotman (1987) reported a passing rate at the Montreal Neurological Institute of 59% after injection contralateral to a clear unilateral seizure onset. Thus, one might conclude from these reports that temporal lobectomy could even have been performed on the wrong side (contralateral to the seizures) without concern for the creation of a postresection amnesia. This high rate of passing following injection contralateral to known dysfunction raises concern regarding the technique's sensitivity to "occult" hippocampal dysfunction contralateral to a primary seizure focus.

In contrast to some epilepsy surgery institutions, our center employs multiple measures to evaluate the functional capacity of the contralateral temporal lobe to sustain memory function (see Chapter 13, this volume). In patients who require intracranial depth electrode placement to accurately identify seizure onset, we may assess hippocampal function during low-level electrical stimulation of the mesial temporal lobe with simultaneous memory testing (Lee, Loring, Smith, & Flanigin, 1990; Loring, Lee, Flanigin, Meador, Smith, Gallagher, & King, 1989). Decreases in memory during stimulation ipsilateral to the proposed surgery are believed to be indicative of potential risk to recent memory. In addition, localized intraoperative hippocampal cooling may be performed if there is residual concern regarding possible postsurgical anterograde amnesia at the time of resection. In these patients, we assess memory performance following thermal inactivation in mesial temporal lobe structures (Flanigin, Schlosberg, Power, & Smith, 1985), and if a significant decline in performance is observed, the hippocampus is not included in the resection. Consequently, with the availability of these additional techniques, the patient potentially is offered two additional chances to demonstrate adequate memory by the temporal lobe contralateral to the surgery.

At MCG, we present the stimuli to be remembered at two discrete times during the procedure (Loring *et al.*, 1990a). To assess early item memory, we present eight common objects (e.g., sea shell, battery) for approximately 4 s each. The object names are repeated twice to the patient, and the patient's eyes are held open as necessary to ensure that the items are presented to the visual field ipsilateral to the hemisphere injected.

After language function has minimally resumed, either by demonstration of spontaneous verbal output or by the ability to execute simple commands, we present additional memory items. The two real objects that are used to assess confrontation naming for language also serve as two memory items. Memory for the nursery rhyme used to assess repetition is obtained. In addition, two visual discrimination items are used to assess nonverbal memory.

After the effects of the medication have worn off, which we define as full return of strength including absence of pronator drift and bradykinesia, normal repetition of the phrase "no if's, and's, or but's," and the ability to execute two-stage commands involving inverted syntax, recognition memory of both the early and late memory items is obtained. Early object memory consists of presentation of the eight target items with 16 randomly interspersed foils. To correct for response bias and guessing, correction scores are obtained by subtracting one-half the incorrect false-positive responses from the total of correct responses. To assess late item memory, the names of five objects are read to the patient if the patient is unable spontaneously to recall the two naming objects. Similarly, if unable spontaneously to remember the nursery rhyme, four nursery rhymes are read to the patient in a recognition format. Multiple-choice recognition assessment is obtained for the two designs with the two targets interspersed with four foils. Again, a correction factor is incorporated.

From our patients who have returned for at least one-year neuropsychological follow-up assessment, we identified 13 patients who failed either their early (i.e., stimuli presented soon after injection) or late (i.e., stimuli presented after minimal return of language) components of our Wada memory testing (Loring, Lee, Meador, Flanigin, Figueroa, & Martin, 1990a). Our failure criterion for the early objects was corrected recognition scores ≤2. Because there were fewer late objects, a corrected recognition score lower than 2 was our failure criterion. Eight of these patients failed the early object recognition but performed sufficiently well on our other measures to include the anterior hippocampus. Six patients failed the late object recognition (four patients from the series failed both early and late components). Not only did these patients fail to develop a serious anterograde amnesia, most of these patients stayed at the same clinical level of performance or displayed some improvement. The hippocampus was spared in the remaining three patients.

The neuropsychological memory tests included the Selective Reminding Test (Buschke & Fuld, 1974), Serial Digit Learning (Hamsher, Benton, & Digre, 1980), a local version of the Rey–Osterrieth Complex Figure (Loring, Meador, Martin, & Lee, 1990b), and Form Sequence Learning (Hamsher, Roberts, & Benton, 1983). No patient displayed a decline on all four memory tasks compared with preoperative levels. On the continuous long-term retrieval score from the Selective Reminding Test, preoperative performance levels by this group of 10 patients was 71.5/144, and postoperative levels were 74.2/144. Preoperative Serial Digit Learning was 14.1/24, and postoperative performance was 16.4/24. Preoperative Complex Figure at 30-min delay performance was 13.4/36, and postoperative CF delay was 18.7/36. Preoperative Form Sequence Learning was 9.5/20, and postoperative performance was 11.9/20. These results indicate that many patients who fail either their early or late components of Wada memory testing may undergo standard temporal lobectomy including anterior hippocampus without the development of a serious anterograde memory deficit.

Data from other surgery centers also indicate that Wada memory failure does not necessarily indicate risk for postoperative amnesia. Novelly and Williamson (1989) repeated Wada memory assessment in 25 patients employing a lower medication dosage. On the repeat evaluation, 21/25 patients obtained a passing score, and these 21 patients underwent temporal lobectomy without development of postsurgical amnesia. Thus, both Novelly and Williamson's and our report indicate the potential for a high degree of false-positive identification for patients at risk for amnesia when Wada memory results are employed.

Girvin, McGlone, McLachlan, and Blume (1987) described three patients who failed the Wada memory test but underwent standard temporal lobectomy by virtue of other clinical variables. The patients had bitemporal EEG abnormalities and displayed verbal and nonverbal memory deficits with borderline to mildly mental retarded IQ levels. Further, MR scans revealed left structural temporal lesions in two of these patients. Anterior hippocampus was resected in all patients without the development of postoperative amnesia.

The timing of stimulus presentation of the material to be remembered is potentially an important variable. If items are presented immediately following injection, the maximal anesthetic effects are present, and, to the degree that the hippocampus is affected by the injection, it is most similar to the state that will be created following surgery. However, presenting objects this soon following injection maximizes the medication effects on other cognitive variables. For example, patients may be aphasic for several minutes, akinetic, and abulic. Therefore, the examiner cannot be certain to what degree the items were attended. When items are presented somewhat later during the procedure, a different problem is present. The new danger is that since the medication effects on the other cognitive variables is less, there is similarly less hippocampal anesthesia. Consequently, these items may not be sufficiently sensitive to certain patients because of reduced medication effects on mesial temporal lobe function. In our report examining postoperative performance in patients failing either the early or late memory items, there was a lack of correspondence between those measures when patients were examined on an individual basis.

In addition to our uncertainty regarding the sensitivity and validity of the Wada test in regard to mesial temporal lobe function, interpretation of Wada memory results can be complicated by inattentiveness, confusion, emotional lability, as well as strong perseverative tendencies (Lee, Loring, Meador, Flanigin, & Brooks, 1988; Lee, Loring, Meador, & Brooks, 1990; Huh, Meador, Loring, Lee, Brooks, & Feldman, 1989). Further, since the anatomic region of primary interest (hippocampal formation) obtains its blood supply from both the internal carotid and posterior cerebral systems, it is not known to what degree the hippocampus is affected in each patient tested. Milner (1975) stated that filling of the posterior artery is not a prerequisite for obtaining memory loss. Consequently, the Wada memory test may primarily assess the competency of the neocortical contribution to recent memory systems.

McGlone and MacDonald (1989) examined differences in pass–fail memory ratings on repeat injection. They found that rating changes frequently were associated with identifiable external factors, such as technically unsatisfactory studies, emotional responsivity, or even failing to wear eyeglasses. Thus, for many reasons, patients may fail Wada memory testing because of factors not directly related to the capacity of the contralateral mesial temporal lobe to sustain memory (see Loring, Lee, Meador, and King, 1991; Loring, Meador, Lee, and King, 1992).

RECOMMENDATIONS

When we observe a strong recognition performance asymmetry (e.g., five or more early objects when injection ipsilateral to seizure onset and two or fewer with contralateral injection), as would be predicted based on an established seizure onset, we conclude that a serious anterograde amnesia will not be produced by including hippocampus in the resection, and our ancillary memory tests are not performed. However, confirming low-risk patients is a different proposition than identifying patients at risk.

When poor memory is obtained following injection ipsilateral to the proposed temporal lobectomy, several options are available depending on the philosophy of the surgical institution in which the patient is being evaluated. The patient may be denied surgery, although this may exclude many candidates who can benefit from surgery. The patients may also undergo resection of the temporal tip, which includes the amygdala but spares hippocampus. However, this may decrease the surgical efficacy regarding seizure control. Some institutions repeat the Wada memory test at the same or lower dose, and if satisfactory performance is obtained on the second assessment, then a standard temporal lobectomy can be performed.

At our institution, we employ a combination of preoperative depth electrode stimulation memory testing and thermal cooling in certain cases. However, more recently, we have begun repeating the Wada memory test. With these approaches, the patient is offered an additional opportunity to demonstrate adequate memory function. Despite poor amobarbital memory performance, if there is sufficient evidence suggesting lateralized temporal lobe pathology (i.e., strictly unilateral seizure onset, presence of a structural lesion by CT/MRI scan, consistent asymmetry of functional measures including limbic evoked potentials, SPECT, PET, and neuropsychological testing), temporal lobectomy including hippocampus may be considered in certain cases, and the Wada memory test discounted. We suggest that Wada memory results not be considered as absolute and be interpreted within the entire clinical context of the preoperative epilepsy surgical evaluation.

ACKNOWLEDGMENTS. We thank Patricia Downs for her assistance in manuscript preparation. We are grateful to our patients who have undergone at times tedious evaluation, including Wada testing, for the chance to manage their intractable seizures.

REFERENCES

Branch, C., Milner, B., & Rasmussen, T. (1964). Intracarotid sodium Amytal for the lateralization of cerebral speech dominance: Observations in 123 patients. *Journal of Neurosurgery, 21*, 399–405.

Buschke, H., & Fuld, P. A. (1974). Evaluating storage, retention, and retrieval in disordered memory and learning. *Neurology, 24*, 1019–1025.

Flanigin, H. F., Schlosberg, A., Power, J., & Smith, J. (1985). Evaluation of memory by localized intraoperative cooling. *Epilepsia, 26*, 543.

Girvin, J. P., McGlone, J., McLachlan, R. S., & Blume, W. T. (1987). Validity of the sodium amobarbital test for memory in selected patients. *Epilepsia, 28*, 636.

Gloning, K. (1977). Handedness and aphasia. *Neuropsychologia, 15*, 355–358.

Hamsher, K. deS., Benton, A. L., & Digre, K. (1980). Serial digit learning: Normative and clinical aspects. *Journal of Clinical Neuropsychology, 2*, 39–50.

Hamsher, K. deS., Roberts, R., & Benton, A. L. (1983). *Form sequence learning*. Unpublished report, Department of Neurology, University of Wisconsin Medical School, Milwaukee Clinical Campus, Milwaukee, Wisconsin.

Hommes, O. R., & Panhuysen, L. H. H. M. (1970). Bilateral intracarotid Amytal injection: A study of dysphasia, disturbance of consciousness and paresis. *Psychiatria, Neurologia, Neurochirurgia, 73*, 447–459.

Huh, K., Meador, K. J., Loring, D. W., Lee, G. P., Brooks, B., & Feldman, D. S. (1989). Attentional mechanisms during the intracarotid amobarbital test. *Neurology, 39*, 1183–1186.

Jones-Gotman, M. (1987). Commentary: Psychological evaluation—testing hippocampal function. In J. Engel, Jr. (Ed.), *Surgical treatment of the epilepsies* (pp. 203–211). New York: Raven Press.

Jones-Gotman, M. (1990, June). Relations of postoperative memory changes to the sodium Amytal test: Results of empirical studies. Panel discussion presented at the Second International Cleveland Clinic Epilepsy Symposium, Cleveland, Ohio.

Lee, G. P., Loring, D. W., Meador, K. J., Flanigin, H. F., & Brooks, B. B. (1988). Severe behavioral complications following intracarotid sodium amobarbital injection: Implications for hemispheric asymmetry of emotion. *Neurology, 38*, 1233–1236.

Lee, G. P., Loring, D. W., Meador, K. J., & Brooks, B. B. (1990). Hemispheric specialization for emotional expression: A reexamination of results from intracarotid administration of sodium amobarbital. *Brain and Cognition, 12*, 267–280.

Lee, G. P., Loring, D. W., Smith, J. R., & Flanigin, H. F. (1990). Material specific learning during electrical stimulation of the human hippocampus. *Cortex, 26*, 433–442.

Loring, D. W., Lee, G. P., Flanigin, H. F., Meador, K. J., Smith, J. R., Gallagher, B. B., & King, D. W. (1989). Verbal memory performance following unilateral electrical stimulation of the human hippocampus. *Journal of Epilepsy, 1*, 79–85.

Loring, D. W., Lee, G. P., Meador, K. J., Flanigin, H. F., Smith, J. R., Figueroa, R. E., & Martin, R. C. (1990a). The intracarotid amobarbital procedure as a predictor of memory failure following unilateral temporal lobectomy. *Neurology, 40*, 605–610.

Loring, D. W., Martin, R. C., Meador, K. J., & Lee, G. P. (1990b). Psychometric construction of the Rey–Osterrieth Complex Figure: Methodological considerations and interrater reliability. *Archives of Clinical Neuropsychology, 5*, 1–14.

Loring, D. W., Meador, K. J., Lee, G. P., Flanigin, H. F., King, D. W., & Smith, J. R. (1990c). Crossed aphasia in a patient with complex partial seizures: Evidence from intracarotid sodium amytal testing, functional cortical mapping, and neuropsychological assessment. *Journal of Clinical and Experimental Neuropsychology, 12*, 340–354.

Loring, D. W., Meador, K.J., Lee, G. P., Murro, A. M., Flanigin, H. F., Smith, J. R., Gallagher, B. B., & King, D. W. (1990d). Cerebral language lateralization: Evidence from intracarotid amobarbital testing. *Neuropsychologia, 28*, 831–838.

Loring, D. W., Lee, G. P., Meador, K. J., and King, D. W. (1991). Controversies in epileptology: Does memory assessment during amobarbital testing predict post-surgical amnesia? *Journal of Epilepsy, 4*, 19–24.

Loring, D. W., Meador, K. J., Lee, G. P., & King, D. W. (1992). *Amobarbital effects and lateralized brain function: The Wada test*. New York: Springer-Verlag.

Luria, A. R. (1979). *Traumatic aphasia*. The Hague: Mouton.

McGlone, J., & MacDonald, B. H. (1989). Reliability of the sodium amobarbital test for memory. *Journal of Epilepsy*, *2*, 31–39.

Milner, B. (1975). Psychological aspects of focal epilepsy and its neurosurgical management. In D. Purpura, J. Penry, & R. Walter (Eds.), *Advances in neurology: Vol. 8, Neurosurgical management of the epilepsies* (pp. 299–321). New York: Raven Press.

Novelly, R. A., & Williamson, P. D. (1989). Incidence of false-positive memory impairment in the intracarotid Amytal procedure. *Epilepsia*, *30*, 711.

Oxbury, S. M., & Oxbury, J. M. (1984). Intracarotid amytal test in the assessment of language dominance. In F. C. Rose (Ed.), *Advances in neurology: Vol. 42. Progress in aphasiology*, (pp. 115–123). New York: Raven Press.

Penfield, W., & Milner, B. (1958). Memory deficit produced by bilateral lesions in the hippocampal zone. *Archives of Neurology and Psychiatry*, *79*, 475–497.

Penfield, W., & Mathieson, G. (1974). Memory: Autopsy findings and comments on the role of the hippocampus in experimental recall. *Archives of Neurology*, *31*, 145–154.

Rasmussen, T., & Milner, B. (1977). The role of early left-brain injury in determining lateralization of cerebral speech functions. *Annals of the New York Academy of Science*, *299*, 355–369.

Rausch, R., Babb, T. L., Engel, J., & Crandall, P. H. (1989). Memory following intracarotid amobarbital injection contralateral to hippocampal damage. *Archives of Neurology*, *46*, 783–788.

Roberts, L. (1969). Aphasia, apraxia and agnosia in abnormal states of cerebral dominance. In P. J. Vinken & G. W. Bruyn (Eds.), *Handbook of clinical neurology: Vol. 4* (pp. 312–326). Amsterdam: North Holland.

Rosenbaum, T., DeToledo, J., Smith, D. B., Kramer, R. E., Stanulis, R. G., & Kennedy, R. M. (1989). Preoperative assessment of language laterality is necessary in all epilepsy surgery candidates: A case report. *Epilepsia*, *30*, 712.

Snyder, P. J., Novelly, R. A., & Harris, L. J. (1990). Mixed speech dominance in the intracarotid sodium Amytal procedure: Validity and criteria issues. *Journal of Clinical and Experimental Neuropsychology*, *12*, 629–643.

Wada, J. (1949). [A new method of determining the side of cerebral speech dominance. A preliminary report on the intracarotid injection of sodium Amytal in man]. *Igaku to Seibutsugaki*, *14*, 221–222. (In Japanese).

Wada, J., & Rasmussen, T. (1960). Intracarotid injection of sodium Amytal for the lateralization of cerebral speech dominance: Experimental and clinical observations. *Journal of Neurosurgery*, *17*, 266–282.

Woods, R. P., Dodrill, C. B., & Ojemann, G. A. (1988). Brain injury, handedness, and speech lateralization in a series of amobarbital studies. *Annals of Neurology*, *23*, 510–518.

12

Functional Hippocampal Assessment with Depth Electrodes

DAVID W. LORING, KIMFORD J. MEADOR, and GREGORY P. LEE

Mesial temporal lobe (MTL) structures, from which seizures commonly originate, are crucial for acquisition of new material into memory. The reason for this relationship is unknown but may be related to the tissue excitability necessary for memory encoding. For information to be encoded into memory and the recent memory systems (i.e., episodic memory) to be constantly updated, a system with sufficient sensitivity and constant, active processing of the environment is necessary to allow continual information updating. However, a balance between the sensitivity and stability of functionally connected cell assemblies is also required (Freeman, 1975). As neurons become excited by background input, the neural gain increases, driving the neurons to an operating point closer to their firing threshold; subsequent input is more likely to trigger a response. However, as sensitivity increases, there is a concomitant increase in instability. Thus, the requirement for a memory system to possess the ability to rapidly lay down memory traces makes it less stable and perhaps predisposed to develop seizures.

When hippocampal tissue is dysfunctional, recent memory systems may be assumed by other brain structures, although memory function may not be at the level expected without temporal lobe pathology. Surgical resection of hippocampus and

DAVID W. LORING • Section of Behavioral Neurology, Department of Neurology, Medical College of Georgia, Augusta, Georgia 30912–3275.   KIMFORD J. MEADOR • Section of Behavioral Neurology, Department of Neurology, Medical College of Georgia, Augusta, Georgia 30912–3200. GREGORY P. LEE • Department of Psychiatry, and Section of Neurosurgery, Department of Surgery, Medical College of Georgia, Augusta, Georgia 30912–4010.

The Neuropsychology of Epilepsy, edited by Thomas L. Bennett. Plenum Press, New York, 1992.

surrounding tissue, therefore, may not produce a significant loss of memory function. However, significant memory impairment may be present following unilateral temporal lobectomy if contralateral mesial temporal dysfunction is present. For example, a patient who became amnestic following unilateral left temporal lobectomy was shown to have extensive atrophy of the right hippocampus at autopsy (Penfield & Mathieson, 1974). Quality of life is not improved by eliminating seizures if a significant residual memory impairment is created.

The ability to identify individuals with significant mesial temporal lobe damage contralateral to the proposed resection remains a principal aspect of the preoperative evaluation of candidates for temporal lobectomy. Final therapeutic decisions for surgical resection are made not only on the basis of epileptic excitability studies but also on measures of focal functional deficits (Engel, Rausch, Leib, Kuhl, & Crandall, 1981).

In this chapter, we review several measures of functional hippocampal integrity that were developed as an adjunct to the Medical College of Georgia Epilepsy Surgery Program. Although these measures differ substantially from each other, they share the common goal of measuring the ability of the temporal lobe contralateral to the proposed resection to sustain memory. If all measures indicate that a patient is at risk for the development of a postsurgical amnestic syndrome, either the patient may be excluded from surgery or a less extensive resection may be performed that spares hippocampus. The functional measures include electrical stimulation of hippocampus during memory testing and evoked potential recording from hippocampus. If memory is significantly disrupted during unilateral hippocampal stimulation, and no afterdischarge develops, we assume that the hippocampus stimulated is contributing to recent memory systems. Similarly, if we observe a large cognitive evoked potential recorded from the hippocampus that displays a polarity inversion across levels of the hippocampus, we also infer that this region is contributing significantly to hippocampal function and, by extension, to recent memory.

FUNCTIONAL HIPPOCAMPAL ASSESSMENT

Intracarotid Sodium Amobarbital Testing

The intracarotid sodium amobarbital (ISA) procedure, introduced by Wada in 1949, is an integral part of the preoperative evaluation of seizure surgery candidates and is primarily designed to assess language dominance. The procedure involves injection of 100–200 mg sodium amobarbital via a catheter placed in the femoral artery into a single internal carotid artery, which pharmacologically inactivates the distribution of the anterior and middle cerebral arteries for several minutes while the patient is presented with multiple cognitive tasks.

The ISA procedure has evolved into the primary technique that most centers use to predict whether the hemisphere contralateral to a unilateral seizure focus is capable of sustaining memory function following temporal lobectomy (e.g., Jones-Gotman, 1987). During the period of hemispheric anesthesia, the contribution of the nonanesthetized regions can be estimated. Several assumptions are required for memory assessment during ISA: (1) mesial temporal lobe regions are critical for the acquisition of new material into memory, (2) inactivation of one temporal region is not in itself capable of producing a generalized anterograde memory defect, only a material-specific memory deficit, and (3) if a preexisting lesion contralateral to the injection exists, an amnesia for the memory items presented during ISA inactivation will have been produced by the temporary bilateral MTL dysfunction.

There are, unfortunately, several limitations to this procedure. Interpretation of performance may be complicated by inattentiveness, mental confusion, emotional lability, and strong perseverative tendencies (Lee, Loring, Meador, Flanigan, & Brooks, 1988; Loring, Meador, Sherman, King, & Gallagher, 1987). Memory performance may be affected by impairment of "supportive" cognitive functions necessary for the formation of new memories. For example, aphasia associated with dominant hemisphere injection may confound interpretation of recent memory performance. Testing memory for many types of material is not feasible because of the medical risk associated with repeated injections. Further, since the hippocampal formation obtains its blood supply from both the internal carotid, via the anterior choroidal, and the posterior cerebral arteries, it remains unknown to what degree the hippocampus is affected in each patient tested. The ISA procedure may primarily test the competency of the neocortical contribution to recent memory acquisition.

Depth Electrode Studies

In patients who require depth electrode placement to accurately identify seizure onset, the contribution of a single hippocampus to memory function can be partially determined by low-level electrical stimulation of mesial temporal lobe structures during memory performance. Depth electrodes are implanted for strictly clinical indications if seizure onset cannot be localized to a single temporal lobe on the basis of scalp and sphenoidal recordings. Electrical stimulation using depth electrodes temporarily disrupts the neural function of the mesial temporal lobe. Consequently, memory assessment during hippocampal stimulation allows an estimate to be obtained regarding the capacity of the hippocampus contralateral to the proposed surgery to support new learning (Brazier, 1966; Chapman, Walter, Markham, Rand, & Crandall, 1967; Sem-Jacobson, 1968; Halgren, Walter, Cherlow, & Crandall, 1978; Loring, Lee, Flanigin, Meador, Smith, Gallagher, & King, 1988a). Hippocampal stimulation during memory performance is potentially superior to the ISA procedure because it eliminates confounding factors resulting from disruption of other cognitive functions inherent in anesthetizing multiple cortical regions.

Early Studies

In a systematic series of studies, Halgren and his colleagues examined memory during electrical stimulation of multiple mesial temporal structures in epilepsy surgery candidates. Simultaneous bilateral stimulation of amygdala, hippocampus, and parahippocampal gyrus sufficient to cause afterdischarge (AD) was initially found to produce amnesia in some patients (Halgren *et al.*, 1978). In the majority of patients (29/36), however, no effect on memory function was observed. In a subsequent study, mesial temporal lobe stimulation accompanied by an AD resulted in a specific deficit in recall of paired associates involving image-mediated words (baseline = 70%, stimulation = 14%) without producing an effect on immediate attention and concentration ability (Halgren & Wilson, 1985). Stimulation below AD threshold resulted in no significant memory impairment (stimulation = 61%). In a third report, however, these authors demonstrated that sub-AD stimulation is capable of disrupting recent memory (Halgren, Wilson, & Stapleton, 1985). Stimulation by a single electrical pulse, synchronized with presentation or recognition of complex visual scenes, resulted in decreased memory performance.

The studies by Halgren demonstrate the efficacy of hippocampal stimulation in disrupting recent memory systems. Nevertheless, the paradigms employed are not commonly used, making it difficult to extrapolate to more standard tests of memory. Given the reported effects of electrical stimulation below AD discharge threshold, we began to examine whether an alternative technique of electrical hippocampal stimulation below AD threshold that was not time-locked to stimulus presentation or recognition would assist in assessing the contribution of each hippocampus to memory. By having the stimulation ongoing and not time-locked to the material to be presented, it could be applied throughout the administration of more commonly employed tests of recent verbal memory.

We chose to administer a verbal memory test for several reasons. Although material-specific forms of recent memory function are well established (e.g., Milner, 1972), verbal memory plays a more prominent role in daily functioning. Further, patient reports have indicated that risk to verbal memory was of greater concern than risk to visual memory. Finally, verbal memory tests can be constructed to allow parallel forms for repeated assessments and allow minor modification in task complexity so as to minimize both floor and ceiling performance effects. If no complications arise, patients with unilateral left seizure onset can undergo unilateral temporal resection without significant additional loss of recent verbal memory, suggesting that homologous regions of the right hemisphere are performing this function. Consequently, we predicted initially that impairment in verbal memory would be observed in all patients when electrical stimulation was applied to the hippocampus contralateral to seizure onset, thereby creating a state of transient bilateral mesial temporal lobe dysfunction. Thus, in right TLE patients, a verbal memory deficit should be observed with left hippocampal stimulation. If the right hemisphere assumes the verbal memory function in patients with left TLE, then stimulation of the right hippocampus should produce a similar reduction in verbal memory performance.

Electrode Implantation

Depth electrodes were stereotactically implanted via a vertex trajectory with one exception, and this patient received a posterior implantation approach (Flanigan, King, & Gallagher, 1984; Flanigan & Smith, 1987). Two of the four electrodes traversed the anterior hippocampi bilaterally (see Fig. 12.1); the remaining two were implanted into amygdalae. The electrodes were six-strand Teflon-coated stainless steel wires with contacts at the loop tip and at 5 to 10-mm intervals along the trees. Proper positioning is critical for both stimulation and recording studies because slight differences in placement can produce large differences in the tissue from which the recordings/stimulations are made. Positioning was confirmed at the time of surgery using x-ray. Further, a postimplantation CT scan was obtained to verify electrode placement and to rule out hemorrhage. At our institution, the electrodes remain implanted so that EEG recording can be made at the time of surgery to compare with surface electrocorticography. Thus, visual confirmation of electrode placement was made on the side of resection.

Depth Electrode Stimulation

Afterdischarge Threshold

A balanced square-wave stimulus (60 Hz, 1 ms/phase) was delivered using constant-current and stimulus isolation units. Three-second trains were employed to determine afterdischarge threshold, and the current was gradually increased from 0.05 mA until AD threshold was determined. The contacts were 10 mm apart and selected to maximally involve hippocampus. For most patients, the contacts were 1–3 or 2–4 (see Fig. 12.1). We preferred to stimulate 1–3, since this would produce

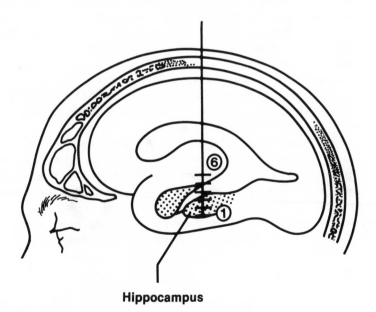

Hippocampus

FIGURE 12.1. Placement of electrodes employing a vertex approach. Note six contact points, with contact 2 being most inferior. (Reproduced with permission of *Annals of Neurology*, Meador *et al.*, 1987.)

greater hippocampal involvement. However, it was sometimes necessary to use contacts 2–4 because stimulation through contact 1 produced a painful irritation of the dura. No other contact pairs were stimulated. Consequently, the electrode sites selected for hippocampal stimulation were based on interpatient variability of contact sites.

Memory Stimulation

The same parameters used to establish AD threshold were used with minor modification. The current was approximately two-thirds of that required to elicit an AD, which was determined on a previous day. However, because AD threshold variability exists over time, the afterdischarge threshold was reestablished prior to memory testing. The level of electrical stimulation was comparable to that required during speech and sensory/motor mapping of the cortex during surgery. The stimulation duration during memory assessment differs from that for AD stimulation. For memory testing, a 7-s train of stimuli, followed by 3 s of no stimulation, was passed between selected contact points separated by 10 mm. In the single patient who received a different electrode implantation approach to record seizure activity that was believed to originate more posteriorly than the typical mesial temporal lobe patient (e.g., electrodes implanted transversely from the occipital region), a 20-mm separation was employed.

In order to protect our patients, we built into our stimulation parameters the means by which ADs could be observed. Although continuous stimulation would produce greater blocking of function, the train sequence of 7 s on and 3 s off was selected so that the ongoing EEG could be monitored to observe possible AD development. Thus, the stimulation trains were designed to disrupt normal activity of the hippocampus during testing without initiating possible recruitment and producing an afterdischarge. If we observed AD development, a smaller amperage was selected. Consequently, ongoing stimulation at or above AD threshold was not inadvertently conducted. The duration of stimulation for each hippocampus for verbal memory was approximately 7–8 min.

This "on/off" interference effect produced by electrical stimulation is analogous to that applied while performing cortical mapping during surgery. During cortical mapping of speech and language zones, the electrical stimulation is applied at selective times while the patient is reciting. Because electrical stimulation during memory testing is ongoing and is not time-locked to the material to be remembered, it can be applied throughout the entire performance of standard memory tests. In the present series of patients (Loring *et al.*, 1988a), the hippocampus contralateral to seizure onset was always stimulated first.

Memory Testing

Verbal memory function was examined using the Brown–Peterson distractor technique. Three words were presented to the patient, and after the patient correctly repeated the words, he or she was asked to count backwards by threes from a different number specified each trial by the examiner. Interpolated distractor intervals of 20–60 s were employed. A problem in memory assessment across a population with impaired memory is that tests aimed at patients with relatively poorer memory are too easy for those patients whose memory is relatively intact. Similarly, tests designed for patients with normal memory are too difficult for the more impaired patients. By varying the distractor length, we could adjust the difficulty of the test to each individual patient. The length of the distractor interval was varied in order to avoid both floor effects, in which the subject could not perform the task, and ceiling effects, in which performance was nearly perfect. We adjusted the length of the distractor interval in 10-s increments to obtain a baseline performance level of approximately 50–75% correct. Three conditions were obtained: (1) baseline, (2) stimulation of hippocampus contralateral to presumed seizure onset, and (3) stimulation of hippocampus ipsilateral to presumed seizure onset.

Performance levels during the baseline and two stimulation conditions in our first series of patients are presented in Table 12.1. A significant main effect for stimulation condition was present ($p < .02$) in addition to a condition-by-group interaction ($p < .004$). We examined the simple main effects of stimulation condition for the left and right seizure-onset groups independently and found no significant stimulation effect in the left-focus patients. In contrast, a significant stimulation effect was present for the right seizure-onset patients ($p < .0005$). A significant effect was also present for the left versus right stimulation condition ($t = 4.34, p < .02$). Left hippocampal stimulation response was significantly impaired relative to base line ($p < .05$). The difference between right stimulation and base line was not significant following the multiple comparison adjustment ($p < .07$).

Electrical stimulation of the left hippocampus interfered with verbal memory performance in patients with demonstrated seizure onset from the right temporal lobe. No significant effect was observed during stimulation in patients with left temporal lobe seizure onset. In addition, our patients with left temporal seizure onset tended to perform more poorly during base line and right hippocampal stimulation than did the right temporal patients.

The effect of left hippocampal stimulation on verbal memory performance is not the result of a confusional state or impaired attentional processing, since stimulation

TABLE 12.1. Means and Standard
Deviations of Hippocampal Stimulation
Memory Performances Expressed
as Percentage Correct

	Left onset	Right onset
Left stimulation	56.4 (13.9)	52.9 (18.0)
Right stimulation	55.6 (13.2)	75.3 (9.6)
Base line	51.8 (15.4)	69.4 (10.4)

was always below AD threshold. Further, even in Halgren's patients, stimulation sufficient to produce an AD did not typically elicit a confusional state. Our patients were able to perform the serial subtractions during stimulation at their baseline levels, indicating no appreciable effect on attention and mental tracking ability. In addition, if stimulation produced an attentional impairment, one would not expect to see it selectively impaired only in patients with right temporal seizure onset.

We did not demonstrate selective impairment of memory during right hippo-campal stimulation in patients with left temporal seizure onset. Patients with left temporal seizure onset, who may rely on the right hemisphere for verbal memory, may have a different organization for verbal memory than subjects with healthy left hippocampi. Although the Brown–Peterson procedure appears sensitive to electrical disruption of left hippocampal function in right temporal patients, the test may not adequately reflect processing of the right temporal lobe when required to perform recent verbal memory functions if the right hemisphere is, in fact, performing verbal memory functions. Alternatively, areas surrounding the epileptogenic hippocampus may be contributing to verbal memory, and consequently, left hippocampal stimula-tion would not be expected to have a disruptive effect. This would be analogous to two-stage versus single-stage lesion experiments, the initial lesion being the brain injury with development of the seizure focus, and the second lesion being the temporal lobectomy. Thus, memory function may have shifted more posteriorly to areas of the hippocampus that are not included in the standard anterior temporal lobectomy.

Electrical stimulation of the right hippocampus may have created the condition in which nonspecific effects of right mesial temporal lobe discharges were no longer observed. Thus, the normal interictal discharges of this region that normally exert distal neuronal disruption may have been either suppressed or contained by stimula-tion. Therefore, stimulation may paradoxically exert a positive influence on verbal memory performance through reduction of the typical negative effects of a right temporal seizure focus.

One patient in our series of temporal lobectomy patients at MCG developed increased memory disruption sufficient to prevent her return to work following right temporal lobectomy. Failure to demonstrate decreased verbal memory during left hippocampal stimulation may have alerted us to the need for additional assessment procedures or a less extensive resection. Unfortunately, she was evaluated before we initiated the hippocampal memory stimulation process. In the patients who have undergone hippocampal stimulation memory testing, the single right-focus patient failing to show at least a 10% reduction of verbal memory during left hippocampal stimulation received a resection of only the temporal tip, and the hippocampus was spared.

These data suggest that low-level electrical stimulation of the hippocampus is capable of producing a verbal memory deficit in patients with right temporal lobe seizure onset. In this capacity, hippocampal stimulation is useful to aid in the localization of seizure onset by demonstrating selective memory impairment in patients with right temporal seizure onset. Further, in the right temporal seizure group, we can infer that no significant reduction in memory function will be present following resection of the right temporal lobe including anterior hippocampus (i.e., memory impairment was present only during left hippocampal stimulation).

We have begun to study visual spatial memory in addition to verbal memory during depth electrode stimulation. In this preliminary series, visual spatial memory was mildly decreased in right seizure patients during right hippocampal stimulation, but no decrease was present in right seizure patients during left hippocampal stimulation. In contrast, visual spatial memory decreased during stimulation of either temporal region in patients with left seizure onset.

Limbic Evoked Potentials

An additional technique of functional hippocampal assessment is to measure evoked potential (EP) activity. The EP is a characteristic shift in electrical fields produced by synchronous brain activity. Evoked potentials are obtained by time-locking the ongoing EEG to a stimulus over repeated trials. For scalp-recorded EPs, a late positive component occurring approximately 300 ms post-stimulus has received the greatest attention by psychologists. The P300 (or P3) is believed to reflect diverse psychological correlates such as expectation, selective attention, motivation, decision making, and orientation to novel stimuli (Pritchard, 1981). The P300, reflecting cognitive processing, is relatively independent of stimulus parameters (e.g., Papanicolaou, Loring, Raz, & Eisenberg, 1985).

The P300 is typically obtained within the context of the "odd-ball" paradigm in which the subject is exposed to two stimuli (e.g., tones) differing on one physical parameter (e.g., frequency). One stimulus occurs predictably with a high probability, and the other occurs infrequently and randomly. The subject's task is to count the number of rare-tone occurrences. The EP to the rare stimulus (i.e., target) is characterized by a negative and positive peak that are absent or greatly reduced compared to the frequent-tone (i.e., nontarget) EP.

Limbic evoked potentials (LEPs) have been reported to occur in the human hippocampus (e.g., Halgren, Squires, Wilson, Rorbaugh, Babb, & Crandall, 1981; Wood, McCarthy, Squires, Vaughn, Woods, & McCallum, 1984; Meador, Loring, King, Gallagher, Gould, & Flanigan, 1987a; Meador, Loring, King, Gallagher, Smith, & Flanigan, 1987b). The LEPs are large-amplitude, time-locked electric field changes recorded from the hippocampus. Limbic EPs are elicited using the same odd-ball stimulation paradigm used to record P300. Thus, the subject listens to a train of auditory tones and counts the number of rare, unpredictable stimuli. The LEPs to the rare target stimuli are characterized by a large-amplitude polarity-inverting wave. These potentials are believed to originate from hippocampal structures because of the polarity inversion across this region, suggesting a local generator.

Since they reflect local neuronal processing, LEPs may be reduced in the temporal lobe corresponding to the seizure onset. Squires, Halgren, Wilson, and Crandall (1983) anecdotally made this observation in a report summarizing both Halgren's initial six patients and six additional depth electrode subjects. From

Halgren's series, Squires *et al.* report a single patient in whom "corresponding to the unambiguous lateralization of the temporal lobe pathology . . ., there was a marked asymmetry in the [LEPs], with essentially no evoked activity seen on the side of the seizure focus. . . . Similar findings were obtained from one subject in the second series. . ." (pp. 223–224). Wood *et al.* (1984) also describe "a tendency for the late endogenous depth potentials to be diminished or less well distributed in the hemisphere in which clinical evaluation has indicated is the site of seizure onset" (p. 709). As support for this description, Squires *et al.* (1983) are cited.

The LEPs were inversely related to the epileptogenic focus, being absent or markedly diminished on the side of the epileptogenic focus and presumed patholog-

Thus, the observation that the LEPs were often absent or greatly attenuated in the hemisphere ipsilateral to seizure onset has been made by two groups (Squires *et al.*, 1983; Wood *et al.*, 1984; Halgren *et al.*, 1982); yet, the strength of this association was not fully studied, and the predictive power of LEP asymmetries is unknown. Our initial series of subjects included seven patients with intractable epilepsy who were undergoing preoperative evaluation for temporal lobectomy (Meador *et al.*, 1987a). On the basis of intracerebral electroencephalographic recordings from bilateral amygdalae and hippocampi, a unilateral temporal lobe seizure onset was found in four patients, bilateral independent temporal lobe seizure onset in two patients, and a non-temporal-lobe seizure onset in one patient.

Limbic EPs were elicited using the odd-ball paradigm described above. Bipolar LEPs were recorded from each hippocampus using progressively ascending pairs of contact points on the hippocampal electrodes (i.e., 1–2, 2–3, 3–4) (see Fig. 12.1). Raters blinded to the side of electrographically proven seizure onset evaluated LEP recordings for the presence of (1) a reproducible, polarity-inverting response, (2) peak-to-peak LEP amplitudes equal to or greater than 25 μV (i.e., from the largest negative to the largest positive deflection), and (3) a peak-to-peak LEP amplitude asymmetry (between the right and left hippocampi) equal to or greater than 50%. Unilaterally absent phase reversals and/or lower-amplitude LEPs were used to predict the side of epileptic ictal focus.

Limbic EPs were obtained to both target and nontarget stimuli but were larger to target stimuli. Well-formed LEPs were characterized by large-amplitude peaks (up to 160 μV peak to peak for targets), usually composed of multiple components. The waveforms were stable over multiple sessions and showed phase reversal in the region of the hippocampus. Limbic EPs were obtained from one or both hippocampi in every patient. On the basis of LEP form and symmetry, raters correctly predicted the side of epileptic focus in all four patients with electrographically proven unilateral focus. In three of the four patients, the LEP on the side of the epileptic focus was absent or markedly decremented as compared to the contralateral LEP. In the fourth patient, LEPs were diminished on the side of seizure onset, but the asymmetry was less marked. Further, LEP amplitudes in two patients with bilateral independent temporal lobe seizure onset were markedly diminished bilaterally. A single patient was found to have a non-temporal-lobe (presumably frontal) seizure onset. In this case, LEPs were well formed, polarity inverting, and high amplitude in both hippocampi.

The LEPs were inversely related to the epileptogenic focus, being absent or markedly diminished on the side of the epileptogenic focus and presumed pathological tissue. Although this association has been noted in sporadic cases, it has not been reported as a consistent finding in a series of patients. The failure of previous studies to discover this association may be related to montage selection. Whereas the present study employed a bipolar montage, prior studies have employed a referential recording system with the individual depth electrode contact points referenced to a distant electrode (e.g., tip of the nose). In general, a bipolar montage will better reflect local electric field changes. Thus, it is possible that the bipolar montage allows better visualization of the local (i.e., medial temporal lobe) potentials. Further, the "indifferent" electrode in a referential montage is not truly inactive. For example, current flow from intracranial sources tends to focus through holes in the skull, thus altering the recorded potential. Additional studies comparing referential and bipolar montages will be necessary to clarify this issue.

An additional problem in the use of LEPs to assess functional hippocampal integrity is the problem of waveform quantification. With standard quantification techniques, there is inherent variability from trial to trial, and at times considerable subjectivity is required during peak identification. Thus, we have begun to quantify our LEPs using spectral analysis of the waveform. Spectral analysis breaks a waveform into its component frequencies and is a measure of the response of the entire system. Thus, spectral power provides a technique to objectively quantify the EP without relying on peak amplitude or latency determination (e.g., Davis & Wada, 1977).

In an independent series of patients with depth electrode implantation, consistently lower spectral power of both low and high bands was recorded in eight patients from the hippocampus associated with electrographically demonstrated unilateral seizure onset as compared to the contralateral side. In this group, the ratio of target LEP spectral power between the "epileptogenic" and "nonepileptogenic" hippocampi averaged 1:3 for whole-band (1–20 Hz) spectral power. This asymmetry was also present on every trial for both low and high components. In contrast, four subjects with bilaterally independent mesial temporal lobe seizure onset demonstrated bilaterally low spectral power with inconsistent left–right power asymmetries. In addition, four subjects with distal or indeterminant seizure foci exhibited high spectral power in both hippocampi. Thus, spectral analysis of LEPs appears useful in the determination of a focal functional deficit and thus in identifying the site of epileptogenic pathology.

Limbic Evoked Potentials and Memory Function

Since patients are at risk for the development of an anterograde memory deficit following unilateral temporal lobe resection, there is an ongoing need for the development of better techniques to predict the relative contribution of each hippocampus to memory mechanisms. Because LEPs appear to be related to local neuronal processing and are decreased ipsilateral to a unilateral seizure onset, they may reflect, in part, the contribution of each hippocampus to memory formation.

To evaluate whether LEPs might be useful as a direct measure of functional hippocampal activity, we examined the relationship between LEPs and neuropsy-chological memory performance (Loring, Meador, King, Gallagher, Smith, & Flanigin, 1988b). Because of protocol variations of the different services providing neuropsychological assessment, patients were administered different tests to assess memory function. To assess verbal memory function, either the Rey Auditory Verbal Learning Test (AVLT) or the Selective Reminding Test (SRT) was administered. For each test, a rating of severity was assigned based on available norms to allow for direct comparisons.

To assess visual spatial memory, either the Visual Retention Test (VRT) or the Rey Complex Figure (CF) was employed. For the VRT, each design was presented for 10 s, and the subject was instructed to draw the design after a delay of 15 s. For the CF, a complex visual spatial form was presented to each subject, and following a copy condition, the subject was asked to draw it from memory. Performance levels were also converted into ratings based on normative tables.

One patient showed well-developed waves bilaterally (Fig. 12.2), five patients showed well-developed waves unilaterally (Fig. 12.3), and two patients had well-formed waves on neither side (Fig. 12.4). The patient with well-developed LEPs had a nontemporal (presumed frontal) seizure onset. All five patients with unilateral LEPs had unilateral seizure onset from the contralateral side. Both patients with bilaterally absent LEPs had bilaterally independent seizure onset. Although our sample size was insufficient to allow statistical treatment of these data, several relationships are suggested. There was no relationship between verbal and nonverbal recent memory function and the side of LEP development. The two patients with bilaterally poorly developed LEPs exhibited the poorest performance on recent memory tests (both verbal and nonverbal). The one patient with bilaterally well-formed LEPs displayed normal verbal and nonverbal memory.

Because they reflect local neuronal processing, LEPs may be a promising

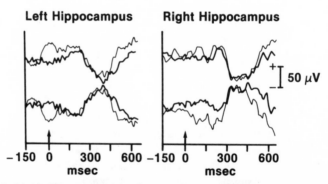

FIGURE 12.2. Limbic EPs to target tones from a patient with bilaterally well-preserved responses. Seizure focus was extratemporal and presumed to be frontal. Repeated trials are superimposed to provide a visual estimate of reproducibility. Arrows indicate stimulus onset. (Reproduced with permission of *Neurology*, Loring *et al.*, 1988.)

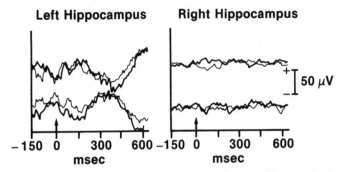

FIGURE 12.3. Limbic EPs to target tones from a patient with electroencephalographically demonstrated right temporal seizure onset. Note presence of polarity-inverting wave recorded from left hippocampus and absence of response in the right hippocampal recordings. (Reproduced with permission of *Neurology*, Loring *et al.*, 1988.)

technique to assess the functional integrity of the hippocampus and its relationship to memory. During evaluation for temporal lobectomy, LEPs have been shown to assist in identifying the temporal lobe from which the seizures are originating. Our data suggest that they may also indicate whether a patient is at risk for postsurgical memory loss. In the one patient with bilaterally well-developed LEPs, both verbal and nonverbal memory function were within normal limits, suggesting that the mesial temporal structures important for memory were intact and functioning well. In the two patients with bilateral poorly developed LEPs, verbal and nonverbal memory were severely impaired, suggesting that bilateral mesial temporal dysfunction resulted in impaired formation of new memories.

No relationship between unilateral LEPs and lateralized neuropsychological memory deficits was observed. One possible explanation is that in these patients with

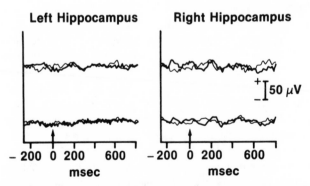

FIGURE 12.4. Limbic EPs to target tones from a patient with bilaterally independent seizure onset. Note absence of polarity-inverting waves from both left and right hippocampi. (Reproduced with permission of *Neurology*, Loring *et al.*, 1988.)

partial complex seizures, temporal lobe dysfunction began in early childhood, thereby allowing a significant functional reorganization. This would diminish the lateralizing power of neuropsychological tests. All patients with unilaterally poor LEPs and contralateral well-developed LEPs had electrographically demonstrated seizure onset ipsilateral to the poorly developed LEPs. All underwent ipsilateral temporal lobectomy, and none developed a postsurgical amnestic state. These data suggest that the contralateral mesial temporal region, which had well-formed LEPs, or the posterior MTL regions not resected supported both verbal and visual–spatial recent memory function.

Identical memory measures were not available for all subjects, unfortunately, thereby necessitating the conversion to ratings based on percentile performance. However, the memory effects appear sufficiently robust. Since the one patient in whom bilateral LEPs were recorded was administered more difficult tests, it appears safe to assume that this subject would have performed at least as well on less difficult tests. Similarly, the two patients with bilaterally absent LEPs received the easier test, suggesting that their performance on the more difficult test would also have been severely impaired.

The potential uses of LEP recordings may include prediction of postoperative memory performance. For example, a unilaterally absent or poorly developed LEP, in conjunction with a contralateral well-developed LEP, suggests little likelihood of postoperative memory deficits when surgery is performed on the side of the decremented LEP. Bilateral poorly developed LEPs may suggest an individual at risk for postsurgical anterograde memory deficits. Finally, bilateral well-preserved waves may also suggest a patient at risk, since both hippocampi may contribute to memory formation, and temporal lobectomy may produce a material-specific (i.e., verbal versus nonverbal) memory deficit.

SUMMARY

Because of the risks to recent memory function associated with unilateral temporal lobectomy, the ability to identify those patients who are poor candidates from a memory/cognitive standpoint remains a primary goal of preoperative neuropsychological assessment. In patients who undergo depth electrode implantation in MTL structures to help identify seizure onset, additional measures can be obtained. The electrodes may also serve as stimulation electrodes. Thus, the contribution of mesial temporal lobe structures to a particular cognitive task (e.g., memory) can be partially measured by determining the degree to which electrical stimulation interferes with performance on that task. Similarly, we can measure the evoked electrical activity of the hippocampus during performance of a simple cognitive task (i.e., counting rare tones) and obtain measures of functional hippocampal integrity from generator sources in that area. Thus, in conjunction with baseline neuropsychological assessment and intracarotid sodium amobarbital testing, memory performance during unilateral electrical hippocampal stimulation and hippocampal LEP recordings may provide a more complete picture of the contribution of each mesial temporal lobe to memory function and thereby identify appropriate candidates for surgery. Examination of the interrelationship between the above variables in larger series of patients will be necessary to determine more precisely the contribution of each measure.

REFERENCES

Brazier, M. A. B. (1966). Stimulation of the hippocampus in man using implanted electrodes. In M. A. B. Brazier (Ed.), *RNA and brain function, memory and learning*. Berkeley: University of California Press.

Chapman, L. G., Walter, R. D., Markham, C. H., Rand, R. W., & Crandall, P. H. (1967). Memory changes induced by stimulation of the hippocampus or amygdala in epilepsy patients with implanted electrodes. *Transactions of the American Neurological Association, 92*, 50–56.

Davis, A., & Wada, J. (1977). Hemispheric asymmetries in human infants: Spectral analysis of flash and click evoked potentials. *Brain and Language, 4*, 23–31.

Engel, J., Jr., Rausch, R., Lieb, J. P., Kuhl, D. E., & Crandall, P. H. (1981). Correlation of criteria used for localizing epileptic foci in patients considered for surgical therapy of epilepsy. *Archives of Neurology, 9*, 215–224.

Flanigin, H. F., & Smith, J. R. (1987). Depth electrode implantation at the Medical College of Georgia. In J. Engel (Ed.), *Surgical treatment of the epilepsies* (pp. 609–612). New York: Raven Press.

Flanigin, H. F., King, D. W., & Gallagher, B. B. (1984). Surgical treatment of epilepsy. In T. Pedley & B. Meldrum (Eds.), *Recent advances in epilepsy, Vol. 2* (pp. 297–339). New York: Churchill-Livingstone.

Freeman, W. Y. (1975). *Mass action in the nervous system*. New York: Academic Press.

Halgren, E., & Wilson, C. L. (1985). Recall deficits produced by afterdischarges in the human hippocampal formation and amygdala. *Electroencephalography and Clinical Neurophysiology, 61*, 375–380.

Halgren, E., Walter, R. D., Cherlow, D. G., & Crandall, P. H. (1978). Mental phenomena evoked by electrical stimulation of the human hippocampal formation and amygdala. *Brain, 101*, 83–117.

Halgren, E., Squires, N. K., Wilson, C. L., Rorbaugh, I. W., Babb, T. L., & Crandall, P. H. (1981). Endogenous potentials generated in the human hippocampal formation by infrequent events. *Science, 210*, 803–805.

Halgren, E., Squires, N. K., Wilson, C. L., & Crandall, P. H. (1982). Brain generators of evoked potentials: The late (endogenous) components. *Bulletin of Los Angeles Neurological Society, 47*, 108–123.

Halgren, E., Wilson, C. L., & Stapleton, J. M. (1985). Human medial temporal-lobe stimulation disrupts both formation and retrieval of recent memories. *Brain and Cognition, 4*, 287–295.

Jones-Gotman, M. (1987). Commentary: Psychological evaluation—testing hippocampal function. In J. Engel (Ed.), *Surgical treatment of the epilepsies* (pp. 203–211). New York: Raven Press.

Lee, G. P., Loring, D. W., Meador, K. J., Flanigan, H. F., & Brooks, B. S. (1988). Severe behavioral complications following intracarotid sodium amobarbital injection: Implications for hemispheric asymmetry of emotion. *Neurology, 38*, 1233–1236.

Loring, D. W., Meador, K. J., Sherman, C. J., King, D.W., & Gallagher, B. B. (1987). Abulia and impaired responsiveness during the intracarotid sodium Amytal procedure. *Journal of Clinical and Experimental Psychology, 9*, 31.

Loring, D. W., Lee, G. P., Flanigin, H. F., Meador, K. J., Smith, J. R., Gallagher, B. B., & King, D. W. (1988a). Verbal memory deficits following unilateral electrical stimulation of the human hippocampus. *Journal of Epilepsy, 1*, 79–85.

Loring, D. W., Meador, K. J., King, D. W., Gallagher, B. B., Smith, J. R., and Flanigin, H. F. (1988b). Relationship of limbic evoked potentials to recent memory performance. *Neurology, 38*, 45–48.

Meador, K. J., Loring, D. W., King, D. W., Gallagher, B. B., Gould, J., & Flanigin, H. F. (1987a). Limbic evoked potentials predict site of epileptic focus. *Neurology, 37,* 494–497.

Meador, K. J., Loring, D. W., King, D. W., Gallagher, B. B., Smith, J. R., & Flanigin, H. F. (1987b). Spectral power of human limbic evoked responses: Relationship to seizure onset. *Annals of Neurology, 22,* 131–132.

Milner, B. (1972). Disorders of learning and memory after temporal lobe lesions in man. *Clinical Neurosurgery, 19,* 421–946.

Papanicolaou, A. C., Loring, D. W., Raz, N., & Eisenberg, H. M. (1985). Relationship between stimulus intensity and the P300. *Psychophysiology, 22,* 326–329.

Penfield, W., & Mathieson, G. (1974). Memory: Autopsy findings and comment on the role of hippocampus in experiential recall. *Archives of Neurology, 31,* 145–154.

Pritchard, W. S. (1981). Psychophysiology of P300. *Psychological Bulletin, 89,* 506–540.

Sem-Jacobsen, C. W. (1968). *Depth electrode stimulation of the human brain and behavior.* Springfield, Ill.: Charles C. Thomas.

Squires, N. K., Halgren, E., Wilson, C., & Crandall, P. (1983). Human-endogenous limbic potentials: Cross-modality and depth/surface comparisons in epileptic subjects. In A. Gaillard & W. Ritter (Eds.), *Tutorials in event related potential research: Endogenous components* (pp. 217–232). New York: North-Holland.

Wood, C., McCarthy, G., Squires, N., Vaughn, H., Woods, D., & McCallum, W. (1984). Anatomical and physiological substrates of event-related potentials. *Annals of the New York Academy of Sciences, 425,* 681–721.

13

Neuropsychological Changes after Anterior Temporal Lobectomy
Acute Effects on Memory, Language, and Music

ANDREW J. SAYKIN, LINDSEY J. ROBINSON,
PAUL STAFINIAK, D. BRIAN KESTER,
RUBEN C. GUR, MICHAEL J. O'CONNOR,
and MICHAEL R. SPERLING

In the first part of this chapter, we present a selective review of neuropsychological changes after anterior temporal lobectomy (ATL). Proposed models for neuropsychological effects of ATL are presented, followed by a review of research on changes in cognitive function, with emphasis on memory and learning, language, and musical processing. Methodological problems that complicate the interpretation of research findings on neuropsychological consequences of surgery are described. In the remainder of this chapter, we present data from a series of recent studies in our laboratory examining changes in memory, language, and musical processing. Patients with medically refractory complex partial seizure disorders who are surgical candidates typically show a mean level of preoperative performance below that of normal control samples. Developmental history, particularly age at first risk factor for

ANDREW J. SAYKIN, LINDSEY J. ROBINSON, PAUL STAFINIAK, D. BRIAN KESTER, and RUBEN C. GUR • Brain Behavior Laboratory, Department of Psychiatry, University of Pennsylvania School of Medicine, Philadelphia, Pennsylvania 19104–4283.   MICHAEL J. O'CONNOR • Division of Neurosurgery, University of Pennsylvania School of Medicine, Philadelphia, Pennsylvania 19104–4283. MICHAEL R. SPERLING • Department of Neurology, University of Pennsylvania School of Medicine, Philadelphia, Pennsylvania 19104–4283.

The Neuropsychology of Epilepsy, edited by Thomas L. Bennett. Plenum Press, New York, 1992.

brain injury and age of onset of seizures, appears to be important for predicting pre- and postoperative neuropsychological function. Before surgery, those with early onset of seizures often have the poorest baseline performance. After surgery, early risk is an important predictor of cognitive outcome. Our finding of less disruption of memory and language 2–3 weeks after surgery in patients with early risks is consistent with the hypothesis that early brain injury is associated with reorganization of function.

NEUROPSYCHOLOGICAL CHANGES AFTER TEMPORAL LOBECTOMY

Anterior temporal lobectomy has become a standard treatment for medically refractory, disabling complex partial seizure disorder (Engel, 1987; Luders, 1991; Porter, 1989; Purpura, Penry, & Walter, 1975; Rasmussen, 1983). Approaches to patient evaluation and criteria for patient selection are discussed in a variety of available sources (e.g., Engel, 1987). Recently, two interdisciplinary panels have recommended guidelines for the surgical treatment of epilepsy (National Association of Epilepsy Centers, 1990; National Institutes of Health, 1990). Although the surgical procedures vary widely across centers (Engel, 1987), ATL typically includes resection of an epileptic focus involving the anterior temporal pole plus significant portions of the hippocampus, amygdala, and uncus. Reports of surgical outcome have emphasized seizure control, with neuropsychological and psychosocial aspects of outcome receiving less attention (Porter, 1989).

Following ATL, alterations have been reported in intellectual, memory, language, musical processing, and occasionally other functions. Although the following discussion is limited to those areas that have received the most attention, other functions have been studied as well. It is not our intention to review comprehensively reports of neuropsychological changes after ATL or attempts at clinical prediction with regard to risk–benefit considerations. For reviews of general neuropsychological outcome the reader is referred to Chelune (1991), Hermann and Wyler (1988a), Ivnik, Sharbrough, and Laws (1987,1988), Jones-Gotman (1987), Milner (1975), and Rausch (1987). The role of preoperative neuropsychological evaluation in surgical epilepsy is reviewed by Dodrill, Wilkus, Ojemann, Ward, Wyler, van Belle, & Tamas (1986), Chelune (in press), Dodrill (1987), Jones-Gotman (1987), Milner (1975), and Rausch (1987).

Models of Change

In addition to the clinical–descriptive aspects of neuropsychological changes after temporal lobe or other surgery, there has been keen interest in the study of these patients as an opportunity to learn more about the cerebral organization and underlying mechanisms of memory and other functions (Engel, Ojemann, Luders, & Williamson, 1987). Neuropsychological observations have been made by many investigators, each typically employing multiple measures. A central theme is whether changes after surgery are behaviorally selective (e.g., decline in verbal but not visual memory) and regionally specific (e.g., decline occurs after left but not right ATL). These can be conceptualized as ipsilateral changes (decline or improvement)—on the same side as the focus and surgery—or as contralateral—changes in functions associated with the nonfocal, unoperated hemisphere. In the study of postoperative changes after ATL, neuropsychological functions can also be characterized as temporal or extratemporal. Tests known to be particularly sensitive to temporal lobe dysfunction serve as measures of temporal function, whereas those tests that are maximally sensitive to dysfunction in other brain regions serve as extratemporal indices (Saykin, Sperling, Reinecke, Kester, O'Connor, Watson, & Gur, 1990). For example, Bornstein, McKean and McLean (1987) reported that left ATL patients demonstrated improvement on measures of left frontal function, indicating an ipsilateral improvement in an extratemporal function. A general model of change after temporal lobectomy would specify predictions for behavioral functions both ipsilateral and contralateral to the seizure focus. Similarly, predictions should be generated for temporal and extratemporal functions, which may show different effects when they are ipsilateral or contralateral to the focus. Thus, changes after ATL could be divided into four basic classes: ipsilateral–temporal, ipsilateral–extratemporal, contralateral–temporal, and contralateral–extratemporal.

Possible changes after surgery are bidirectional: there may be decrements or improvements in function. For models that predict selective improvements, the mechanism requires clarification. For example, it has been suggested that contralateral improvement results from the release of the intact hemisphere from the irritative effects of the seizure focus. But many issues remain to be investigated, such as the relative disruption of preoperative function caused by the ictal focus and clinical seizures, subclinical focal seizure activity (Bridgman, Malamut, Sperling, Saykin, & O'Connor, 1989), and the ongoing effects of interictal epileptiform activity. Of course, other factors such as test-retest effect, medication, affective state, and motivation may also have a significant influence. Prediction of postoperative decline or improvement is complicated by many factors, discussed below, one of which is the possibility that for those patients with early brain insult, representation of function has been reorganized.

Cognitive Function

Several groups have reported outcome data for intellectual functioning in temporal resection. Short-term results (2–4 weeks after surgery) have often indicated decline in IQ scores following left lobectomy. In an early study Meyer (1959) reported a 10-point decline in Verbal and Performance IQs for the left temporal (LT) group but no change in the right temporal (RT) patients. Blakemore and Falconer (1967) reported ipsilateral declines in IQ scores: a 16-point decline in VIQ following LT lobectomy and a 7-point decline in PIQ following RT lobectomy. Milner (1975) found a 15-point decline in Full-Scale WAIS IQ in the early postoperative period after left lobectomy but only a 5-point decline following right lobectomy. It is noteworthy that long-term follow-up in seizure-free patients indicated a return to baseline level of intellectual functioning for both groups.

Short-term changes in IQ scores were also reported by the Maudsley group (Powell, Polkey, & McMillan, 1985). Their patients showed average Verbal and Performance IQ scores prior to surgery (both RT and LT groups). A 6-point decline was noted in VIQ after left lobectomy, with no change for the RT group. Performance IQ subtests showed a 2-point decline after right lobectomy and no change after left lobectomy. These authors reported that, as a group, changes in intelligence and memory were "small and nonsignificant" in contrast to previous reports from the same center of significant deterioration. They attributed the difference to improved selection over the prior Maudsley series and concluded that temporal lobectomy is an acceptably safe procedure regarding cognitive side effects. However, some individual patients were noted to show significant deterioration (two cases had >20-point decline in Verbal IQ after left lobectomy). Novelly, Augustine, Mattson, Glaser, Williamson, Spencer, & Spencer (1984) did not find any long-term decline in VIQ or PIQ scores. Patients receiving nondominant resections tended to show significant improvement in IQ scores; for dominant resections, there was no change.

The influence of age of onset of seizures on intellectual functioning was examined in several studies, and the results indicate its importance. In a prior (1982–1985) Graduate Hospital series (Saykin, Gur, Sussman, Gur, & O'Connor, 1989), correlations between preoperative IQ scores and age of onset were $r(28) = .64, .59$, and .50 for FSIQ, VIQ, and PIQ, respectively (all $p < .01$). This replicated early reports of lower IQ associated with early onset (Sullivan & Gahagan, 1935; Klove & Matthews, 1974).

Memory and Learning

Several models have been proposed to organize observations of memory changes after ATL (Saykin, Sperling, Robinson, Stafiniak, Kester, Gur, O'Connor, submitted). Following left ATL, material-specific verbal decline has been reported for recall of short story passages, word lists, and digit supraspan. Following RT resection, decline has been reported in recall of geometric designs and the Rey–Osterrieth Complex Figure and in recognition of unfamiliar faces, unfamiliar musical passages, and recurring nonsense figures. In patients with large right hippocampal resections, replication of block-tapping sequences, subject-ordered pointing to abstract designs, and tactually and visually guided maze learning had been found to be impaired postoperatively (see Jones-Gotman, 1987, for review).

Implicit in the neuropsychological literature are three models for change after temporal lobe resection. The material-specific "ipsilateral deficit" (model 1) indicates that the hemisphere on which the resection is performed influences the type of material affected by surgery (Milner, 1970, 1975). Left ATL has been associated with a decline in verbal memory, and right lobectomy has been associated with a decrease in nonverbal, particularly visual, memory (Jones-Gotman, 1987). For example, Ojemann and Dodrill (1985) reported a 22% decline in Wechsler Memory Scale memory passages at 1 month after LT resections and 11% decline at a year.

Model 2, "contralateral improvement," extends the ipsilateral deficit model by incorporating evidence of postoperative improvement in memory functions associated with the contralateral hemisphere (Cavazzuti, Winston, Baker, & Welch 1980; Rausch & Crandall, 1982; Novelly et al., 1984). Ipsilateral deficit (Ojemann & Dodrill, 1985) and contralateral improvement in memory have been related to postoperative seizure control, with better memory outcome noted in patients who become seizure-free (Rausch & Crandall, 1982; Novelly et al., 1984). In the Bornstein et al. (1987) study of a small surgical series, both LT and RT groups improved on a dexterity test with the hand ipsilateral to the side of surgery, suggesting that contralateral improvement may include extratemporal function, in this case psychomotor function.

The third model, "developmental hemispheric asymmetry," incorporates two additional factors (Saykin et al., 1989). The developmental aspect indicates that memory changes are influenced by age at onset of seizures or presumed early brain injury. The asymmetry component is based on evidence that the left, compared to right, medial temporal lobe (MTL) is better able to simultaneously support both verbal and nonverbal memory after contralateral resection. Model 3 predicts that (1) early risk factors for CNS dysfunction are associated with less postoperative deficit and greater improvement, and (2) greater change (decline or improvement) is seen after left resection and for verbal compared to visual material.

Olfactory perception and memory have also been studied by several groups (Henkin, Comiter, Fedio, & O'Doherty 1977; Rausch, Serafetinides, & Crandall, 1977). Eskenazi, Cain, Novelly, and Friend (1983) administered unilateral olfactory tests to temporal lobe seizure patients and found minor bilateral reduction of absolute sensitivity, although most were within normal limits. After surgery, patients showed impairment of odor identification and recognition memory, but primarily in the nostril ipsilateral to surgery.

Language

Most of the literature on language dysfunction in patients with temporal lobe epilepsy (TLE) and after ATL has focused on naming (Heilman, Wilder, & Malzone, 1972; Burnstine, Lesser, Hart, 1990; Ojemann, Creutzfeldt, Lettich, & Haglund, 1988), which is known often to be disrupted after temporal lesions (Benson, 1979). Naming deficits can occur interictally in nonoperated left TLE patients (Mayeux, Brandt, Rosen, & Benson, 1980). After dominant ATL, declines in naming have been reported in some (Heilman et al., 1972; Loring, Meador, Martin, & Lee, 1988) but not other (Hermann & Wyler, 1988b) studies. The time interval between surgery and retest may influence these differences.

It is unclear to what extent the three models presented for memory pertain to language and other domains. It is well established that there can be a dissociation between components of language processing in aphasia (Goodglass & Kaplan, 1983). There is also evidence for selective deficits in components of language in the context of developmental disorders (Dennis, 1988). There has been comparatively less attention to changes in language other than naming after dominant ATL. Examination of effects of ATL on language functions such as fluency, repetition, and reading, which are considered to be maximally sensitive to extratemporal regions, would help to clarify the specificity of naming changes. Handedness, hemispheric speech dominance, and age of brain insult may influence the effects of surgery. Early brain damage, left-hand motor dominance, and partial or complete transfer of speech dominance to the right hemisphere should lead to less impairment after left ATL. Thus, there may be material-specific ipsilateral and contralateral changes and influences of developmental factors such as early CNS insult. In cases of early lesions, linguistic function may become anomalously developed or reorganized within the left hemisphere, transferred to the right hemisphere, or shared by both hemispheres.

Musical Processing

Most studies of musical processes after brain damage suggest greater involvement of the right hemisphere (Benton, 1977; Carmon, Lavy, Gordon, & Portnoy, 1975; Critchley & Henson, 1977; Gordon, 1983; Henschen, 1926; McKee, Humphrey, & McAdam, 1973; Zatorre, 1984). Early case reports suggested selective left hemispheric involvement for some tasks including rhythm discrimination, reading musical notation, and detailed musical analysis (Henschen & Schaller, 1925). In studies addressing temporal lobe resections specifically, decline in perception and discrimination were noted for some types of musical stimuli following right but not left temporal lobectomy. Milner (1962) studied patients with the Seashore Measures of Musical Talents (Saeveit, Lewis, & Seashore, 1940). Right temporal lobectomy patients declined on four of six subtests: decrement was primarily identified on Timbre and Tonal Memory, but Loudness and Time also showed some decline. Left temporal patients did not show postoperative changes. These findings were replicated by Berlin, Chase, Dill, and Hagepanos (1965). Shankweiler (1966), using short musical excerpts, and Zatorre (1985), using electronically generated tones, found similar lateralized changes in musical processing.

Overall, the convergence of evidence, particularly for subjects without formal musical training, suggests that musical processes are primarily mediated by the right hemisphere. The temporal region appears to be particularly involved, although there are very little data that directly address the regional specificity of musical processing within the right hemisphere. In beginning to address the issue of specificity, Zatorre (1985) examined discrimination and recognition processes and found that damage to Heschl's gyri on either side may add to the musical discrimination deficit associated with RT lesions. In the same study, he found that patients with right frontal lesions showed a response bias but normal performance level. Recognition of tonal melodies was impaired after both RT and LT resection. In a later report addressing melodic and harmonic discrimination, Samson and Zatorre (1988) found that left ATL sparing Heschl's gyrus did not cause impairment, whereas right temporal and frontotemporal resections were associated with a discrimination deficit relative to normal controls.

In terms of the models presented above, most aspects of musical processing should probably be considered ipsilateral to the right hemisphere and contralateral to the left hemisphere. Tentatively, musical processing might be considered more temporal than extratemporal.

Can Changes Be Predicted?

Having considered some of the literature on neuropsychological changes after temporal resection, we turn now to the question of prediction. Very few studies have tried to predict changes.

Javornisky (1981) evaluated preoperative neuropsychological and neurological variables as predictors of postoperative memory outcome in a small sample (LT = 7; RT = 11) but found no significant relationships. Much of the variance in postoperative memory was accounted for by preoperative scores.

Powell, Polkey, & McMillan (1985) reviewed several potential predictors: intactness of the unoperated hemisphere, intactness of the unoperated temporal lobe, clinical outcome of lobectomy (change in seizure frequency), age at operation, time since operation, sex, and the nature of the resection (size and structures removed). They reported that patients who showed no deterioration or most improvement tended to be younger, lower in preoperative intellectual ability, and to have had an earlier age at first seizure and onset of regular seizures.

McMillan, Powell, Janota, and Polkey (1987), in a later report from the same group, examined neuropathology as a predictor of cognitive changes 1 month after temporal resection ($n = 40$). Hippocampal sclerosis, compared to tumor-like malformations, was associated with febrile convulsions, an earlier onset of regular seizures, poorer preoperative intelligence, and a tendency toward greater postoperative cognitive improvement. Patients with damage in the amygdala had a worse outcome in verbal and nonverbal memory. Absence of any tissue pathology did not predict poor cognitive outcome.

Data from several reports have suggested an association between preoperative cognitive and memory performance levels and degree of decrement or improvement after surgery (Ivnik et al., 1988, Ojemann & Dodrill, 1985; Powell et al., 1985; Rausch, 1987). This issue was specifically addressed by Chelune, Naugle, Luders, & Awad (in press), who reported that for left temporal patients higher preoperative performance on language and memory measures was associated with larger postoperative decrements. However, patients with right-sided surgery did not show this relationship.

The age of earliest brain insult, whether seizure onset, onset of underlying etiology, or another event, appears to be predictive of acute memory and language outcome. Data from our first series (Saykin et al., 1989) suggested that age of onset of seizures is a useful predictor of the pattern of memory change after ATL. Data from a second series, described in more detail below, suggest that age at first risk factor is a strong predictor of vulnerability to acute deficits in naming after left ATL (Stafiniak, Saykin, Sperling, Kester, Robinson, O'Connor, & Gur, 1990).

Taking a different strategy, some centers have used electrical stimulation mapping, either intraoperatively or with chronically implanted subdural grid or strip electrodes, to map zones involved in language and memory function. The model driving this approach is that there is heterogeneity in representation of language and memory functions, that the areas involved in these functions can be mapped through individualized testing, and that sparing implicated cortical areas will reduce the likelihood of postoperative impairment. For example, Ojemann and Dodrill (1985) reported that verbal memory decline after LT resection could be predicted with 80% accuracy by using intraoperative mapping of areas essential to naming or storage aspects of memory. Another technique used to predict language and memory impairment after surgery is the intracarotid amobarbital (ICA) procedure or "Wada test." Although stimulation mapping and the ICA procedure are widely used clinically to reduce the risk of postoperative aphasia or amnesia, there has been little systematic research addressing the reliability and validity of the stimulation mapping or ICA procedures.

Methodological Considerations

Interpretation of the body of research reviewed above is complicated by a variety of methodological issues. These include differences in patient selection, test selection, timing of evaluations, surgical procedures, medical management, use and selection of a control group, and statistical approach to the data.

Subject variables potentially related to postoperative neuropsychological changes include age, gender, handedness, and education and training. Age of onset of seizures and age at first risk factor for brain injury are strongly associated with cognitive, memory, and language changes (Saykin et al., 1989; Stafiniak et al., 1990; Saykin et al., submitted). Early brain insults can trigger changes in representation of cortical function including intra- or interhemispheric transfer or changes in the pattern of interhemispheric relations (Liederman, 1989). Frequently, these clinical-demographic variables are ignored, or if they are presented, there is no attempt to analyze the influence of these factors. In addition to the general effect of education on neuropsychological performance, there is likely to be a complex interaction between how a given task is performed and the level of training and expertise an individual has in that specific domain. For example, there is evidence that individuals with musical training may be activating different regions and utilizing different strategies to process and interpret musical stimuli than those without such training (Bever & Chiarello, 1974; Johnson, 1977; Keller & Bever, 1980).

Specific selection criteria used in the decision to operate vary across centers (Engel, 1987). Some series may include patients with lateral temporal involvement, whereas others restrict patients to medial temporal foci only. Similarly, some include patients with extratemporal involvement. Preoperative imaging studies suggesting structural or metabolic abnormalities may be variously used and weighted in the surgical decision. Also, there is variability in the manner and extent to which preoperative neuropsychological findings are included in the decision to operate or in modifications of surgical procedure.

Another problem rendering cross-center comparisons difficult is the selection of neuropsychological measures. Fortunately, most centers include the Wechsler Adult Intelligence Scale–Revised (WAIS-R) and Wechsler Memory Scale (WMS). These provide a general overview of cognitive and memory function, although by itself the

WMS visual design subtest may be a relatively weak marker of right temporal lobe function. Beyond the Wechsler scales there is great heterogeneity in test batteries for both breadth and depth of coverage of higher functions. Little attention has been given to the intercorrelations and factor structure of test batteries used to assess cognitive outcomes. Psychometric properties of tests warrant greater attention. Test reliability and task difficulty are important for identifying the selectivity of deficits (Chapman & Chapman, 1978), and the sensitivity and specificity of tests to baseline deficits and change after surgery need to be determined. The ecological validity or generalizability to patients' "real-world" functioning has often been neglected. There have been few attempts to integrate neuropsychological assessment with patient and family perception of postoperative function (e.g., Chapter 8, this volume). What, for example, is the agreement between patient and family perception of memory capability after surgery and actual psychometric performance on tests of memory? Also, what is the relationship of neuropsychological changes to those on affective and psychosocial scales? Changes in level of anxiety and depression may influence aspects of test performance, but this relationship is infrequently analyzed in neuropsychological reports.

The timing of postoperative reevaluations probably also accounts for many differences between studies. For example, we observed anomia in some patients who had dominant ATL when tested 2–3 weeks after surgery (Stafiniak, Saykin, Sperling, Kester, Robinson, O'Connor, & Gur, 1990), but the deficit had largely resolved by 1-year follow-up (Stafiniak, Saykin, Sperling, Robinson, Gur, & O'Connor submitted). Others have noted anomia at 1 month (Loring et al., 1988) but not 6 months (Hermann & Wyler, 1988b), suggesting that this deficit may be present shortly after surgery but may be minimal or not detectable by 6 months. The course of recovery of neuropsychological functions between 1 and 6 months warrants further study. The recent Consensus Conference on Surgery for Epilepsy (National Institutes of Health, 1990) specifically recommends longitudinal assessment of neuropsychological and psychosocial outcome, including use of family interviews; it stipulates that this "assessment must be done repeatedly for several years." Many clinicians believe that recovery is complete by 1 year. Although this may often be true, there are no prospective data establishing the stabilization of neuropsychological and psychosocial function by 12 months.

Although there are well-established multivariate methods for analysis of repeated testing with correlated dependent measures (e.g., Morrison, 1976), many reports have relied on univariate t or F tests or nonparametric methods. This may lead to inflation of type I error in some cases but may also potentially lead to a failure to detect more subtle differences because of a loss of power. The a priori specification of appropriate models for change after surgery should increase the efficiency of experimental designs in this area. Some early reports used two-group (LT, RT) posttest-only designs. Given the magnitude of individual differences in preoperative impairment in seizure surgery patients, failure to control for baseline performance is a serious flaw.

Particularly troubling in surgical reports, with a few exceptions, is the absence of control groups. Short of a randomized clinical trial, which is difficult for ethical reasons in the case of a treatment with established efficacy, it is proposed that nonoperated patients with partial epilepsy, as closely matched as possible to those undergoing surgery, would be suitable control subjects. This is a compromise relative to a randomized trial, but it may be the best control group available. Most reports also do not include healthy normal controls, which would permit determination of normal performance distributions and hence the degree of baseline impairment in patients prior to surgery. Normal controls are also helpful (as illustrated below) in providing norms for standardizing various tests, so that they share a commensurate scale (e.g., z-transformation). This permits direct comparison of, for example, verbal and visual memory. Greater use of control groups would clarify expected test–retest effects, including statistical regression to the mean.

A word about matching of patients and controls: elsewhere, we have argued that patients with schizophrenia should not be matched to controls on variables such as IQ or education (Saykin, Gur, Gur, Mozley, Mozley, Resnick, Kester, & Stafiniak, 1991). Because schizophrenia itself interferes with cognitive processes and ability to attain one's educational potential, matching on these variables would constitute the "matching fallacy" described by Meehl (1970). This problem is also relevant to intractable epilepsy. Matching on variables such as IQ, which may be related to the process or outcome of the disease, may lead to biased comparisons, that is, contrasting overachieving patients with underachieving controls. It is proposed that matching on parental socioeconomic status (SES) may provide a better marker for expected baseline performance.

Multiple medical and surgical issues need to be considered in the data analysis or controlled for, including resection size and location, type of operative procedure and anesthesia, medication changes, seizure frequency and outcome, and tissue pathology. Models using multivariate techniques such as multiple linear regression (MLR) can use weighted combinations of these independent variables to enhance prediction. Dodrill et al. (1986) use multivariate procedures to predict seizure outcome. However, these techniques can readily be applied to prediction of neuropsychological outcomes. For example, we have employed a MLR prediction model for acute memory changes incorporating preoperative baseline performance levels, age at first risk, seizure outcome, and tissue pathology (Saykin et al., submitted). Separate models were developed for ipsilateral and contralateral memory; each accounted for a significant amount of the variance in memory outcome.

NEUROPSYCHOLOGICAL STUDIES OF A SURGICAL SERIES FROM THE GRADUATE HOSPITAL IN PHILADELPHIA

The Comprehensive Epilepsy Center (CEC) at Graduate Hospital is a tertiary care facility affiliated with the University of Pennsylvania where approximately 300–400 new outpatients are evaluated each year and over 1,000 patients receive continuing care. The CEC is clinically staffed by four faculty neurologists, one neurosurgeon, and three neurology fellows. Approximately 110 new patients per year are admitted for intensive video-EEG monitoring, of whom 50–60% are considered for epilepsy surgery. Referral sources are regional and local, from private and academic sources.

Results of three studies of acute neuropsychological changes after ATL are summarized below. Each attempts to address some of the methodological issues described above. Subjects for each of the three studies were consecutive patients meeting inclusion criteria for that study. Descriptive statistics for the parent sample of 64 patients who underwent surgery is provided in Table 13.1. Detailed methods for each study are available in the separate reports and from the authors.

Surgical patients ($n = 64$) in this series, aged 16 to 50 years, were treated with ATL for complex partial seizures or secondarily generalized seizures. Seizures occurred at least monthly and were refractory to conventional anticonvulsant therapy. The duration of epilepsy was at least 2 years. All patients completed intensive clinical localization studies prior to surgery, as described by Sperling and O'Connor (1989). Patients were excluded from this series if they had extratemporal foci, persistent interictal psychosis, progressive neurological disorder, or were unavailable for neuropsychological reevaluation 2–3 weeks after surgery ($n = 2$). Surgery included removal of the amygdala and anterior 2–3 cm of the hippocampus (Sperling & O'Connor, 1989). The resection line was typically 4.5–5 cm from the tip of the temporal lobe for dominant ATL and 5.5–6.0 cm in nondominant ATL. Patients remained on preoperative medications at nontoxic therapeutic levels at the time of postoperative follow-up.

We also administered the neuropsychological battery to a carefully screened normative sample ($n = 32$). Controls were recruited from a pool of healthy subjects

TABLE 13.1. Demographic and Clinical Characteristics of the Sample

	Control ($n = 32$)	RT ($n = 32$)	LT ($n = 32$)
Age	27.12 ± 8.24	33.19 ± 6.96	29.78 ± 6.80
Education	14.12 ± 1.58	13.42 ± 2.68	12.91 ± 2.04
Sex (M/F)	16/16	17/15	18/14
Handedness (R/L)	32/0	27/5	25/7
VIQ	111.27 ± 15.10	92.15 ± 14.52	93.52 ± 12.28
PIQ	110.70 ± 14.05	90.52 ± 13.88	91.40 ± 14.38
FSIQ	112.12 ± 14.98	91.11 ± 14.43	91.84 ± 12.86
Age at first risk	—	7.20 ± 8.65	7.64 ± 9.35
Age at onset of regular seizures	—	14.03 ± 8.20	13.31 ± 9.51
Size of resection (cm)			
Lateral temporal	—	5.73 ± 0.58	4.87 ± 0.71
Hippocampus	—	2.26 ± 0.47	2.11 ± 0.34
Test–retest interval (median)	—	113 days	129 days
Surgery-to-retest interval (median)	—	18 days	18 days
Length of postsurgery follow-up (median)	—	25 months	27 months

who volunteered for protocols at the Mental Health Clinical Research Center at the University of Pennsylvania (Saykin et al., 1991). They were sociodemographically balanced to patients with respect to age, education, gender, and ethnicity. Potential controls were excluded if they had any past or present history of neurological or psychiatric disorder, learning disability, or alcohol or other substance abuse. All were right-handed and had normal neurological examinations.

In our center all patients are administered a comprehensive neuropsychological battery before and 2–3 weeks after surgery and at 1-year follow-up. Controls were tested once to provide normative data, but 1-year reevaluations are being performed on a subsample. The neuropsychological battery is presented in Table 13.2. Functions assessed by the battery include intellectual skills (abstraction, verbal and spatial cognition), memory and learning (verbal and nonverbal), receptive and expressive language, auditory and visual information processing and attention, musical perception, as well as lateralized sensory processing (auditory, visual, tactile) and motor skills. The battery administered 2–3 weeks after surgery is an abbreviated protocol that includes about two-thirds of the baseline battery. The complete baseline battery is repeated at 1-year follow-up. The full Wechsler Adult Intelligence Scale–Revised (WAIS-R; Wechsler, 1981) is administered at baseline and 1 year.

For the memory and language studies, all raw test scores were adjusted for age, education, and gender, demographic variables known to influence neuropsychological performance in some domains (Heaton, Grant, & Matthews, 1986). This adjustment was performed using a multiple linear regression (MLR) procedure as described by Saykin et al. (1991). To equate the scaling of tests for profile construction, raw scores were transformed to z-scores using parameters derived from the normative sample. Baseline and postoperative change score profiles were then analyzed by multivariate analysis of variance (MANOVA). The MANOVA was used to evaluate the level and shape of memory, language, and music baseline and change score profiles. Where there were significant function × group interactions, MANOVA within-subject contrast procedures were used to decompose such effects to establish selective areas of deficit or improvement beyond any generalized changes (Saykin et al., 1991). In the memory study, factor analysis was also used as described below.

Below, we present an overview of studies of acute changes in memory, language, and musical processing after ATL. The reader is referred to the specific reports for further details.

Study 1: Memory, Construct Validity, and Laterality Effects

Material-Specific Memory Battery

The memory battery we employed, summarized in Table 13.2, includes parts of the WMS (Wechsler, 1945; Russell, 1975) and the California Verbal Learning Test (CVLT; Delis, Kramer, Kaplan, & Ober, 1983). The WMS Logical Memory passages subtest was scored with a half-point partial-credit system (Gangarosa, Saykin, Malamut, & Gur, 1988) to enhance reliability. In addition to these published tests, we developed or modified the following paired verbal and visual memory tests:

TABLE 13.2.   Neuropsychological Battery with Tests Grouped by Function

Abstraction and mental flexibility
    A. Wisconsin Card-Sorting Test (Heaton, 1981)
Verbal cognitive
    A. Vocabulary (WAIS-R; Wechsler, 1981)[a]
    B. Information (WAIS-R)
    C. Reading recognition (WRAT-R; Jastak & Wilkinson, 1984)
Spatial–constructional ability
    A. Block design (WAIS-R)
    B. Drawings to command and copy (quantitative scoring)
Semantic memory and verbal learning
    A. Logical Memory (WMS, Russell, 1975 form)
    B. California Verbal Learning Test (CVLT; Delis et al., 1983)
    C. Paired-Associate Learning (WMS; Wechsler, 1945)
    D. Digit Sequence Learning (Modified Hebb Digit Task)
    E. Low-Imagery Word Recognition (see text)
Visual–spatial memory
    A. Figural Reproduction (WMS; Russell, 1975)
    B. Facial Recognition Memory Test (see text)
    C. Spatial Sequence Learning (Modified Corsi Block Task)
Language
    A. Phonemic Fluency (CFL; Benton & Hamsher, 1978)
    B. Semantic Fluency (Animal Naming, BDAE; Goodglass & Kaplan, 1983)
    C. Boston Naming Test (BDAE; Kaplan, Goodglass, & Weintraub, 1983)
    D. Comprehension of Complex Ideational Material (BDAE)
    E. Sentence Repetition (MAE; Benton & Hamsher, 1978)
Musical perception
    A. Tonal Memory (Seashore; Saeveit et al., 1940 revision, split-half)
    B. Musical Aptitude Profile (MAP; Gordon, 1965)[b]
Information processing and attention
    A. Continuous Performance Test (CPT; Gordon, 1986)
       Task Conditions: (a) Simple RT; (b) Vigilance; (c) Distractibility
    B. Digit Span (WAIS-R; forward and reversed)
    C. Digit Symbol (WAIS-R)
    D. Trail Making (parts A and B; Reitan & Wolfson, 1985)
    E. Stroop Color–Word Test (Golden, 1978)
Fine motor speed and sequencing
    A. Finger Tapping (Reitan & Wolfson, 1985)
    B. Finger Sequencing (Luria; Golden, Hammeke, & Purisch, 1980)
Sensory function
    A. Hastead–Reitan sensory–perceptual exam (Reitan & Wolfson, 1985)
       Double Simultaneous Stimulation: auditory, tactile, visual; graphesthesia

[a]Full WAIS-R administered at baseline and 1-year follow-up.
[b]Subsample only.

Facial Recognition Memory. The Facial Memory test requires the subject to examine (for 1 min) a page containing 20 photocopies of unfamiliar faces taken from a university yearbook. The subject is then asked to identify those target faces from of 40 faces (on two pages) that includes 20 distractors. Following a 30-min de subject has to make the same discrimination from new distractors. The score of the number of items correct (out of 40) minus the number incorrect (as a correction for guessing). This test is similar to that shown by Milner (1968) to be sensitive to right temporal lobe damage. However, it includes more items and uses partially degraded stimuli, which render it more difficult. Scores for the normative group (M ± S.D.) were: immediate 27.66 ± 7.21; delayed 27.59 ± 7.00.

Low-Imagery Word Recognition Memory. This test is a verbal analogue of the Facial Recognition Memory test. It requires the subject to examine a page containing 20 low-imagery words for 1 minute. These are abstract words to which it is difficult to form visual associations. The subject is then asked to identify those 20 words from a set of 40 words that includes 20 distractors. Following a 30-min delay, the subject has to make the same discrimination from new distractors. Normative scores: immediate 25.97 ± 8.55; delayed 24.72 ± 9.38.

Spatial Sequence Learning Task. A nine-block board based on Corsi's original apparatus (Milner, 1971) is employed. Subjects are asked to repeat a nine-block sequence tapped out (one block per second) by the examiner. The task is repeated, using the same sequence for each trial, until the subject correctly duplicates the sequences on two consecutive trials or until 15 trials are completed. Scores include number of trials to reach criterion (two consecutive correct trials) and maximum number of items correctly repeated. Normative scores: trials-to-criterion 5.39 ± 3.43; maximum number correct 8.88 ± 0.70.

Digit-Sequence Learning Task. Subjects are asked to repeat verbally a 12-digit supraspan sequence read by the examiner (one digit per second) until two consecutive correct trials or 15 unsuccessful trials are completed. Scores are the same as for the Spatial Learning Task. Normative scores: trials-to-criterion 7.91 ± 3.89; maximum number correct 11.88 ± 0.70.

Construct Validity: Confirmation of the Structure of Memory Change

The material-specific deficit model implies that there are two relatively independent sources of variation in memory change scores (verbal and visual). Establishment of construct validity is part of the process of validating psychometric tests, which involves evaluation of their correlations with other tests measuring theoretically related and unrelated abilities (Cronbach & Meehl, 1955). A recent report has examined construct validity of verbal and nonverbal memory tests in an epilepsy surgery sample using ANOVA (Lee, Loring, & Thompson, 1989). Specific abilities can be clustered into higher-order categories or factors by multivariate procedures that address the pattern of test intercorrelations. In the case of ATL, because the material-specific model leads to specific predictions regarding change, analyses can most meaningfully be performed on post–pre change scores.

We tested the construct validity of the material-specific model using confirmatory factor analysis (PROC FACTOR; SAS, 1987). Patients' change scores (post–

minus presurgery) for each memory test were entered. For tests with both immediate and delayed components, each was given a weight of 0.5. For tests with multiple scores, such as trials to completion and maximum correct, the component scores were equally weighted. The memory change scores were subjected to initial factor extraction by principal components analysis. Number of factors retained was determined by the Mineigen criterion. To enhance interpretability, factors were rotated by the Varimax method, which preserves factor independence.

Factor loadings, indicating the correlation between memory test change scores and each factor, are shown in Table 13.3. Two factors were extracted that together accounted for 60.2% of the variance in change scores. For Factor I, all five of the verbal memory tests had high loadings, whereas the three visual memory tests had very low or negative loadings. For Factor II, the reverse pattern was observed: the visual memory tests had high loadings, and the verbal memory tests had low or negative loadings. These results confirmed the presence of material-specific changes in memory for verbal (Factor I) and visual (Factor II) material. The factor loadings for the eight tests suggest that the best markers of verbal change are verbal learning measures, whereas the best markers of visual memory change are facial recognition and spatial learning. In contrast to Lee *et al.* (1989), we were able to demonstrate construct validity for visual as well as verbal memory and learning after ATL.

Testing Models of Memory Change

After confirming that there were two major underlying dimensions of memory change, verbal and visual memory, we used composite z-scores of verbal and visual memory tests for further analyses of postoperative change by MANOVA. This procedure yielded two primary dependent variables, verbal and visual memory, which reduced the number of univariate comparisons and hence the probability of

TABLE 13.3. Factor Structure
of Memory Change Scores[a]

Memory change scores	Factor 1	Factor 2
California Verbal Learning	**.83**	−.08
Digit Learning	**.77**	.12
WMS Paired Associates	**.72**	.17
WMS Story Passages	**.70**	−.18
Low-Imagery Word Recognition	**.59**	.08
Facial Memory	.16	**.79**
Spatial Learning	−.18	**.74**
WMS Designs	.09	**.63**

[a]Memory change scores were calculated as post–preoperative z-score for each test. Immediate and delayed memory scores were averaged where applicable. Initial factor extraction was by principal components analysis with retention determined by Mineigen criterion. Results were then subjected to orthogonal rotation using the Varimax method. Tests were reordered by magnitude of loadings.

type I error. The composite variables gave equal weight to each of the original memory tests for each type of material.

Prior to surgery, patients performed worse than controls ($z = 0$, by definition) across both verbal and spatial memory [both $p < .001$], but there were no significant differences between the RT and LT groups. As illustrated in Fig. 13.1, verbal memory declined after left lobectomy, and visual memory declined after right-sided surgery [interaction: pre–post × verbal–visual × right–left; $F(1,62) = 24.58$, $p < .0001$]. These changes are consistent with model 1 (material-specific). Also, as predicted by model 2 (contralateral improvement), the LT group showed a decline in verbal memory and improvement in visual memory, whereas the RT group declined in visual memory and improved in verbal memory.

To examine model 3 (developmental factors and hemispheric asymmetry), the LT and RT groups were stratified by age at first risk (using age 5 as cutoff). Groups were composed as Early Risk (ER; age ≤ 5 years) and No Early Risk (NER). Early risk factors included perinatal distress, febrile convulsions, meningitis, encephalitis, head trauma, tumor, and arteriovenous malformation.

Figure 13.2 shows the pre- and postoperative memory results for the four groups. MANOVA was performed with focus (RT, LT) and risk group (ER, NER) as between-group factors and material (verbal–visual) and surgery (pre–post) as within-subject (repeated) factors. The interaction predicted by model 3 was highly significant. Across focus groups and type of material, ER patients showed less ipsilateral decline and more contralateral improvement [interaction: pre–post × risk group; $F(1,60) = 9.98$, $p < .003$]. Material-specific memory changes were significant for both the ER and NER groups, but the pattern was much stronger for the NER group (interaction: pre–post × verbal–visual × focus side; for ER group $p < .02$; for the NER group $p < .0001$).

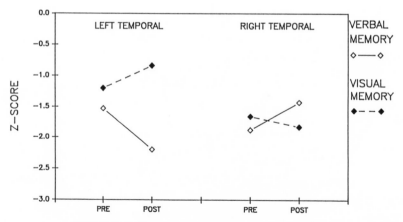

FIGURE 13.1. Change in memory after right and left ATL.

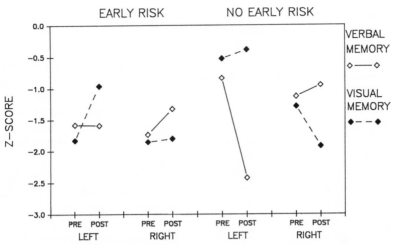

FIGURE 13.2. Relationship of early risk factors (age ≤5 years) to changes in memory after temporal lobectomy. Early risk factors included perinatal distress, febrile convulsions, meningitis, encephalitis, head trauma, tumor, and arteriovenous malformation.

Comment

Overall, these findings for memory, which indicate the relative independence of changes in verbal and visual memory, support earlier reports (Milner, 1970, 1975) of a "double dissociation" (Teuber, 1955) between verbal and visual memory, with verbal memory lateralized to the left medial temporal region and visual memory to the homologous right MTL (Milner, 1975), and of the construct validity of material-specific memory processes. Additionally, our results support the importance of developmental factors and hemispheric asymmetry (model 3). The pattern of memory change appears strongly influenced by the patients' age of onset of seizures (Saykin *et al.*, 1989) and age at first risk factor (Saykin *et al.*, submitted). Also, the magnitude of change, whether improvement or decline, is greater after left resection. By incorporating age at first risk for CNS pathology and predicting greater change after left ATL and for verbal material, the developmental–hemispheric asymmetry model accounts for more of the variance in acute memory change after ATL than either prior model.

Study 2: Language

Our studies of language processes before and after ATL have concentrated on changes in naming after dominant ATL (Stafiniak *et al.*, 1990) and the specificity of those changes with regard to other language functions (Saykin *et al.*, in press). As in the memory studies, we have been particularly interested in the role of early brain injury (i.e., seizures or other risk factors) in predicting language changes after surgery. Left-handed patients were excluded from the language studies.

To evaluate the specificity of changes in naming relative to other language functions (Saykin *et al.*, in press), we analyzed measures of confrontation naming, phonemic and semantic fluency, repetition, comprehension, and reading recognition administered before and 2–3 weeks after ATL. Demographic adjusted z-transformed baseline and change score data were analyzed by MANOVA, as described above. With MANOVA contrasts, change scores for each of the six language tests were contrasted with the mean of the remaining five functions in the profile (SAS, 1987; PROC GLM Contrast Procedure, Mean Option).

Language change score profiles for the four groups are presented in Fig. 13.3. Overall, in the language study, we were able to confirm the following hypotheses: (1) before ATL there is generalized impairment in language skills relative to normative performance; (2) after dominant ATL there is a selective deficit in naming relative to other language functions; and (3) decline in naming occurs primarily in LT patients without early risk factors.

Comment

Why is naming a selective area of language deficit? We have suggested (Saykin *et al.*, in press) that confrontation naming could be viewed as a functional system/ network (Luria, 1980; Mesulam, 1981) that includes visual recognition, selection and retrieval from lexical-semantic store, and productive speech. Resection of the hippocampal "node" of this system could interfere with retrieval (Halgren, Wilson,

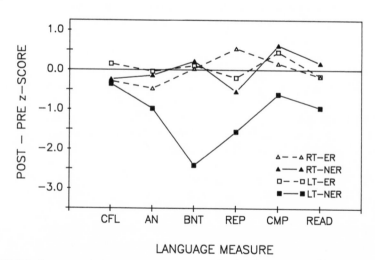

FIGURE 13.3. Language change profiles (post–pre z-scores) after ATL by risk group and focus. ER, early risk; NER, no early risk; CFL, phonemic fluency (letters CFL); AN, animal naming; BNT, Boston naming; REP, sentence repetition; CMP, comprehension; READ, oral reading recognition.

& Stapleton, 1985; Ojemann, *et al.*, 1988). Similarly, a disconnection between visual input and the hippocampus may be responsible for dysnomia. Studies of naming in patients undergoing operations restricted to either lateral neocortex or medial temporal structures (Wieser, 1988) should help to clarify the mechanism of anomia.

Relation of Changes in Language to Changes in Memory

There has been considerable recent interest in the relationship of language and memory in epilepsy. Hermann, Wyler, Steenman, and Richey (1988) reported that language performance could account for verbal memory deficits before surgery. Two recent presentations have examined the relationship between postoperative changes in memory and language (Stanulis & Valenstein, 1988; Chelune, Awad, & Luders, 1989). Stanulis and Valenstein (1988) suggested that decline in verbal memory after dominant resections may be secondary to decline in language, particularly naming. By contrast, Chelune *et al.* (1989), although also reporting an association between verbal memory loss and changes in naming (BNT) and VIQ, stated "it is more likely that the degree of verbal memory loss following LTL determines whether a given patient will show an improvement or a loss in verbal intelligence and naming rather than the converse."

We examined this issue in our series of left ATL patients. Prior to surgery, naming (BNT) and composite verbal memory scores were not correlated. After left ATL, decline in naming was highly correlated with decline in verbal memory ($r = .68, p = .0001$) and to a lesser extent with decline in visual memory ($r = .38, p < .04$). The relationship between changes in naming and verbal memory for the LT group is illustrated in Fig. 13.4. Note that the NER subgroup accounts for most of the relationship. For RT patients, change scores for naming and memory were unrelated.

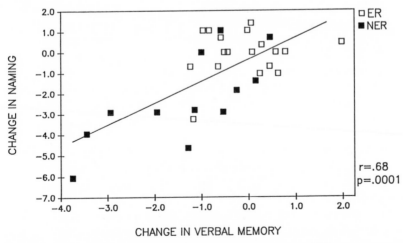

FIGURE 13.4. Relationship of changes in verbal memory after left temporal lobectomy to changes in naming on the Boston Naming Test (Pearson $r = .68$, $p = .0001$). Change scores are post–pre z-scores.

Comment

Unlike Hermann *et al.* (1988), we did not find language performance to account for verbal memory deficits before surgery. We did find a significant correlation between confrontation naming and verbal memory after resection. This reflected the correlation between change scores for these two domains. Extending the position by Chelune *et al.*, it seems possible that the postoperative decline in naming is another form of verbal memory deficit, associated with impairment in retrieval, a function attributed to the MTL system (Halgren *et al.*, 1985; Heit, Smith, & Halgren, 1988). Because the overall verbal memory deficit after ATL probably represents a combination of dysfunctional consolidation (Milner, 1970) and retrieval capacities (Halgren *et al.*, 1985; Heit *et al.*, 1988), the extent of relationship to naming changes may provide an estimate of the relative contribution of disordered retrieval. Judging by the amount of shared variance (46%) between the two sets of change scores, our data suggest approximately equal contributions.

Study 3: Musical Processing

Changes in memory and language after temporal lobectomy have received considerable attention, but there have been comparatively fewer studies of musical processing. As reviewed above, most studies of musical processes after ATL report greater involvement of the right hemisphere, although there has been some suggestion of left hemisphere involvement. We have suggested (Kester, Saykin, Sperling, O'Connor, Robinson, Gur, 1991) that some of the differences between reports may have been caused by varying definitions of "musical processing," differences in the type of musical stimuli (e.g., single notes versus complex excerpts; low versus high familiarity and recognizability), and subject's level of musical training. Also, many studies did not include a normal control group.

We examined the selectivity of changes in musical processing while attempting to address some of the above methodological issues by administering a standardized comprehensive battery of musical measures, The Musical Aptitude Profile (MAP; Gordon, 1965), before and 2–3 weeks after surgery (Kester *et al.*, 1991). Subjects in this study were 21 consecutive right-handed, left hemisphere speech dominant patients treated with ATL (RT, $n = 12$; LT, $n = 9$). Healthy controls ($n = 12$) were also studied at comparable intervals. Only subjects without musical training were included.

The MAP consists of seven subtests that measure three domains of musical processing: Tonal Imagery (Melody and Harmony), Rhythm Imagery (Tempo and Meter), and Musical Sensitivity (Phrasing, Balance, and Style). In the first four subtests the subject must listen to pairs of musical passages and make a same/different discrimination. For the last three subtests, the Sensitivity section, the subject must make a higher-level judgment as to the "more musically sound" of the two passages. The correct answer was established by consensus of a panel of professional musicians. The reader interested in details of the development, validity, and psychometric properties of the MAP is referred to the test manual (Gordon, 1965). We also included a 15-item split-half version of the Seashore Tonal Memory Test, which has been in use in our lab. Normative performance for the sample of 12 controls tested twice (number of errors out of 15 items): baseline 1.56 ± 0.88; retest 1.67 ± 1.12. The test–retest Pearson reliability for controls on the 15-item short form appeared quite adequate ($r = .85$, $p = .004$). For normative data on the MAP, see Gordon (1965) and Kester *et al.* (1991).

The MAP data were analyzed by MANOVA similar to that used in the language study, described above, with diagnosis (RT, LT, control) as the between-group factor and subtest (Melody, Harmony, Tempo, Meter, Phrasing, Balance, Style) as the within-subject factor. Postoperative changes were analyzed by MANOVA on the retest–baseline difference score profiles. The change-score profiles for the RT and LT groups and controls (in *T*-score units) are shown in Fig. 13.5.

Prior to operation, patients showed overall poorer performance than controls ($p < .001$), but there were no differences between the RT and LT foci groups. The RT group was impaired at baseline relative to controls on the Tonal Memory short form. After surgery, there was a significant main effect for diagnosis ($p < .02$), but not subtest. On planned contrasts, the RT group demonstrated an overall decrement in comparison to the LT group ($p = .04$) and controls ($p = .007$), who showed either no change or improvement. Analysis of individual subtests indicated that whereas RT patients declined, controls improved on the Tempo and Meter subtests ($p = .008$ and $p = .005$, respectively). The RT declined and LT improved on the Style subtest ($p < .03$). Thus, the decrement was primarily noted for rhythmic processes and tasks requiring aesthetic judgment and was not noted for tonal processes. The LT and controls showed no decline.

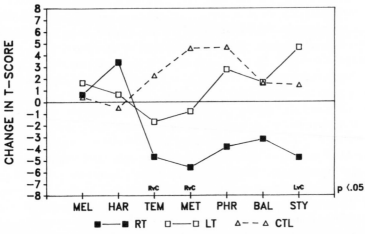

FIGURE 13.5. Change scores for the Musical Aptitude Profile (retest–baseline *T* scores) for RT, LT, and control groups. Negative numbers represent a decline in performance. MEL, Melody; HAR, Harmony; TEM, Tempo; MET, Meter; PHR, Phrasing; BAL, Balance; STY, Style.

No changes were noted on the Tonal Memory short form for any of the groups. This differed from Milner's (1962) finding of decline after right lobectomy. However, the Tonal Memory short form does appear to have some validity given the lower performance of the RT group compared to controls both before and after surgery.

The effects of ATL were selective with regard to side of surgery and musical process. These results support the role of the right hemisphere in music generally, but differ from previous studies which have mostly pointed to change in tonal (melodic and harmonic) processing. Further studies of localized brain injury and rhythmic and aesthetic processes appears warranted. The similar level of preoperative impairment on the MAP for both RT and LT patients relative to controls indicates an adverse effect of refractory TLE on musical processing independent of lateralization of seizure focus. In view of the reasonably consistent evidence of greater right hemispheric involvement in music processes, for RT patients baseline impairment may represent direct interference in right hemispheric processing, whereas for LT patients baseline deficits may be caused by interference from contralateral LT epileptogenic tissue. It would be of interest to determine whether developmental factors influence change in musical functions, as they do language-mediated functions. Our present RT sample size has not permitted the examination of possible influences of early risk factors in the musical domain. Because we have noted changes related to early insults in visual memory, a function for which the right hemisphere appears specialized, it seems reasonable that music could be similarly affected.

SUMMARY AND CONCLUSIONS

In the beginning of this chapter we described a number of methodological problems that complicate the interpretation of many of the studies; nonetheless, some general conclusions can be drawn regarding previous research on the neuropsychological effects of ATL. A framework of three models was suggested for viewing neuropsychological changes. The models incorporate ipsilateral decline, contralateral improvement, and developmental and hemispheric asymmetry factors.

The largest acute decrements in IQ are reported after LT resection. Usually, there is a return to baseline level of functioning at long-term follow-up. Memory findings have generally supported the ipsilateral decline/contralateral improvement model, with decrements in verbal memory and improvements in nonverbal/visuospatial memory following LT resection and the opposite pattern following RT resection. Some studies have also suggested improvement in nonmemory functions associated with contralateral and ipsilateral extratemporal regions (e.g., psychomotor function). Acute dysnomia may occur after dominant ATL but appears to resolve within 6–12 months after surgery. Relatively little attention has been paid to the effects of ATL on other aspects of language functioning. Nondominant ATL results in declines in some aspects of musical processing, though this effect is mediated by variables such as extent of musical training and nature of the specific musical task.

Attempts to identify preoperative predictors of neuropsychological outcome have yielded inconsistent findings, perhaps because of small sample sizes and other methodological problems. However, it appears that cognitive/memory decline is associated with higher preoperative level of cognitive functioning and late onset of seizures or risk factors; conversely, neuropsychological improvement is associated with seizure-free status after surgery, lower baseline functioning, and history of early risks or seizure onset.

In the second part of the chapter, a series of studies from the Comprehensive Epilepsy Center in Philadelphia were reviewed that address acute (2- to 3-week) postoperative changes in memory, language, and music. A major interest of our group has been the influence of developmental variables, particularly age at first known risk factor and seizure onset, on pre- and postoperative neuropsychological function in adult surgical epilepsy patients. At a general level, the findings from our laboratory on effects of ATL can be summarized as follows:

Before surgery, patients with medically refractory TLE tend to perform below controls on functions ipsilateral and contralateral to their seizure focus. Both LT and RT patients perform less adequately than controls on verbal (language and verbal memory) and nonverbal (visual–spatial memory and musical processing) tests relative to sociodemographically balanced healthy controls. These group differences at baseline assessment may represent generalized effects of seizure disorder associated with multiple factors such as ictal and interictal abnormalities, acute and cumulative effects of medication, interference with education, etc. In addition, developmental factors appear to play a significant role. In our series, the lower baseline performance of TLE patients in IQ scores, memory, and language is primarily accounted for by the patients with evidence of early brain insult, whether seizure onset or other early risks. This tendency of unilateral TLE patients to show bilateral neuropsychological dysfunction complicates preoperative assessment with regard to contributing to diagnostic lateralization, and developmental factors should be considered in clinical interpretation for individual patients.

After surgery, developmental factors take on additional importance as predictors. We have observed an acute decline in function ipsilateral to the side of surgery primarily in patients who do not have early risks. By contrast, contralateral improvement is associated with the presence of early risks as well as with relief from seizures. The ipsilateral decrement and contralateral improvement fit the models of change implicit in much of the recent literature. However, our data suggest that incorporating developmental factors improves prediction. It would therefore be useful if reports of prediction by the ICA procedure and electrical stimulation mapping considered early risk factors. Additionally, evidence that ipsilateral and contralateral effects on memory are more pronounced after left ATL suggests a hemispheric asymmetry in response to surgery. Whether this is an artifact of our ability to measure functions of the right hemisphere requires further investigation.

Future studies of patients undergoing ATL should relate neuropsychological changes, both acute and long-term, to measures of brain anatomy and regional electrophysiological and metabolic activity. Correlation of cognitive changes with data from studies of resected tissue using emerging quantitative histological and neurophysiological techniques is an exciting development that should help to clarify the underlying mechanisms. There is little doubt that models of neuropsychological

286 ANDREW J. SAYKIN *et al.*

change after ATL will be refined as additional predictor and outcome variables are added during the "Decade of the Brain."

ACKNOWLEDGMENTS. We thank Drs. Peter Bridgman, Martha Morrell, Catherine Phillips, and Barbara Watson for help with clinical evaluations of patients; Drs. Raquel Gur and David Mozley for neuropsychiatric screening of normal controls; Drs. Barbara Malamut and Edward Moss and Lyn Harper Mozley, M.S., for their assistance and comments; Drs. Larry Muenz, Helena Kraemer, and Donald Morrison for statistical advice; Dr. Nicholas Gonatas for neuropathological evaluations; and Drs. Fawzi Habboushe and Edwin Gordon for their help with the study of musical processing. This work was supported in part by NIH grant RO1-NS-28813 and NIMH grant MH-43880.

REFERENCES

Benson, D. F. (1979). Neurologic correlates of anomia. In H. Whitaker & H. Whitaker (Eds.), *Studies in neurolinguistics* (pp. 293–328). New York: Academic Press.

Benton, A. L. (1977). The amusias. In M. Critchley & R. A. Henson (Eds.), *Music and the brain* (pp. 378–397). Springfield, Ill.: Charles C. Thomas.

Benton, A. L., & Hamsher, K. deS. (1978). *Multilingual aphasia examination.* Iowa City: University of Iowa.

Berlin, C. I., Chase, R. A., Dill, A., & Hagepanos, T. (1965). Auditory findings in patients with temporal lobectomies. *American Speech and Hearing Association, 7*, 386.

Bever, T. G., & Chiarello, R. F. (1974). Cerebral dominance in musicians and non-musicians. *Science, 185*, 537–539.

Blakemore, C., & Falconer, M. (1967). Long-term effects of anterior temporal lobectomy on certain cognitive functions. *Journal of Neurology, Neurosurgery and Psychiatry, 30*, 364–367.

Bornstein, R., McKean, J., & McLean, D. (1987). Effects of temporal lobectomy for treatment of epilepsy on hemispheric functions ipsilateral to surgery: Preliminary findings. *International Journal of Neuroscience, 37*, 73–78.

Bridgman, P., Malamut, B., Sperling, M. R., Saykin, A. J., & O'Connor, M. J. (1989). Memory during subclinical hippocampal seizures. *Neurology, 39*, 853–856.

Burnstine, T. H., Lesser, R. P., Hart, J., Uematsu, S., Zinreich, S., Krauss, G., Fisher, R., Vining, E., & Gordon, B. (1990). Characterization of the basal temporal language area in patients with left temporal lobe epilepsy. *Neurology, 40*, 966–970.

Carmon, A., Lavy, S., Gordon, H., & Portnoy, Z. (1975). Hemispheric differences in rCBF during verbal and non-verbal tasks. In D. H. Ingvar & N. A. Lassen (Eds.), *Brainwork* (pp. 4414–4423). Copenhagen: Alfred Benzon.

Cavazzuti, V., Winston, K., Baker, R., & Welch, K. (1980). Psychological changes following surgery for tumors in the temporal lobe. *Journal of Neurosurgery, 53*, 618–626.

Chapman, L. J., & Chapman, J. P. (1978). The measurement of differential deficits. *Journal of Psychiatric Research, 14*, 303–311.

Chelune, G. J. (in press). The role of neuropsychological assessment in the presurgical evaluation of the epilepsy surgery candidate. In A. Wyler & B. Hermann (Eds.), *The surgical treatment of epilepsy.* New York: Demos.

Chelune, G. J. (1991). Using neuropsychological data to forecast postsurgical cognitive outcome. In H. Luders (Ed.), *Surgery of epilepsy* (pp. 477–485). New York: Raven Press.

Chelune, G. J., Awad, I. A., & Luders, H. (1989). Verbal memory deficits following temporal lobectomy: Independent or confounded by language? *Epilepsia, 30*, 712.

Chelune, G. J., Naugle, R. I., Luders, H., & Awad, I. A. (in press). Prediction of cognitive change as a function of preoperative ability status among temporal lobectomy patients seen at six-month follow-up. *Neurology*.

Critchley, M. & Henson, R. A. (Eds.). (1977). *Music and the brain*. Springfield, Ill.: Charles C. Thomas.

Cronbach, L. J., & Meehl, P. E. (1955). Construct validity in psychological tests. *Psychological Bulletin*, *52*, 281–302.

Delis, D. C., Kramer, J. H., Kaplan, E., & Ober, B. A. (1983). *California Verbal Learning Test, research ed*. Cleveland, OH: The Psychological Corporation.

Dennis, M. (1988). Language and the young damaged brain. In T. Boll & B. K. Bryant (Eds.), *Clinical neuropsychology and brain function: Research, measurement, and practice* (pp. 89–123). Washington, DC: American Psychological Association.

Dodrill, C. B. (1987). Commentary: Psychological evaluation. In J. Engel (Ed.), *Surgical treatment of the epilepsies* (pp. 197–201). New York: Raven Press.

Dodrill, C. B., Wilkus, R., Ojemann, G., Ward, A., Wyler, A., Van Belle, G., & Tamas, L. (1986). Multidisciplinary prediction of seizure relief from cortical resection surgery. *Annals of Neurology*, *20*, 2–12.

Engel, J. (Ed.). (1987). *Surgical treatment of the epilepsies*. New York: Raven Press.

Engel, J., Ojemann, G. A., Luders, H. O. & Williamson, P. D. (1987). *Fundamental mechanisms of human brain function*. New York: Raven Press.

Eskenazi, B., Cain, W., Novelly, R., & Friend, K. (1983). Olfactory function in temporal lobectomy patients. *Neuropsychologia*, *21*, 365–374.

Gangarosa, M. E., Saykin, A. J., Malamut, B. L., & Gur, R. C. (1988). New scoring systems for Wechsler Memory Scale: Interrater reliability. *Journal of Clinical and Experimental Neuropsychology*, *10*, 43.

Golden, C. J. (1978). *Stroop Color and Word Test: A manual for clinical and experimental uses*. Chicago: Stoelting.

Golden, C. J., Hammeke, T. A., & Purisch, A. D. (1980). *Luria–Nebraska Neuropsychological Battery (manual)*. Los Angeles: Western Psychological Services.

Goodglass, H., & Kaplan, E. (1983). *The assessment of aphasia and related disorders, 2nd ed*. Philadelphia: Lea & Febiger.

Gordon, E. (1965). *The Musical Aptitude Profile (manual)*. New York: Houghton Mifflin.

Gordon, H. W. (1983). Music and the right hemisphere. In A. W. Young (Ed.), *Functions of the right hemisphere* (pp. 65–86). New York: Academic Press.

Gordon, M. (1986). *The Gordon diagnostic system (manual)*. DeWitt, NY: Gordon Systems.

Halgren, E., Wilson, C. L., & Stapleton, J. M. (1985). Human medial temporal lobe stimulation disrupts both formation and retrieval of recent memories. *Brain and Cognition*, *4*, 287–295.

Heaton, R. K. (1981). *Wisconsin Card-Sorting Test (manual)*. Odessa, NY: Psychological Assessment Resources.

Heaton, R. K., Grant, I., & Matthews, C. G. (1986). Differences in neuropsychological test performance associated with age, education and sex. In I. Grant & K. M. Adams (Eds.), *Neuropsychological assessment of neuropsychiatric disorders*. New York: Oxford University Press.

Heilman, K. M., Wilder, B. J., & Malzone, W. F. (1972). Anomic aphasia following anterior temporal lobectomy. *Transactions of the American Neurological Association*, *97*, 291–293.

Heit, G., Smith, M. E., & Halgren, E. (1988). Neural encoding of individual words and faces by the human hippocampus and amygdala. *Nature*, *23*, 773–775.

Henkin, R., Comiter, H., Fedio, P., & O'Doherty, D. (1977). Defects in taste and smell following temporal lobectomy. *Transactions of the American Neurological Association*, *102*, 146–150.

Henschen, S. E. (1926). On the function of the right hemisphere of the brain in relation to the left in speech, music and calculation. *Brain*, *49*, 110–123.

Henschen, S. E., & Schaller, W. F. (1925). Clinical and anatomical contributions on brain pathology. *Archives of Neurological Psychiatry*, *13*, 226–249.

Hermann, B., & Wyler, A. (1988a). Neuropsychological outcome of anterior temporal lobectomy. *Journal of Epilepsy*, *1*, 35–45.

Hermann, B., & Wyler, A. (1988b). Effects of anterior temporal lobectomy on language function: A controlled study. *Annals of Neurology, 23,* 585–588.

Hermann, B., Wyler, A., Steenman, H., & Richey, E. (1988). The interrelationship between language function and verbal learning/memory performance in patients with complex partial seizures. *Cortex, 24,* 245–253.

Ivnik, R. J., Sharbrough, F. W., & Laws, E. R. (1987). Effects of anterior temporal lobectomy on cognitive function. *Journal of Clinical Psychology, 43,* 128–137.

Ivnik, R. J., Sharbrough, F. W., & Laws, E. R. (1988). Anterior temporal lobectomy for control of partial complex seizures: Information for counseling patients. *Mayo Clinic Proceedings, 63,* 783–791.

Jastak, S., & Wilkinson, G. (1984). *Wide Range Achievement Test–Revised (manual).* Wilmington: Jastak Associates.

Javornisky, J. (1981). Neuropsychological and neurological presurgery measures as predictors of memory performance following temporal lobectomy. *Dissertation Abstracts International, 43,* 551.

Johnson, P. (1977). Dichotically-stimulated ear differences in musicians and nonmusicians. *Cortex, 13,* 259–299.

Jones-Gotman, M. (1987). Commentary: Psychological evaluation, testing hippocampal function. In J. Engel (Ed.), *Surgical treatment of the epilepsies* (pp. 203–211). New York: Raven Press.

Kaplan, E. F., Goodglass, H., & Weintraub, S. (1978). *The Boston Naming Test.* Philadelphia: Lea & Febiger.

Keller, L., & Bever, T. (1980). Hemispheric asymmetries in the perception of musical intervals as a function of musical experiences and family handedness background. *Brain and Language, 10,* 24–38.

Kester, D. B., Saykin, A. J., Sperling, M. R., O'Connor, M. J., Robinson, L. J., & Gur, R. C. (1991). Acute effect of anterior temporal lobectomy on musical processing. *Neuropsychologia, 29,* 703–708.

Klove, H., & Matthews, C. (1974). Neuropsychological studies of patients with epilepsy. In R. Reitan & J. Davidson (Eds.), *Clinical neuropsychology* (pp. 237–265). Washington, DC: Winston.

Lee, G. P., Loring, D. W., & Thompson, J. L. (1989). Construct validity of material-specific memory measures following unilateral temporal lobe ablations. *Psychological Assessment: Journal of Consulting and Clinical Psychology, 3,* 192–197.

Liederman, J. (1989). Misconceptions and new conceptions about early brain damage, functional asymmetry, and behavioral outcome. In D. L. Molfese & S. J. Segalowitz (Eds.), *Brain lateralization in children: Developmental implications* (pp. 375–399). New York: Guilford Press.

Loring, D. W., Meador, K. J., Martin, R. C., & Lee, G. P. (1988). Language deficits following unilateral temporal lobectomy. *Journal of Clinical and Experimental Neuropsychology, 11,* 41.

Luders, H. (Ed.). (1991). *Surgery of epilepsy.* New York: Raven Press.

Luria, A. R. (1980). *Higher cortical functions in man.* New York: Basic Books.

Mayeux, R., Brandt, J., Rosen, J., & Benson, F. (1980). Interictal memory and language impairment in temporal lobe epilepsy. *Neurology, 30,* 120–125.

McKee, G., Humphrey, B., & McAdam, D. W. (1973). Scaled lateralization of alpha activity during linguistic and musical tasks. *Psychophysiology, 10,* 441–443.

McMillan, T. M., Powell, G. E., Janota, I., & Polkey, C. E. (1987). Relationships between neuropathology and cognitive functioning in temporal lobectomy patients. *Journal of Neurology, Neurosurgery and Psychiatry, 50,* 167–176.

Meehl, P. (1970). Nuisance variables and the ex post facto design. In M. Radner & S. Winokur (Eds.), *Minnesota studies in the philosophy of science.* Minneapolis: University of Minnesota Press.

Mesulam, M.-M. (1981). A cortical network for directed attention and unliateral neglect. *Annals of Neurology, 10,* 309–325.

Meyer, V. (1959). Cognitive changes following temporal lobectomy for relief of temporal lobe epilepsy. *Archives of Neurology and Psychiatry, 81,* 299–309.

Milner, B. (1962). Laterality effects in audition. In V. B. Mountcastle (Ed.), *Interhemispheric relations and cerebral dominance* (pp. 177–195). Baltimore: Johns Hopkins Press.

Milner, B. (1968). Visual recognition and recall after right-temporal lobe excision in man. *Neuropsychologia, 6,* 191–209.

Milner, B. (1970). Memory and the medial temporal regions of the brain. In K. Pribram & D. Broadbent (Eds.), *Biology of memory* (pp. 29–50). New York: Academic Press.

Milner, B. (1971). Interhemispheric differences in the localization of psychological processes in man. *British Medical Bulletin, 27*, 272–277.

Milner, B. (1975). Psychological aspects of epilepsy and its neurosurgical management. In D. Purpura, J. Penry, & R. Walter (Eds.) *Advances in neurology. Vol. 8* 299–321. New York: Raven Press.

Morrison, D. F. (1976). *Multivariate statistical methods, ed. 2*. New York: McGraw-Hill.

National Association of Epilepsy Centers. (1990). Recommended guidelines for diagnosis and treatment in specialized epilepsy centers. *Epilepsia, 31*(Supplement 1), S1–S12.

National Institutes of Health. (1990). NIH consensus conference: Surgery for epilepsy. *Journal of the American Medical Association, 264*(6), 729–733.

Novelly, R., Augustine, E., Mattson, R., Glaser, G., Williamson, P., Spencer, D., Spencer, S. (1984). Selective memory improvement and impairment in temporal lobectomy for epilepsy. *Annals of Neurology, 15*, 64–67.

Ojemann, G., & Dodrill, C. (1985). Verbal memory deficits after left temporal lobectomy for epilepsy. *Journal of Neurosurgery, 62*, 101–107.

Ojemann, G. A., Creutzfeldt, O., Lettich, E., & Haglund, M. M. (1988). Neuronal activity in human lateral temporal cortex related to short-term verbal memory, naming, and reading. *Brain, 111*, 1383–1403.

Porter, R. J. (1989). Editorial reply. *Annals of Neurology, 25*, 509–510.

Powell, G., Polkey, C., & McMillan, T. (1985). The new Maudsley series of temporal lobectomy. I: Short-term cognitive effects. *British Journal of Clinical Psychology, 24*, 109–124.

Purpura, D. P., Penry, J. K., & Walter, R. D. (1975). *Neurosurgical management of the epilepsies (Advances in neurology, Vol. 8.)* New York: Raven Press.

Rasmussen, T. (1983). Surgical treatment of complex partial seizures: Results, lessons, and problems. *Epilepsia, 24*(Supplement 1), S65–S76.

Rausch, R. (1987). Psychological evaluation. In J. Engel (Ed.), *Surgical treatment of the epilepsies* (pp. 181–195). New York: Raven Press.

Rausch, R., & Crandall, P. H. (1982). Psychological status related to surgical control of temporal lobe seizures. *Epilepsia, 23*, 191–202.

Rausch, R., Serafetinides, E., & Crandall, P. (1977). Olfactory memory in patients with anterior temporal lobectomy. *Cortex, 13*, 445–452.

Reitan, R., & Wolfson, D. (1985). *The Halstead–Reitan Neuropsychological Test Battery: Theory and clinical interpretation*. Tucson, AZ: Neuropsychology Press.

Russell, E. W. (1975). A multiple scoring method for assessment of complex memory functions. *Journal of Consulting and Clinical Psychology, 43*, 800–809.

Saeveit, J. G., Lewis, D., & Seashore, C. G. (1940). Revision of the Seashore Tests of Musical Talent. *University of Iowa Aims Progressive Research, 65*, (whole issue).

Samson, S., & Zatorre, R. (1988). Melodic and harmonic discrimination following unilateral cerebral excision. *Brain and Cognition, 7*, 348–360.

SAS Institute. (1987). *SAS/STAT software, version 6.03*. Cary, NC: SAS Institute.

Saykin, A. J., Gur, R. C., Sussman, N. M., Gur, R. E., & O'Connor, M. J. (1989). Memory before and after temporal lobectomy: Effects of laterality and age of onset. *Brain and Cognition, 9*, 191–200.

Saykin, A. J., Sperling, M. R., Reinecke, L. J., Kester, D. B., O'Connor, M. J., Watson, B., Gur, R. C. (1990). Neuropsychological prediction of seizure outcome in anterior temporal lobectomy candidates. *Journal of Clinical and Experimental Neuropsychology, 12*, 71.

Saykin, A. J., Gur, R. C., Gur, R. E., Mozley, P. D., Mozley, L. H., Resnick, S. M., Kester, D. B., Stafiniak, P. (1991). Neuropsychological function in schizophrenia: Selective impairment in memory and learning. *Archives of General Psychiatry, 48*, 618–624.

Saykin, A. J., Sperling, M. R., Robinson, L. J., Stafiniak, P., Kester, D. B., Gur, R. C., O'Connor, M. J. (submitted). Memory changes after anterior temporal lobectomy: Relation to early risk factors, seizure outcome, and pathology.

Saykin, A. J., Stafiniak, P., Robinson, L. J., Gur, R. C., O'Connor, M. J., Sperling, M. R. (in press). Language before and after temporal lobectomy: Specificity of acute changes and relation to early risk factors. *Epilepsia*.

Shankweiler, D. (1966). Effects of temporal-lobe damage on perception of dichotically presented melodies. *Journal of Comparative and Physiological Psychology*, *62*, 115–119.

Sperling, M. R., & O'Connor, M. J. (1989). Comparison of depth and subdural electrodes in recording temporal lobe seizures. *Neurology*, *39*, 1497–1504.

Stafiniak, P., Saykin, A. J., Sperling, M. R., Kester, D. B., Robinson, L. J., O'Connor, M. J., & Gur, R. C. (1990). Acute naming deficits following dominant temporal lobectomy: Prediction by age at 1st risk for seizures. *Neurology*, *40*, 1509–1512.

Stafiniak, P., Saykin, A. J., Sperling, M. R., Robinson, L. J., Gur, R. C., O'Connor, M. J. (submitted). Recovery from anomia after dominant temporal lobectomy: A 1 year follow-up.

Stanulis, R. G., & Valenstein, R. J. (1988). Material-specific memory deficits: Language or memory? *Epilepsia*, *29*, 681.

Sullivan, E. B., & Gahagan, L. (1935). On intelligence of epileptic children. *Genetic Psychology Monograph*, *17*, 309–376.

Teuber, H.-L. (1955). Physiological psychology. *Annual Review of Psychology*, *6*, 267–296.

Wechsler, D. (1945). A standardized memory scale for clinical use. *Journal of Psychology*, *19*, 87–95.

Wechsler, D. (1981). *Wechsler Adult Intelligence Scale–Revised, manual*. Cleveland, OH: The Psychological Corporation.

Wieser, H. G. (1988). Selective amygdalo-hippocampectomy for temporal lobe epilepsy. *Epilepsia*, *29* (Supplement 2), 100–113.

Zatorre, R. J. (1984). Musical perception and cerebral function: A critical overview. *Music Perception*, *2*, 196–221.

Zatorre, R. J. (1985). Discrimination and recognition of tonal melodies after unilateral cerebral excisions. *Neuropsychologia*, *23*, 31–41.

14

The Neuropsychology of Corpus Callosotomy for Epilepsy

\or "Split Brain" Operation

KIMBERLEE J. SASS, SUSAN S. SPENCER,
MICHAEL WESTERVELD, and DENNIS D. SPENCER

Corpus callosotomy as a palliative treatment for medically refractory epilepsy is an uncommon neurosurgical procedure. It is performed when no resectable seizure focus is identified and isolation of ictal seizure phenomena to one hemisphere would lead to a significant diminution of personal injury risk and/or an appreciable increase in adaptive function. Most patients tolerate the procedure well, but mild declines in isolated areas of function are common, and severe declines can sometimes occur (Campbell, Bogen, & Smith, 1981; Gur, Gur, Sussman, O'Connor, & Vey, 1984; Novelly & Lifrak, 1985; Rayport, Ferguson, & Corrie, 1984; Sass, Novelly, Spencer, & Spencer, 1987, 1990; Sass, Spencer, Novelly, & Spencer, 1988b; Sass, Spencer, Spencer, Novelly, Williamson, & Mattson, 1988a; Sass, Westerveld, Novelly, Spencer, & Spencer, 1989).

Postcallosotomy functional declines occur because surgical disconnection isolates language to one hemisphere and interrupts callosally mediated compensatory mechanisms. When the brain develops normally, the two cerebral hemispheres become functionally dissimilar. One hemisphere, typically the left, becomes dominant for language and motor function. The other becomes proficient in visual–spatial information processing. When the cerebral hemispheres are surgically disconnected, language is isolated from aspects of visual–spatial function and motor control of one side of the body. The resulting changes in function are predictable.

Central nervous system disease or injury may permanently arrest the neural

KIMBERLEE J. SASS, MICHAEL WESTERVELD, and DENNIS D. SPENCER • Section of Neurological Surgery, Department of Surgery, Yale University School of Medicine, New Haven, Connecticut 06510. SUSAN S. SPENCER • Department of Neurology, Yale University School of Medicine, New Haven, Connecticut 06510.

The Neuropsychology of Epilepsy, edited by Thomas L. Bennett. Plenum Press, New York, 1992.

development that mediates functional specificity, but overt behavior may be disrupted only for a short time. The reestablished behaviors reflect functional reorganization of the cerebral hemispheres. Functional reorganization may be intrahemispheric or interhemispheric in nature. Surgical disconnection will disrupt interhemispheric compensatory mechanisms. If functional reorganization, like normal development, is governed by rules that are ultimately discernable, the behavioral sequelae of cerebral disconnection also may be predictable, even when disease has caused significant functional reorganization of the cerebral hemispheres. This chapter presents a model for predicting the behavioral outcome of corpus callosotomy and the empirical data from which this model was developed.

NEUROPSYCHOLOGICAL OUTCOME OF CALLOSOTOMY

Altered neuropsychological function following corpus callosotomy can be attributed to four etiologies: (1) surgical practices (complications and neighborhood effects); (2) disconnection phenomena (transient and chronic); (3) interruption of longstanding compensatory mechanisms; and (4) altered seizure control. Some deficits (e.g., those attributable to surgical practices) are unpredictable, and others (e.g., disconnection phenomena) occur reliably. Methods for predicting impairments attributable to interruption of longstanding compensatory mechanisms and altered seizure control are being developed. Although impairments that originate from these different sources are discussed separately in the following sections, they typically do not appear in isolation.

Surgical Complications and Neighborhood Effects

Discussion of surgically induced neurological impairments during corpus callosum section is rare in the related literature. There have been no controlled studies relating surgical variables (e.g., duration and intensity of retraction) and neurological outcome. However, numerous events, planned (e.g., ligating arteries) and unplanned (e.g., venous infarction), can alter neurological functioning. During exposure and section, the surgeon encounters the sagittal sinus, bridging veins, pericallosal artery, callosal marginal artery, anterior cerebral artery, and its branches. Manipulation of the mesial aspect of the cerebral hemispheres can result in infarction or intraparenchymal hemorrhage if the cerebral vasculature is disturbed. Intraventricular collections of even small amounts of blood can cause obstructive hydrocephalus. If the surgical procedure involves an intraventricular approach, the hypothalamus can be affected by manipulation within the ventricle. Posteriorly, the thin fibers of the hippocampal commissure abut those of the corpus callosum, and the fornical bodies lie in close proximity. Infection is also possible. The neuropsychological literature contains reports of ventriculitis, meningitis, obstructive hydrocephalus, and death following cerebral disconnection. These complications have been avoided in recent series, but hematoma, isolated venous infarction, and wound infection still occur.

In addition to these surgical complications, focal areas of injury can occur to adjacent structures. The retraction that provides access to the callosum can injure the paracallosal brain structures (e.g., cingulate gyrus, fornix, and hypothalamus) mechanically or through vascular compromise. The most common are injuries that occur to the cortical area representing motor control of the leg, the cingulate and the fornical bodies.

Since its development, the surgical procedure has been revised many times to minimize complications. The one-stage commissurotomy involving the entire corpus callosum, hippocampal commissure, one limb of the fornix, and the anterior commissure (Wilson's first series) was found to have a high rate of complication. As a result, Wilson modified the procedure for his second series of patients. He tried frontal commissurotomy, which included the anterior commissure and the rostral half of the corpus callosum. Subsequently, he introduced a two-stage division of the corpus callosum and hippocampal commissure using an extraventricular approach. Although this modification represented a significant improvement, the procedure was refined even further by Spencer, who introduced lateral patient positioning, which allowed gravity to facilitate exposure of the corpus callosum and minimized the need for retraction.

Disconnection Phenomena (Acute and Chronic)

Immediately following surgery, a number of signs of impaired neurological function appear, some of which abate rapidly, whereas others persist indefinitely. These impairments, which occur to some degree in most patients, are distinguished from the interruption of interhemispheric recovery mechanisms (discussed below) which occurs in only some patients. Disconnection phenomena vary depending on the disconnection procedures.

Acute Disconnection

"Acute disconnection phenomena" refer to an ill-defined number of pathognomonic signs that appear immediately after surgery and variously include mutism, akinesia or apathy, unilateral weakness, forced grasping, buccofacial apraxia, fixed gaze, and disinhibition. These signs are highly variable and depend in part on the surgical procedure. They are more common following forebrain commissurotomy, which involves section of the anterior commissure, corpus callosum, and hippocampal commissure. They occur less often after total callosotomy, which spares the anterior commissure and permits transfer of the caudal orbitofrontal and rostral temporal fibers. If portions of the hippocampal commissure are spared, transfer of information occurs between medial temporal areas. Acute disconnection phenomena are sometimes absent entirely following anterior two-thirds callosotomy, which spares connections from the posterior parietal cortex, superior temporal and inferotemporal cortex, insula, and occipital cortex.

The etiology of acute disconnection phenomena is unproven, but many assume they are caused by retraction. Novelly and Lifrak (1985) argued against the retraction hypothesis with regard to unilateral weakness. They reviewed prior reports (Bogen, 1969; Geoffroy, Lassonde, Delisle, & Decarie, 1983) and concluded that "the occurrence of left upper limb paresis/motor dyspraxia in these patients reflects the effect, not of retraction acting in isolation, but of the severing of the commissures in the presence of a prior structural lesion in the right hemisphere." Data from the Yale Epilepsy Surgery Program support the conclusion that some patients with focal injury of the neocortex incur permanent declines in motor function after callosotomy (discussed in detail later in this chapter). However, the permanence of these declines suggests that they differ in etiology from the transient unilateral weakness that is much more common. Transient unilateral weakness in patients without focal areas of neocortical injury favors the retraction hypothesis as an explanation for this acute disconnection phenomenon.

Mutism and akinesia are rarely observed following anterior callosotomy or staged total callosotomy. Bogen (1979) suggested that, when present, mutism was a transient reaction to the disorganization of cognitive processes ordinarily coordinated by interhemispheric communication through the corpus callosum. Wilson, Reeves, Gazzaniga, and Culver (1977) agreed that the interruption of interhemispheric communication was important to the etiology of mutism and akinesia but argued that retraction was equally important, suggesting that these factors interacted. Currently there is no accepted model for predicting acute disconnection phenomena.

Chronic Disconnection

"Chronic disconnection phenomena" refer to behavioral abnormalities that result not from cortical injury but from isolation of neural input, information-processing, and/or output systems. This isolation has been demonstrated in many combinations of sensory–motor channels. The basic paradigm involves demonstration that (1) information selectively presented to one hemisphere cannot be acted on by the other hemisphere; (2) by using a response that is within the behavioral repertoire of the stimulated hemisphere, knowledge of the information can be demonstrated; (3) there is no paresis or sensory defect that could account for the phenomena. Several examples follow.

Input Requiring a Verbal or Written Response. Following corpus callosum section, a patient may be unable to name a common object placed in the hand ipsilateral to the speech-dominant hemisphere, but, using that hand, he may choose the correct item from among several others. He may be unable to name which of the fingers of the nondominant hand have been touched or manipulated, but he may correctly identify the digits by using the thumb on the same hand. He may be unable to identify odors selectively presented to the nostril ipsilateral to the nondominant hemisphere, but, using the nondominant hand, he may be able to select from a group of items the one having that odor. When different words are presented simultaneously to each ear, the patient may only identify the one presented contralateral to the dominant hemisphere.

He may be unable to write spontaneously or to take dictation with the hand ipsilateral to the speech-dominant hemisphere. He may be unable to read words presented to the hemifield contralateral to the nondominant hemisphere. He may be unable to follow commands with his nondominant hand but can perform the behavior requested when imitated.

Input Requiring Analysis of Complex Visual Information. The patient may experience considerably more difficulty reproducing graphic stimuli with the hand ipsilateral to the nondominant hemisphere. This includes drawing geometric forms and building objects. Also, difficulty can occur with tasks that require a verbal response to visual stimuli (e.g., picture completion).

Lateralized Input Requiring a Motor Response by a Contralateral Limb. When one hand is posed, the patient may be unable to reproduce its configuration with the contralateral limb. While holding an object in one hand, the patient may be unable to select the same item from a group of facsimiles using the other hand. When one hand is touched, the patient may not be able to identify the location of the stimulation with the opposite hand.

Observation of Intermanual Conflict. Following callosotomy, it is not uncommon to observe a patient begin to perform a task with one hand only to have the other hand interrupt or attempt to alter the performance. This occurs most frequently during dressing, when a patient will button a shirt with one hand and simultaneously unbutton it with the other. Patients report that this process can occur for 10 min or more. Other examples reported by our patients include reaching into a drawer with one hand, only to have the other hand close the drawer. They have reported that when rising from a chair to walk, one side of the body may resist, causing them to fall back into the chair. Less commonly, actual physical conflict between the hands is observed. Typically this occurs in response to a situation of intermanual conflict. As one hand begins to disrupt the work of the other, the latter grabs or strikes the former. The situation is sometimes resolved by the dominant hand securing the nondominant hand and forcing it under the nondominant leg. As a further variant of this phenomenon, the patient develops a conscious disregard for the nondominant limb. It is not uncommon in such situations to observe the patient insulting aloud his nondominant side.

Failure to Demonstrate Disconnection Phenomena. If surgical disconnection was complete and absolute, patients would be expected to perform at the level of chance during the paradigms described in the preceding sections. Frequently, patients perform with limited success on tasks where total failure would be predicted on the basis of surgical disconnection. There are several explanations for the failure to demonstrate disconnection phenomena. The first is that disconnection phenomena are most common after forebrain commissurotomy. Total callosotomy spares the anterior commissure, permitting information transfer of the caudal orbitofrontal and rostral temporal areas. Also, many surgeons use an extraventricular approach to the callosum. This does not permit visualization of the landmarks that identify the furthest extent of the callosum. As a result, the surgeon may inadvertently spare a small portion of the anterior and posterior fibers. Sparing even a small portion of callosum will avoid many disconnection phenomena. When callosotomy is limited to the anterior two-thirds, interhemispheric communication in all three modalities (i.e., vision, hearing, touch) is routinely demonstrated.

Studies of patients with seizure disorders suggest that the amount of control over the ipsilateral limb, the degree of language representation within the nondominant hemisphere, and the visual–spatial capabilities of the dominant hemisphere vary considerably. Therefore, it is not safe to assume that behaviors are represented in their normal cortical areas. Early-onset CNS injury may result in development of behavior, such as language comprehension, in areas where it is not normally resident. This may foil attempts to isolate stimuli to areas where such information is not processed normally.

Patient considerations are also important in evaluating disconnection phenomena. Longstanding brain dysfunction or neighborhood damage at the time of surgery may leave the patient without the abilities to perform the sophisticated tasks by which disconnection phenomena are revealed. Isolation of neural input to a single hemisphere, which is a requirement for the demonstration of many disconnection phenomena, is occasionally accomplished by tachistoscopic or dichotic listening devices. Fully one-third of our sample obtained Full-Scale IQ indices of less than 80 prior to surgery. Complicated testing procedures are not adequately completed by these patients. Similarly, the directions for tasks used to reveal disconnection phenomena are primarily verbal in nature. Yet, it is generally accepted that the comprehension of complex verbal information, such as paragraph-length instructions, is a function of the dominant hemisphere. Not all patients can extrapolate enough information from the instructions to perform the given tasks with their nondominant limbs.

Finally, patients can be adept in the use of secondary cues when performing the tasks noted above. For example, when asked to identify an object placed in a nondominant hand, the patient may drop the object to the table, producing a sound that is helpful in identifying the object. They may press the object tightly into their hands, producing a painful sensation, which is projected both ipsilaterally and contralaterally. Through this painful stimulation, information about the general structure of the object (e.g., whether or not it has corners) can be transmitted to the ipsilateral hemisphere. Such "cross-cuing," provides a means of extracallosal information transfer.

Interruption of Longstanding Compensatory Mechanisms

In addition to disconnection phenomena, some patients incur declines in neurological function attributal to the interruption of compensatory mechanisms that are maintained by the callosum. Campbell *et al.* (1981) first reported declines in visuospatial processing after callosotomy for patients who had right hemisphere structural abnormalities. They concluded that the left hemisphere facilitated recovery from a right hemisphere injury through compensatory mechanisms mediated by the callosum. With callosotomy, the compensatory mechanisms were interrupted, and deficits associated with right hemisphere dysfunction appeared. This phenomenon was referred to as reinstatement.

Subsequently, the notion of reinstatement was refined by Novelly and Lifrak (1985), who demonstrated that impairments indicative of focal injury sometimes followed callosotomy in patients with no structural lesions. Conversely, some patients with structural lesions show minimal postoperative deficits and occasionally improvements. They suggest that recovery after seizure onset could involve compensatory mechanisms that were totally within the ipsilateral hemisphere, totally within the contralateral hemisphere, or interhemispheric. Callosotomy would cause declines only when compensatory mechanisms were interhemispheric.

Because interhemispheric compensatory mechanisms (ICMs) cannot be demonstrated directly, it has been difficult to provide empirical support for the contention that interruption of such mechanisms causes many of the permanent declines observed after callosotomy. The majority of research in this area has focused on the identification of anomalous clinical findings that predict postsurgical declines and appear to represent markers of ICMs.

The hypothesis that anomalous clinical findings may identify ICMs was proposed by Sass et al. (1988a) in a review of Yale's initial callosal series. Sass reported the neurological and neuropsychological outcome for the initial 22 patients. Three mentally retarded patients were unable to complete the neuropsychological examination, and one additional patient was lost to follow-up. These factors reduced the sample size to 18 patients.

Before and after surgery, these patients underwent an examination tailored to their individual needs and abilities. Virtually all of them were examined using the following measurement instruments: hand dynamometer, Lafayette Pegbord, Speech Sounds Perception Test, Controlled Word Production Test, Russell adaptation of the Wechsler Memory Scale, and the Wechsler Adult Intelligence Scale. A T-score transformation was performed, using data obtained from a larger group of neurologically impaired patients who completed the same measures. Gender effects were controlled during T-score transformation of motor scores. A composite index was obtained by calculating the mean of these scores.

The good-outcome group included patients whose postsurgical gains equaled or exceeded losses (i.e., mean postsurgical change in T-scores equal to or greater than 0). The fair-outcome group included patients whose postsurgical losses exceeded gains, but whose degree of change was mild (i.e., mean postsurgical change in T-scores was between -0.1 and -4.9). The poor-outcome group included patients whose postsurgical losses exceeded gains, and whose average degree of change was at least moderate (mean postsurgical declines in T-scores exceeded 5.0).

When these patients were grouped according to age of seizure onset and degree of CNS impairment, several important relationships were identified. All patients with poor outcome had seizure onset after age 6 years. In contrast, 7 of 11 patients with good outcome had seizure onset prior to age 6 years. Patients with early-onset left hemisphere disease of significant proportion such that the right hemisphere became dominant for speech, memory was absent in the left hemisphere during IAP examination, the left hand became preferred for writing, and the right upper extremity became paretic reliably obtained good outcome. Improvements were also common in patients with normal strength or mild hemiparesis and bilateral memory on the intracarotid amobarbital test. These two types of patients, those with severe lateralized injury that occurs well before age 6 years (see Case 1 of the illustrative cases reviewed at the end of this chapter) and those with minimal CNS dysfunction that is associated with no anomalous clinical findings (see Illustrative Case 2) were hypothesized to have developed without interhemispheric compensatory mechanisms. Recovery in the severely impaired patients appears to be mediated by the hemisphere contralateral to the injury. Mildly impaired patients appear to recover by ipsilateral mechanisms.

A third group of patients, in whom declines were common, consisted of those with anomalous clinical findings. Patients whose language-dominant hemisphere was ipsilateral to the dominant hand had significant language impairments following callosotomy. Postoperative sequelae for right hemisphere speech-dominant, right-handed individuals included verbal dysfluency, dysnomia, conductive dysphasia, and alexia with or without agraphia (see Illustrative Case 3). In these patients, who all had signs of left hemisphere dysfunction, recovery of language functions appeared to be mediated by the interaction of the two hemispheres. In contrast, the postoperative impairment in the single left hemisphere dominant, left-handed patient was limited to dysgraphia. This latter impairment did not appear to represent the interruption of interhemispheric compensatory supports for writing but occurred because the speech-dominant hemisphere was isolated from the hemisphere dominant for manual abilities.

Further exploring the significance of anomalous clinical findings, Sass *et al.* (1989) reported that the failure to demonstrate memory capabilities in the left hemisphere during the intracarotid amobarbital procedure (IAP) in right hemisphere speech-dominant patients was associated with a significant postoperative decline in upper extremity motor function. Nine patients with right hemisphere speech dominance were studied before and after callosotomy, using a hand dynamometer to measure strength. Two of these patients, who both had normal strength prior to surgery, demonstrated memory in their left hemisphere during IAP examination. Of the remaining seven, all of whom failed to demonstrated memory in the left hemisphere during IAP examination, one was densely hemiparetic, three were mildly hemiparetic, and three had average strength. After surgery, the two patients with intact left hemisphere memory and one densely hemiparetic patient were unchanged. Patients with mild hemiparesis developed dense right hemiparesis, but the left side was unchanged. Patients with average strength prior to surgery incurred motor declines bilaterally. Declines in upper extremity motor function also occurred in left speech-dominant patients, but these were not predicted by the failure to demonstrate memory from the right hemisphere or the presence of mild hemiparesis prior to surgery (see Illustrative Case 4).

Effects of Altered Seizure Control

Even though surgical procedures differ, seizure control is similar. Seventy to 80% of patients enjoy control of secondarily generalized seizures. After total callosotomy, complex partial seizures are also controlled in 25–50% of patients. A few patients are cured, and several (25% in most series) have more intense partial seizures (simple or complex) postsurgically. More intense focal seizures (MIFS) have included violent unilateral or bilateral asymmetric tonic and/or clonic activity, intense body rotation, fear during the motor activity, prolonged duration, postictal hemiparesis, and severe headache (Spencer, Spencer, Glaser, Williamson, Mattson, 1984). An extensive literature documents behavioral impairments associated with epileptic foci; therefore, it is reasonable to hypothesize that poor seizure control, particularly the occurrence of more intense partial seizures, may impair neuropsychological function.

Sass *et al.* (1988b) investigated the relationship of seizure outcome and memory difficulties following corpus callosotomy. Seven patients studied had only partial seizures after surgery. Four had simple and complex partial seizures, and nine continued to have generalized seizures. These patients completed the logical memory and visual reproduction sections of the Wechsler Memory Scale and subtests comprising the Attention/Concentration factor of the Wechsler Adult Intelligence Scale (Digit Span, Arithmetic, Digit Symbol). Three factor indices, representing attention, verbal memory, and visual memory, were computed using factor scores derived from analyses of a larger comparison group of neurologically impaired patients who completed the same measures. No significant changes in memory were related to seizure classification. However, when patients who did not have MIFS ($n = 15$) were contrasted with those who did ($n = 6$), a statistically significant improvement in visual memory was observed postoperatively for the former group only. This suggests that improved seizure control can enhance memory function.

THEORETICAL CONSIDERATIONS

The findings of postcallosotomy studies suggest that some postsurgical functional declines are unavoidable (e.g., acute and chronic disconnection phenomena) or unpredictable (e.g., surgical complications), but others can be predicted from the patient's presentation (e.g., interruption of ICMs). The demonstration that variability in surgical outcome is predicted by anomalous clinical findings has implications regarding the brain's accommodation of focal injury. Specifically, this implies that recovery from focal injury to one hemisphere sometimes depends on acquisition of new behaviors by the other, but at other times this does not occur. Deriving a model from the callosotomy data that accounts for this variability and generates specific predictions regarding callosotomy outcome requires identification of those cases in which functions are acquired by the hemisphere that is congenitally nondominant for that function. Selecting such cases with a high degree of confidence is difficult, however. Even though the right hemisphere may be dominant for visual–spatial function, these abilities are present bilaterally. A relative improvement in visual–spatial ability of the hemisphere congenitally nondominant for such function is virtually impossible to identify. Similarly, the transfer of manual dominance can be difficult to detect, since left-handedness can occur as a natural variant in healthy individuals. Because language is mediated by the left hemisphere in virtually all right-handed adults and the majority of left-handed adults, the demonstration of right hemisphere speech dominance, particularly in patients with history of left hemisphere disease, is a compelling sign of cortical reorganization of functions. Therefore, the model of the brain's accommodation of focal injury initially focused on right hemisphere speech-dominant patients. This model indicates that the nature of language recovery after focal injury is age dependent, but recovery of motor skills may not be.

Age-Related Changes in Language Recovery following CNS Injury

Critical Phase I: Birth to First Utterance

Before the child makes his first utterance at about the age of 1 year, both cerebral hemispheres appear to be capable of mediating language. This conclusion is suggested by studies of hemispherectomy performed on patients whose disease began prior to age 1 year and who were left with hemiplegia. Although a few infantile hemiplegics obtained normal levels of functioning in all areas, they were typically spared the information-specific impairments expressed by hemispherectomy patients who were not hemiplegic since infancy. The capacity of one hemisphere to acquire the abilities of the other at a level equivalent to those abilities typically mediated by the intact hemisphere appears to end when language develops.

Critical Phase II: First Utterance to Age 6 Years

The development of language is hypothesized to provoke the specialization of visual–spatial abilities in the contralateral hemisphere. With the development of visual–spatial capabilities, the neural circuitry available for language acquisition diminishes. From the time the child utters his or her first word until the next critical period, focal injury may encourage the development of the abilities by the contralateral hemisphere, but the development will be imperfect.

Critical Phase III: Age 6 Years to 12 Years

By the age of 6 years, the lateralization of language is well established. After this time, a lesion within the dominant hemisphere will not provoke acquisition of language by the nondominant hemisphere as a primary source of recovery. Instead, language functions appear to be maintained by intrahemispheric transfer. The mechanics remain obscure, however.

Critical Phase IV: 13 Years through Adulthood

Extensive evaluation of adults following corpus callosum section suggests that behavioral competence continues to develop through adulthood. Studies of the lateralization of language demonstrated continued development in receptive capabilities by the nondominant hemisphere, but expressive capabilities remain limited. It is probably fair to conclude that in the adult bisected brain, capabilities already possessed by the disconnected hemisphere continue to develop in degree, but no new behavioral competencies are acquired. Therefore, recovery of damage to language mechanisms after puberty is hypothesized to be mediated by ipsilateral cortical areas (see Illustrative Case 5).

Absence of Age-Related Changes in Recovery of Motor Skills

If the processes that mediated language recovery were similar to those that mediated recovery of motor skills, motor declines after callosotomy would be common for those whose injury occurred after age 6 and before puberty. However, the data indicate that some patients with injuries that occurred at birth suffered motor declines after surgery. Conversely, BB (Illustrative Case 3), who developed seizures at age 8 years and had a severe decline in language abilities, did not decline in motor skills. Instead, motor declines were predicted by the severity of the injury, as evidenced by the degree of hemiparesis and the memory findings of the IAP. Right hemisphere speech-dominant patients with average strength and adequate memory in the left hemisphere did not decline after surgery. Nor did those with absent left memory and severe hemiparesis. Right hemisphere speech-dominant patients with mild hemiparesis and absent left hemisphere memory evidenced a unilateral decline. Those with average strength and absent left hemisphere memory declined bilaterally. These findings suggest a dissociation of language and motor findings. Furthermore, they suggest that different variables may be important in functional reorganization. Specifically, language recovery appears to be age related, but motor recovery appears to be related to the severity of the injury.

ILLUSTRATIVE CASES

Illustrative Case 1

PD was a 39-year-old left-hand-dominant Caucasian female whose birth was uneventful. At 6 months of age, she developed a dense right hemiparesis. Her seizures began at age 6 years. Computed tomographic scanning showed a low-density lesion in the left temporal area, which probably represented an old infarct. The intracarotid amobarbital procedure documented right hemisphere speech dominance, intact right memory, and absent left memory.

In addition to a dense right hemiparesis, this patient exhibited moderate left (dominant) upper extremity motor impairments, impaired visual perception, poor visual and verbal memory, and intellectual impairment (VIQ = 86; PIQ = 78). Total callosotomy was accomplished in two stages without complication. Six years post-surgery, this patient exhibited improved left upper extremity motor function and improved visual perception. Intellectual functions did not change substantially. Verbal memory mildly declined.

This patient with severe lateralized neurological deficit, characterized by dense right hemiparesis, right speech dominance, and absent left memory on IAP examination, incurred no more than a mild decline in verbal memory following total callosotomy. A number of abilities typically mediated by the right hemisphere improved following surgery. The source of the improvements is speculative, but the most plausible explanation is that the more intact right hemisphere was isolated from the left and spared the negative consequences of frequent seizure activity. In this patient, the right hemisphere appears to have completely acquired behaviors ordinarily mediated by the left hemisphere (e.g., language and manual dominance). Since it acquired them completely, the callosum was divided with no alteration in function.

Illustrative Case 2

JL was a 23-year-old right-hand-dominant Caucasian male whose birth and development were unremarkable. He completed high school and joined the Air Force at age 18 years. While playing flag football, he collided with another player and lacerated his head in the left parietal area. A few weeks later, his seizures began. Radiographic examination (CT and MRI) was normal. The intracarotid amobarbital procedure showed left hemisphere speech dominance and adequate memory bilaterally. Interictal EEG showed a preponderance of left frontal abnormalities. Ictal scalp EEG was characterized by high-amplitude paroxysmal activity that was bilaterally synchronous and frontally predominant.

Neuropsychological examination showed mild bilateral motor impairments, an isolated visual perceptual deficit involving face recognition, intact speech and language, and intact visual memory. Verbal information acquisition was moderately impaired, and verbal intellectual functions were relatively inferior (VIQ = 92; PIQ = 102).

The patient underwent anterior two-thirds corpus callosotomy, which resulted in a significant improvement in seizure control. Six months following surgery, neuro-psychological examination revealed precisely the same findings as seen prior to surgery, with the exception of a mild improvement in verbal memory.

This case involves a patient with a later age of seizure onset (18 years), who presented with no signs of anomalous cortical organization. He was left speech dominant, demonstrated memory bilaterally, and had average motor function in both upper extremities. He tolerated anterior callosotomy with no increased deficit.

Illustrative Case 3

Patient BB was a right-hand-dominant Caucasian male, the product of a normal pregnancy and high forceps delivery. He achieved developmental milestones at normal ages. Seizures began at age 8 years in the absence of a clear precipitating event. A CT scan, angiography, visual fields, and physical examination were unremarkable. The intracarotid amobarbital procedure documented right hemisphere speech dominance and adequate memory in each hemisphere. Surface EEG demonstrated bitemporal and right occipital spike foci and left hemisphere slowing. Depth electrode study documented seizures originating from both occipital areas and the left temporal lobe.

Neuropsychological examination documented a mild dysnomia and verbal memory difficulties, but his speech was clear. Phoneme perception (i.e., speech sounds perception) and written language skills were within normal limits. At age 16 years, his written language age equivalents were as follows: reading recognition 15 years 1 month; reading comprehension 15 years 3 months; spelling 16 years 4 months. Impaired nonverbal reasoning was observed (Verbal IQ = 94: Performance IQ = 86), a paradoxical finding reported for many right hemisphere speech-dominant males whose seizures begin during later childhood.

Because seizure foci were present bilaterally, and these involved a prominent occipital component, the patient underwent posterior two-thirds corpus callosotomy. The CT demonstrated no postsurgical abnormalities.

Four months following posterior callosotomy, neuropsychological examination documented mild declines in some language functions. Speech and confrontational naming were unchanged, but phoneme comprehension was impaired, and written language skills had declined (reading recognition) 10 years 7 months; reading comprehension 10 years 11 months; spelling 13 years 3 months). Verbal memory was unchanged, but intellectual functions declined (VIQ = 75: PIQ = 77).

After surgery, the EEG demonstrated frequent independent spikes in the left occipital, right occipital, and temporal areas. Daily seizures continued, so the patient underwent anterior callosotomy 7 months after the initial operation.

Sixteen months following total callosotomy, changes were apparent in the patient's speech and writing. When speaking, agrammatisms were common. He used the wrong tense for verbs and often used plural nouns when singular nouns were appropriate. Less difficulty was observed for repetition. Common phrases were repeated adequately, and repetition of uncommon phrases was only intermittently impaired. Writing was laborious and impaired for paragraph-length material but intact for simple phrases.

Other areas of language were unchanged by the completion of the surgery. Verbal comprehension was intact for simple phrases and only mildly impaired for complex material. Phoneme comprehension and confrontational naming were unchanged. Measures of reading and spelling remained below the presurgical base line, but they were no worse than after partial section (reading recognition 12 years 6 months; reading comprehension 12 years 5 months; spelling 12 years 2 months).

Neither memory nor intellectual functions declined after completion of the callosotomy (Verbal IQ = 75; Performance IQ = 76; Full-Scale IQ = 74).

For Patient BB, each surgical procedure appeared to affect language functions. Section of the splenium affected receptive abilities (e.g., phoneme comprehension, reading recognition, reading comprehension, spelling) and intellectual functions. Anterior section affected expressive functions (speech and writing) without further impairment of receptive functions or intelligence. Interested readers can refer to a more complete summary of language impairments following callosotomy (Sass *et al.*, 1990).

Like Patient PD (Case 1), BB probably developed right hemisphere speech dominance because of injury to his left hemisphere. However, these patients differ along the dimensions of the severity of their CNS dysfunction and the age at which it occurred. PD was densely hemiparetic since age 6 months and had no memory within the left hemisphere on IAP examination. BB had relatively normal development to age 8 years, normal strength in both upper extremities, and memory in both hemispheres during IAP examination. PD's recovery from severe lateralized injury appears to have been mediated entirely by the right hemisphere. BB appears to have recovered from less severe lateralized injury, occurring later in development, by the interaction of the two cerebral hemispheres via the corpus callosum. Therefore, sectioning the callosum resulted in minimal deficit for PD but severe deficit for BB.

Illustrative Case 4

CP was a 29-year-old left-hand-dominant Caucasian female who developed generalized seizures at 1 month of age. Radiographic examination (CT and MRI) revealed no abnormalities. The intracarotid amobarbital procedure documented right speech dominance, intact right hemisphere memory, but absent left memory. Interictal scalp EEG monitoring revealed frequent multifocal left hemispheric independent spikes, sometimes with bilateral synchrony but without independent right abnormalities. Ictal scalp EEG documented bilateral high-frequency onset with rhythmic buildup. These features were somewhat greater on the left. Clinical neuropsychological examination documented mild right hemiparesis, impaired visual perception, dysarthria, impaired verbal and visual memory, and intellectual impairment (VIQ = 79; PIQ = 63).

Anterior two-thirds callosotomy was accomplished without complication. The patient was examined neuropsychologically at 1 month, 6 months, and 3 years following surgery. During each evaluation, the patient demonstrated dense right hemiparesis, which represented a severe decline from the presurgical level of function. No changes were observed in left upper extremity motor function, visual perception, speech and language, verbal memory, visual memory, or intellectual functioning (the last measure was obtained only at 6-month follow-up: VIQ = 77; PIQ = 69).

This case presents a permanent marked increase in unilateral motor impairment, following anterior-two thirds callosotomy. Like Patients PD (Case 1) and BB (Case 3), this patient was right speech dominant. Like Patient PD, she had no memory in the left hemisphere by IAP examination. Both PD and CP incurred their injuries during infancy, but PD's were more severe. PD obtained a right-hand dynamometer index of 0.0, and CP obtained an index of 13.2. BB incurred his injury later in childhood and continued to have good strength (left-hand dynamometer index = 45), suggesting that his injury was the mildest of the three.

After surgery, PD showed no change in motor function and improvements in visual–spatial function. CP showed a marked and permanent decline in motor function and no improvements in visual–spatial function. This suggests that recovery from the lateralized injury in PD was mediated entirely by the right hemisphere. BB incurred a severe, persisting language impairment but no motor impairment, suggesting that his injury involved only his language mechanisms, and recovery was mediated by the interaction of the two hemispheres. CP appeared to evidence both forms of recovery. Her language functions, which did not change, appear to have been mediated entirely by the right hemisphere. However, recovery from the moderate injury to her motor system was mediated by the interaction of the two hemispheres via the callosum, in the same manner that BB recovered from injury to his language area.

These three cases support the dissociation of language dominance and manual dominance. Development of both functions appears to be within the capability of the congenitally nondominant hemisphere if the necessary conditions prevail. However, the functions can be developed independently by the congenitally nondominant hemisphere by two processes that can be present simultaneously. One involves total acquisition of the function by the nondominant hemisphere, and the other involves interaction of the two cerebral hemispheres.

Illustrative Case 5

NG was a 22-year-old right-hand-dominant Caucasian female. Her history was negative for neurological dysfunction until age 13 years, when she was rendered unconscious by a blow to the left frontal area that occurred during a bicycle accident. Six months later secondary generalized seizures began. These seizures were characterized by abrupt vocalization, loss of contact, contortion of the right side of the mouth, extension of the right arm with posturing of the fingers, and extension of the left leg. Postictal confusion was brief. An intracarotid amobarbital procedure documented left speech dominance and bilateral memory capabilities; CT and MRI were within normal limits.

Interictal scalp EEG documented a left frontal spike-and-wave focus and a sharp slow focus that was intermittently observed throughout the left hemisphere. Ictal scalp EEG documented no clear area of seizure onset. Neuropsychological examination documented average intellectual functioning (VIQ = 87; PIQ = 75; FSIQ = 80), intact visual memory, and normal motor function. Verbal memory was moderately impaired.

The patient had as many as 10 seizures per day. Because these were unlocalized, the patient underwent anterior two-thirds corpus callosotomy at age 22 years. During the first two postoperative days, she exhibited difficulty with visual tracking, a right facial weakness, and a mild buccofacial apraxia. She spontaneously moved all four extremities, showed no weakness or forced grasping. Neither visual or tactile neglect was elicited. By postoperative day 4, the patient's neurological examination was within normal limits. Neuropsychological examination on postoperative day 12 documented impaired manual dexterity bilaterally and intermittent left suppression of double simultaneous tactile stimulation. Otherwise, motor function, visual perception, speech and language, memory, and intellectual functions were unchanged.

Anterior callosotomy failed to control the patient's seizures, so she was evaluated for completion of the section at age 23. She was studied by depth electrode implantation and cortical recording. The EEG during seizures documented a left frontal onset.

The cortical recording provided the opportunity for mapping through stimulation studies. The motor areas of shoulder, upper arm, hand, thumb and first two fingers, mouth, lips, and tongue were identified. The primary sensory regions for forearm, hand, and mouth were also noted. Broca's area and several areas associated with halting speech were identified.

With a frontal lobe onset identified anterior to the primary motor cortex and language areas, she underwent a prefrontal lobectomy. During the acute postoperative period, she was mute. She could not produce even monosyllabic vocalizations. Writing was severely impaired as well. As the patient resolved, she had considerable difficulty responding verbally to commands or questions. However, lengthy grammatically intact sentences were intermittently observed during casual conversation. Conduction and comprehension were generally intact. The speech apraxia was accompanied by buccofacial apraxia, ideational apraxia, and right facial paresis. The language impairment improved considerably, but it was still apparent at the time of discharge, approximately 2 weeks after surgery. A CT scan obtained during the acute postoperative period excluded surgical complications.

Although this patient has rare partial seizures, she is substantially improved. Neuropsychological examination documented intact motor function and visual perception. A mild dysnomia and visual and verbal memory impairments were present. However, the Verbal IQ had improved (VIQ = 93), and the PIQ was unchanged (PIQ = 94).

One year following the second surgery, normal motor function and visual perception were observed. Speech, language, and memory had returned to the presurgical level. The Verbal IQ was relatively unchanged (VIQ = 89), but the Performance IQ dramatically improved (PIQ = 126).

There is little question that the language impairment was related directly to the dominant prefrontal lobectomy. Because the connections between the frontal lobes had been surgically disconnected prior to the prefrontal lobectomy, it is reasonable to conclude that the recovery from the severe language deficit was mediated by ipsilateral cortical areas. This case supports the model that after puberty, the primary source of recovery from focal injury is ipsilateral. Second, the dramatic improvement in the PIQ accompanied by smaller improvements in memory and the complete absence of persisting declines indicates that combined lobectomy and callosotomy may be an attractive surgical alternative in carefully selected cases.

PREDICTION OF CALLOSOTOMY OUTCOME

On the basis of the information presented in this chapter, the following conclusions have been drawn about the prediction of postcallosotomy neuropsychological outcome.

Patients with severe lateralized disease that occurs prior to age 6 years tend to tolerate the procedure quite well. These patients have dense hemiplegia and absent memory during IAP evaluation. When the left hemisphere has been injured, the patient also will have right hemisphere speech dominance.

Patients with minimal disease and no anomalous clinical findings also tend to tolerate the procedure well. These patients typically present with late-onset seizure development (after age 12 years), left hemisphere speech dominance, bilateral memory during IAP evaluation, and adequate motor function bilaterally.

Recovery from seizure onset after age 6 years and prior to age 12 years often involves interhemispheric compensatory support for language, which places the patient at risk for postcallosotomy declines. Right hemisphere speech-dominant, right-handed patients incur severe speech and language impairments. Left hemisphere speech-dominant, left-handed patients develop an isolated defect in writing.

Right hemisphere speech-dominant patients with mild hemiparesis who fail to demonstrate memory in the left hemisphere during IAP evaluation typically show worsening of their preoperative hemiparesis. Right hemisphere speech-dominant patients with average strength who fail to demonstrate memory in the left hemisphere typically experience bilateral motor declines.

Corpus callosotomy in left speech-dominant patients who fail to demonstrate left hemisphere memory during the intracarotid amobarbital procedure may develop an amnestic disorder of profound proportions. Although corpus callosotomy seems theoretically to be contraindicated in such circumstances, there is no empirical validation of this hypothesis.

Some postsurgical declines result from poor seizure control, particularly the occurrence of MIFs. Research that has as its goal the prediction of seizure control after callosotomy also may lead to other means of predicting postcallosotomy neuropsychological declines.

REFERENCES

Bogen, J. E. (1969). The other side of the brain. I. Dysgraphia and dyscopia following cerebral commissurotomy. *Bulletin of the Los Angeles Neurological Society, 34*, 73–105.

Bogen, J. E. (1979). The callosal syndrome. In K. M. Heilman & E. Valenstein (Eds.), *Clinical neuropsychology* (pp. 308–359). New York: Oxford University Press.

Campbell, A. L., Jr., Bogen, J. E., & Smith, A. (1981). Disorganization and reorganization of cognitive and sensorimotor functions in cerebral commissurotomy: Compensatory roles of the forebrain commissures and cerebral hemispheres in man. *Brain, 104*, 493–511.

Geoffrey, G., Lassonde, M., Delisle, F., & Decarie, M. (1983). Corpus callosotomy for control of intractable epilepsy in children. *Neurology, 33*, 891–897.

Gur, R. E., Gur, R. C., Sussman, N. M., O'Connor, M. J., & Vey, M. M. (1984). Hemispheric control of the writing hand: The effect of callosotomy in the left-hander. *Neurology, 34*, 904–908.

Novelly, R. A., & Lifrak, M. D. (1985). Forebrain commissurotomy reinstates effects of preexisting hemisphere lesions: An examination of the hypothesis. In A. G. Reeves (Ed.), *Epilepsy and the corpus callosum*, (pp. 451–500). New York: Plenum Press.

Rayport, M., Ferguson, S. M., & Corrie, W. S., (1984). Mutism after corpus callosum section for intractable seizure control. *Epilepsia, 5*, 665.

Sass, K. J., Novelly, R. A., Spencer, D. D., & Spencer, S. S. (1987). Focal deficits associated with anticonvulsant toxicity reappear following callosotomy: A case study. *Journal of Clinical and Experimental Neuropsychology, 9*, 77.

Sass, K. J., Spencer, D. D., Spencer, S. S., Novelly, R. A., Williamson, P. D., Mattson, R. H. (1988a). Corpus callosotomy for epilepsy II. Neurologic and neuropsychological outcome. *Neurology, 38*, 24–28.

Sass, K. J., Spencer, S. S., Novelly, R. A., & Spencer, D. D. (1988b). Mnestic and attention impairments following corpus callosum section for epilepsy. *Journal of Epilepsy, 1*, 61–66.

Sass, K. J., Westerveld, M., Novelly, R. A., Spencer, D. D. & Spencer, S. S. (1989). Intracarotid Amytal procedure findings predict post-callosotomy motor weakness in right speech dominant patients. *Epilepsia, 30*, 711–712.

Sass, K. J., Novelly, R. A., Spencer, D. D., & Spencer, S. S. (1990). Post callosotomy language impairments in patients with anomalous cerebral dominance. *Journal of Neurosurgery, 72*, 85–90.

Spencer, S. S., Spencer, D. D., Glaser, G. H., Williamson, P. D., & Mattson, R. H. (1984). More intense focal seizure types after callosal section: The role of inhibition. *Annals of Neurology, 16*, 686–693.

Spencer, S. S., Spencer, D. D., Williamson, P. D., Sass, K., Novelly, R. A., & Mattson, R. H. (1988). Corpus callosotomy for epilepsy I. Seizure effects. *Neurology, 38*, 19–24.

Wilson, D., Reeves, A., Gazzaniga, M., Culver, C. (1977). Cerebral commissurotomy for control of intractable seizures, *Neurology, 27*, 708–715.

Index